Peripartum Care of the Pregnant Patient

Ashish C. Sinha • Ioana F. Pasca
Editors

Peripartum Care of the Pregnant Patient

A Question-and-Answer Review for Anesthesiologists and Obstetricians

Springer

Editors
Ashish C. Sinha
Department of Anesthesiology
Loma Linda University
Loma Linda, CA, USA

Ioana F. Pasca
Department of Anesthesiology, Critical Care, and Neurocritical Care
Loma Linda University at Riverside University Health System
Loma Linda, CA, USA

ISBN 978-3-031-62755-2 ISBN 978-3-031-62756-9 (eBook)
https://doi.org/10.1007/978-3-031-62756-9

This Springer imprint is published by the registered company Springer Nature Switzerland AG
The registered company address is: Gewerbestrasse 11, 6330 Cham, Switzerland

Preface

Welcome to our review of obstetric anesthesiology, a dynamic field at the intersection of obstetrics and anesthesiology. The provision of safe and effective anesthesia care during pregnancy and childbirth is a paramount concern for both mothers and their unborn babies. As such, the knowledge and expertise required of both obstetricians and obstetric anesthesiologists are unique and multifaceted.

This textbook aims to serve as a comprehensive resource for students, residents, and practitioners alike, offering an exploration of the principles, practices, and challenges encountered in obstetric anesthesiology. Through a question-and-answer format, readers will engage in an interactive learning experience, delving into key topics ranging from the physiological changes of pregnancy to the management of obstetric emergencies.

Each chapter is designed to address common uncertainties faced by clinicians in the field, providing evidence-based answers supported by current research and clinical guidelines. Moreover, special attention is given to practical considerations, including the nuances of patient assessment, anesthesia techniques, and postpartum care.

Furthermore, this textbook intends to foster essential critical thinking using questions and answers, providing information needed for delivering optimal care in diverse clinical scenarios. By elucidating complex concepts in a clear question-and-answer format, it is our hope that readers will gain confidence in their abilities to navigate the complexities of obstetric anesthesia with proficiency and compassion. Multiple references are scattered throughout the book for readers who may want to do a deeper dive into the subject matter.

We extend our sincere gratitude to the contributors from all over the world who generously shared their time, expertise, and insights to make this textbook possible. Additionally, we express our appreciation to the readers whose dedication to advancing their knowledge drives innovation and excellence in obstetric anesthesiology. We thank our families, Kavita, Ishan, and Anamika Sinha as well as Teo, Abigail, Lucas, and Sofia Pasca, for supporting us through this project and allowing us the time away from them required to complete this textbook. We also thank the many indirect contributors to this textbook who helped with the editorial process including Gian Ignacio, Malin Cannon, and Dinorah Hamilton from Riverside University Health System; and Gregory Sutorius and Nishanthini Vetrival from Springer Nature Publishing. Our anesthesia chief Gary Stier, MD and our obstetrics chief Ronald Johnson, MD have been instrumental to the success of this project allowing us time and resources plus an environment that encourages collaboration and innovation.

As the landscape of obstetrics and anesthesia continues to evolve, this textbook serves as an easy resource for those committed to the highest standards of care for mothers and their newborns. May it inspire curiosity, spark intellectual inquiry, and ultimately enhance the practice of obstetric anesthesiology for the betterment of maternal and fetal health worldwide.

Loma Linda, CA, USA
Moreno Valley, CA, USA
Riverside, CA, USA
Visalia, CA, USA
Ashish C. Sinha

Loma Linda, CA, USA
Moreno Valley, CA, USA
Riverside, CA, USA
San Diego, CA, USA
Ioana F. Pasca

Contents

Contributors

Ayman Ads Los Angeles General Medical Center, Los Angeles, CA, USA

John V. Agapian Riverside University Health System, Moreno Valley, CA, USA

Loma Linda University, Loma Linda, CA, USA

University of California Riverside, Riverside, CA, USA

Aymen Alian Department of Anaesthesiology, Yale University, New Haven, CT, USA

Ashley Almajan Riverside University Health System, Moreno Valley, CA, USA

Ashley Beem Loma Linda OBGYN Residency Program, Linda School of Medicine, Loma Linda, CA, USA

Riverside University Health System, Moreno Valley, CA, USA

Nidhi Bhatia Department of Anesthesia & Intensive Care, PGIMER, Chandigarh, India

Mira Bishawi Riverside University Health System, Moreno Valley, CA, USA

John Bouz Riverside University Health System, Moreno Valley, CA, USA

Nisha Branch Lewis Katz School of Medicine at Temple University, Philadelphia, PA, USA

Justin Calvert Department of Anaesthesiology, Riverside University Health System Medical Center, Moreno Valley, CA, USA

Jessica Chan Kaweah Health Medical Center, Visalia, CA, USA

Peter Cheng Riverside University Health System, Moreno Valley, CA, USA

Loma Linda University, Loma Linda, CA, USA

Thomas Cho Riverside University Health System, Moreno Valley, CA, USA

Jonathan Molina Cifuentes Yale School of Medicine, New Haven, CT, USA

Lenorre Clarke Riverside University Health System, Moreno Valley, CA, USA

Loma Linda University, Loma Linda, CA, USA

Alicia Cryer University of Pennsylvania at Chester County Hospital, West Chester, PA, USA

Christopher Dextras Yale School of Medicine, New Haven, CT, USA

Michael Douglas Department of Anesthesiology and Perioperative Medicine, Riverside University Health System, Moreno Valley, CA, USA

Sara Edwards Riverside University Health System, Moreno Valley, CA, USA

Kristen L. Fardelmann Yale School of Medicine, New Haven, CT, USA

Asaf Gans Department of Anesthesia and Perioperative Medicine, Mayo Clinic, Jacksonville, FL, USA

Katherine Ghobrial Riverside University Health System, Moreno Valley, CA, USA

Nigel Gillespie Department of Anesthesia and Perioperative Medicine, Mayo Clinic, Jacksonville, FL, USA

Maria Acosta de Gonzalez Loma Linda University Health, Loma Linda, CA, USA

Antonio Gonzalez-Fiol Division of Obstetric Anesthesia, Yale School of Medicine, New Haven, CT, USA

Anju Grewal Department of Anaesthesiology and Critical Care, AIIMS Bathinda, Bathinda, Punjab, India

Anjeleena Kumar Gupta Institute of Anaesthesiology, Pain and Perioperative Medicine, Sir Ganga Ram Hospital, New Delhi, India

Sunanda Gupta Anaesthesiology, Geetanjali Medical University, Udaipur, Rajasthan, India

Ming J. Huang Anesthesiology Loma Linda School of Medicine, Loma Linda, CA, USA

Riverside University Health System, Moreno Valley, CA, USA

Alan Iwahashi Loma Linda University Medical Center, Loma Linda, CA, USA

Aditi Jain Department of Anaesthesia and Intensive Care, Government Medical College and Hospital, Chandigarh, India

Kajal Jain Department of Anesthesia and Intensive Care, Postgraduate Institute of Medical Education and Research, Chandigarh, India

Ronald B. Johnson Department of Gynecology and Obstetrics, Loma Linda University School of Medicine, Loma Linda, CA, USA

Riverside University Health System—Medical Center, Moreno Valley, CA, USA

Shilpa Kasodekar PD Hinduja Hospital and Medical Research Centre, Khar, Mumbai, Maharashtra, India

Hemanth Kumar Department of Anaesthesiology and Critical Care, AIIMS Bathinda, Bathinda, Punjab, India

Benjamin Kuo Department of Anesthesiology, Riverside University Health System, Moreno Valley, CA, USA

Department of Anesthesiology and Perioperative Medicine, University of California, Irvine, Orange, CA, USA

Avery Lahodny Riverside University Health System, Moreno Valley, CA, USA

Loma Linda University, Loma Linda, CA, USA

Chelsea Lee Riverside University Health System, Moreno Valley, CA, USA

Donald Lee Department Anesthesiology, Cedars-Sinai Medical Center, Los Angeles, CA, USA

Jae Woong Lee Department of Anaesthesiology, Yale University, New Haven, CT, USA

Trenton G. Lum Department of Anesthesiology and Perioperative Medicine, Riverside University Health System, Moreno Valley, CA, USA

Sumana Mahata Riverside University Health System, Moreno Valley, CA, USA

Hanna Mandell Universirty of California Riverside, Riverside, CA, USA

Avoumia Marcus A.T. Still University School of Osteopathic Medicine, Mesa, AZ, USA

Erin I. Martin University of California San Diego, San Diego, CA, USA

Wyatt McGilvery A.T. Still University Health Osteopathic Medicine in Arizona, Mesa, AZ, USA

PJ McGuire Yale New Haven Hospital, New Haven, CT, USA

Jehan M. Momin University of California San Diego, San Diego, CA, USA

Avrodet Mourkus University of California Riverside, Riverside, CA, USA

Aparajita Nathroy PD Hinduja Hospital and Medical Research Centre, Khar, Mumbai, Maharashtra, India

Hinduja Hospital Khar, Mumbai, Maharashtra, India

Brandon Ngo UC Riverside School of Medicine, Riverside, CA, USA

Kenneth Nguyen Riverside University Health System, Moreno Valley, CA, USA

Scott Nguyen Riverside University Health System, Moreno Valley, CA, USA

Sindhuja R. Nimma Department of Anesthesia and Perioperative Medicine, Mayo Clinic, Jacksonville, FL, USA

Shashank Paliwal Department of Anaesthesiology, All India Institute of Medical Sciences, Bathinda, Punjab, India

Bashu Dev Parajuli Department of Anaesthesiology, Tribhuvan University Teaching Hospital, Maharajgunj Medical Campus, Institute of Medicine, Maharajgunj, Kathmandu, Nepal

Seema Partani Partani ENT Hospital, Udaipur, Rajasthan, India

Ioana F. Pasca Riverside University Health System, Moreno Valley, CA, USA

Department of Anesthesiology, Critical Care, and Neurocritical Care, Loma Linda University at Riverside University Health System, Loma Linda, CA, USA

University of California San Diego, San Diego, CA, USA

University of California Riverside, Riverside, CA, USA

Christopher Patty Kaweah Delta Health Care District, Visalia, CA, USA

Jack Peace Lewis Katz School of Medicine at Temple University, Philadelphia, PA, USA

Gabrielle Pina Loma Linda University, Loma Linda, CA, USA

Riverside University Health System, Moreno Valley, CA, USA

Gegal Pruthi Department of Anaesthesiology and Critical Care, AIIMS Bathinda, Bathinda, Punjab, India

Christia Del Rosario Department of Gynecology and Obstetrics, Loma Linda University School of Medicine, Riverside University Health System—Medical Center, Moreno Valley, CA, USA

Ivan Rybkin Riverside University Health System, Moreno Valley, CA, USA

Charles Schoepflin Riverside University Health System, Moreno Valley, CA, USA

Loma Linda University, Loma Linda, CA, USA

Yudhyavir Singh AIIMS, New Delhi, India

Ashish C. Sinha Department of Anesthesiology, Riverside University Health System, Moreno Valley, CA, USA

Loma Linda University, Loma Linda, CA, USA

University of California Riverside, Riverside, CA, USA

Kaweah Health Medical Center, Visalia, CA, USA

Sarah Smithson Riverside University Health System, Moreno Valley, CA, USA

Loma Linda University, Loma Linda, CA, USA

Leonard J. Soloniuk Riverside University Health System, Moreno Valley, CA, USA

Loma Linda University, Loma Linda, CA, USA

Gary Stier Anesthesiology, Internal Medicine, Critical Care/Loma Linda University, Loma Linda, CA, USA

Riverside University Health System Medical Center, Moreno Valley, CA, USA

Katharine Stolz Riverside University Health System, Moreno Valley, CA, USA

Bowei Su Department of Anaesthesiology, Riverside University Health System Medical Center, Moreno Valley, CA, USA

Rashmi Thapa Department of Anaesthesiology, Tribhuvan University Teaching Hospital, Maharajgunj Medical Campus, Institute of Medicine, Maharajgunj, Kathmandu, Nepal

Jeffery Thomas Riverside University Health System, Moreno Valley, CA, USA

Akshay Toshniwal Department of Anaesthesiology, Geetanjali Medical College and Hospital, Geetanjali University, Udaipur, Rajasthan, India

Minh Chau Joe Tran VA Loma Linda Health Care, Loma Linda, CA, USA

Alexandra Vacaru Loma Linda University, Loma Linda, CA, USA

Joshua Vasquez Western University of Health Sciences College of Osteopathic Medicine of the Pacific, Pomona, CA, USA

Joseph Villaluz University of California Irvine, Irvine, CA, USA

Allen Wang University of California, Davis, Sacramento, CA, USA

Mark Zakowski Department Anesthesiology, Cedars-Sinai Medical Center, Los Angeles, CA, USA

The History of Obstetric Anesthesia

Jehan M. Momin, Erin I. Martin, and Leonard J. Soloniuk

Questions

1. **On January 19, 1847, James Young Simpson, professor of Midwifery at University of Edinburgh, Scotland, famously first used a modern anesthetic in obstetrics by administering ___ to a patient in labor.**
   A. Nitrous oxide
   B. Diethyl ether
   C. Propofol
   D. Halothane
2. **In 1853, Queen Victoria requested inhalational analgesia for the birth of her eighth child by anesthesiologist John Snow resulting in which of the following?**
   A. Proof of the safety and efficacy of chloroform
   B. Increased public acceptance of labor analgesia
   C. Evidence that analgesia was harmful for mother and baby
   D. Widespread rejection of inhalational analgesia
3. **In 1906, *Dämmerschlaf,* meaning "twilight sleep," was introduced by administering a combination of an opioid, usually morphine, along with scopolamine. This technique was made possible by what technical invention?**
   A. Spinal needle
   B. Intravenous access

J. M. Momin · E. I. Martin
University of California San Diego, San Diego, CA, USA
e-mail: eim002@health.ucsd.edu

L. J. Soloniuk (✉)
Loma Linda University, Loma Linda, CA, USA

Riverside University Health System, Moreno Valley, CA, USA
e-mail: l.soloniuk@ruhealth.org

A. C. Sinha, I. F. Pasca (eds.), *Peripartum Care of the Pregnant Patient*,
https://doi.org/10.1007/978-3-031-62756-9_1

   C. Oral opioids
   D. Hypodermic syringe and needle
4. **In the latter part of the nineteenth century, physicians were increasingly concerned with the effects of anesthetics on the newborn. Which anesthesiologist is responsible for developing a simple system to evaluate the newborn infant that is still used to this day?**
   A. Virginia Apgar
   B. Ralph Waters
   C. Paul Zweifel
   D. Elizabeth Blackwell
5. **In the early twentieth century, with the development of regional anesthesia, including caudal, spinal, epidural, paravertebral, and pudendal nerve blocks, anesthesiologists and obstetricians were eager to adopt these techniques with their primary advantage being which of the following?**
   A. Ability for surgeons to administer analgesia
   B. Reduced risk of aspiration
   C. More reliable analgesic properties
   D. Relative absence of drug effects on the fetus
6. **With the development of the pencil point spinal needle, the incidence of which side effect implicated in many early spinal anesthetics was significantly reduced?**
   A. Nerve injury
   B. Incomplete block
   C. Headache
   D. Hypotension
7. **When was the first demonstrated use of neuraxial anesthesia for surgery?**
   A. 1898
   B. 1901
   C. 1921
   D. 1933
8. **The curved-point needle for neuraxial anesthesia was invented by:**
   A. Johannes Friedrich August von Esmarch
   B. August Karl Gustav Bier
   C. Ralph L. Huber
   D. Edward Boyce Tuohy
9. **Who developed the modern form of the epidural needle that is used contemporarily?**
   A. Edward Boyce Tuohy
   B. Jess Bernard Weiss
   C. Oral Bascom Crawford
   D. Jürgen Sprotte
10. **The first epidural catheters were made with which material?**
   A. Silk
   B. Cotton
   C. Rayon

D. Nylon

11. **For the first use of epidural labor analgesia in 1931, which local anesthetic was used?**
A. Cocaine
B. Dibucaine (cinchocaine)
C. Procaine (Novacaine)
D. Lidocaine (lignocaine)

12. **Who first described the efficacy of programmed intermittent epidural boluses (PIEB) for the maintenance of labor analgesia?**
A. Bhavani-Shankar, Malov, and colleagues of Brigham and Women's Hospital, Boston, in 2000
B. De Eccher, Martino, and colleagues, Bologna, Italy, in 2002
C. Chua and Sia of Singapore General Hospital in 2004
D. Fettes, Moore, and colleagues, in 2006

13. **Patient-controlled epidural analgesia (PCEA) allows patient-initiated activation of a bolus of epidural medication to treat labor pain. In comparison with continuous epidural infusions, studies have shown that PCEA decreases breakthrough pain requiring provider intervention, reduces total local anesthetic dose, maintains analgesia, and increases patient satisfaction. PCEA is commonly administered with a basal infusion in addition to boluses on patient demand.**

Patient-controlled epidural analgesia (PCEA) for labor analgesia was introduced by:
A. D.R. Gambling and colleagues of University of British Columbia, Vancouver, Canada, in 1988
B. F.M. Ferrante and colleagues of Brigham and Women's Hospital, Boston, MA, in 1991
C. Cynthia A. Wong and colleagues of Northwestern University Feinberg School of Medicine, Chicago, Illinois, in 2006
D. Uma Srivastava and colleagues of SN Medical College Agra, India, in 2009

14. **The use of ether for surgical anesthesia was first publicly demonstrated on 16 October 1846 at Massachusetts General Hospital in Boston, Massachusetts. When was the date of the first use of ether for childbirth pain?**
A. January 19, 1847
B. February 18, 1847
C. April 7, 1847
D. November 8, 1847

15. **When asked by a pregnant patient for a medication to help with childbirth pain, a physician in sixteenth-century CE Edinburgh, Scotland, would be expected to:**
A. Prescribe small beer
B. Prescribe medicinal whisky and white willow bark tea
C. Prescribe tincture of opium
D. Refer the patient to the authorities to be burned at the stake

16. **Who was the first anesthesiologist in China to administer and study labor epidural analgesia?**
    A. Wu Lien-teh (1879–1960)
    B. Buwei Yang Chao (1889–1981)
    C. Li Zhisui (1919–1995)
    D. Guang-Bo Zhang (b. 1928)
17. **Who was the first woman in Japan to receive intravenous analgesia for childbirth?**
    A. Ginko Ogino (1851–1913)
    B. Tsuda Umeko (1864–1929)
    C. Akiko Yosano (1878–1942)
    D. Toshiko Tamura (1884–1945)
18. **Who was the first to use spinal cocaine for labor analgesia?**
    A. James Young Simpson (Edinburgh)
    B. Oskar Kreis (Germany)
    C. Stanislav Sigismund Kilkovich (Russia)
    D. August Bier (Germany)
19. **Who pioneered the use of nitrous oxide for labor analgesia?**
    A. Humphry Davy (England)
    B. Horace Wells (United States)
    C. Arthur Ernest Guedel (United States)
    D. Stanislav Klikovich (Russia)
20. **Lidocaine was introduced into clinical practice by:**
    A. Benjamin Ward Richardson (1828–1896) of London in 1896
    B. Heinrich Friedrich Wilhelm Braun (1862–1934) of Leipzig in 1905
    C. Otto Eisleb (1887–1948) of Germany, in 1928
    D. Torsten Gordh (1907–2010) of Karolinska Hospital, Stockholm, in 1949

Answers and Explanations

1. **B**. Of foremost importance in the history of obstetrical anesthesia was the administration of inhalational analgesia in the form of (**B**) diethyl ether by Dr. James Young Simpson to a woman with a severely deformed pelvis for delivery [1].
2. **B**. During the nineteenth century, there was great moral, religious, and medical opposition to labor analgesia. Many physicians, including Dr. Simpson's greatest critic, Dr. Charles D. Meigs, professor of midwifery at Jefferson Medical College in Philadelphia, believed labor pain to be inextricably linked to uterine contractions, and thus, any medicine that alleviates pain would negatively impact contractions. Dr. Simpson firmly disagreed, believing labor pain lacks physiologic value. It was not until 1853 when Dr. John Snow famously and successfully administered chloroform to Queen Victoria during the birth of her child that there became increased public acceptance of labor analgesia (**B**). The medical community continued to remain skeptical [2, 3].

3. **D**. The same year Dr. John Snow administered chloroform to Queen Victoria, Scottish physician Alexander Wood is credited with the invention of the hypodermic syringe and hollow bore needle (**D**). His advancement simplified the administration of opioids, which was vital in twilight sleep during labor [2, 4].
4. **A**. With increased use of morphine during labor, physicians noted cases of neonatal respiratory depression, asphyxia, and stillbirth. In 1953, Virginia Apgar (**A**) published a simple, consistent, and rapid method to evaluate the newborn including five criteria each starting with the letter of her last name: **A**ppearance, **P**ulse, **G**rimace, **A**ctivity, and **R**espiration. Notably, Apgar was the first female to achieve professorship at Columbia University. To date, every newborn in a modern hospital is evaluated with the Apgar scoring system at 1 and 5 min following birth [2].
5. **D**. At the time, the chief advantage of regional anesthesia was viewed as the absence of systemic drug effects given to the mother on the fetus (**D**). Prior to the 1900s, the survival of the mother had been the primary marker of success of obstetrical and anesthetic care. However, with rapidly declining maternal risk, the condition of the newborn infant became the new standard for evaluating obstetrical outcomes. It was noted that infants born to mothers receiving spinal anesthesia had higher Apgar scores than those receiving general anesthesia [2].
6. **C**. The earliest spinal anesthetics were performed with large-bore, sharp, cutting needles, resulting in a high postdural puncture headache (PDPH) rate. The introduction of pencil-point needles, a close-ended tip with a lateral orifice, significantly decreased the rate of PDPH [5].
7. **A.** In 1885, J. Leonard Corning, a neurologist from New York, accidently administered a spinal anesthetic to a dog. Although he contemplated the use of spinal anesthesia in surgery, he did not proceed with its use for surgery. On August 16, 1898, spinal anesthesia was first performed by Dr. August Bier and his colleagues. "Cocainization of the spinal cord" was performed by introducing 15 mg of cocaine intrathecally, resulting in a pain-free experience during a lower-extremity surgery (**A**). In 1901, French physician Jean-Anthanase Sicard, a radiologist, described injecting dilute solutions of cocaine through the sacral hiatus to treat severe sciatic pain, the first demonstration of epidural analgesia (**B**). In 1921, a Spanish surgeon, Fidel Pagés, described a lumbar approach to epidural anesthesia, the first described use of an epidural anesthesia for surgery (**C**). In 1933, an Italian surgeon, Archile Mario Dogliotti, resurrected and popularized the ideas of Pagés, performing abdominal surgeries with single-shot lumbar epidural anesthesia (**D**) [5–8].
8. **C**. Friedrich von Esmarch (1823–1908) was a German surgeon who was a preeminent authority on battlefield medicine and hospital management. He developed the Esmarch bandage (used, e.g., for Bier blocks) and was a mentor to August Bier (**A**). August Bier (1861–1949) was a German surgeon who was the first to demonstrate spinal anesthesia and, also, developed intravenous regional anesthesia (the Bier Block). (**B**). Ralph L. Huber (1890–1953) was a University of Oregon graduate and a dentist in Seattle, WA, USA, who developed a needle with a long, sharp, curved tip. It was designed to lessen the pain of an injection

and decrease the risk of depositing skin plugs into underlying tissues (**C**). Edward B. Tuohy (1908–1959) trained at the Mayo Clinic and was an advocate for neuraxial block techniques for anesthesia. To minimize the risk of skin plugging, Tuohy designed a variant of the Huber needle with a stylet (**D**) [9, 10].

9. **B**. Tuohy modified the needle developed by Ralph L. Huber and added a stylet, hoping to further decrease the risk of skin plugging. However, his needle was still sharp as the intended application was continuous spinal anesthesia (**A**). Weiss, the Chief of Obstetric Anesthesia at the Brigham and Women's Hospital in Boston, dulled the tip of the Tuohy needle and added wings, creating the epidural needle that is in widespread use today (**B**). Crawford preferred a straight-tip needle for epidural access and developed the Crawford needle with a blunt, flat (60°) tip (**C**). Jürgen Sprotte developed the Sprotte Spezial needle for epidural catheter placement, utilizing a blunt, pencil-point tip with a lateral aperture for catheter placement (**D**) [8].
10. **A**. The first catheters used for epidural placement were silk ureteral catheters adapted for anesthetic use [8].
11. **B**. In 1931, Romanian obstetrician Eugene Aburel injected dibucaine through a silk ureteral catheter to achieve analgesia for laboring women [8].
12. **C**. There was recognition in the late 1990s and early 2000s that continuous epidural infusions for labor analgesia lost efficacy over the duration of the infusion and that there appeared to be more effective analgesia with intermittent boluses. The first study documenting the efficacy of programmed intermittent epidural boluses (PIEB) via an automated pump was published by Chua and Sia in 2004 [11].
13. **A**. Patient-controlled epidural analgesia (PCEA) was established as a preferred mode of epidural drug delivery since it was introduced by Gambling in 1988 [12].
14. **A**. The use of ether as an anesthetic spread around the world in an amazingly rapid fashion. James Young Simpson of Edinburgh administered the first use of ether analgesia for childbirth on January 19, 1847 (**A**). Adam Hammer, who worked as a doctor for the poor in Mannheim, was the first doctor in the German-speaking world to use ether analgesia for childbirth on February 18, 1847 (**B**). On April 7, 1847, the first obstetric anesthetic in the United States was administered by Nathan Cooley Keep M.D. to Fanny Longfellow, the wife of the poet Henry Wadsworth Longfellow (**C**). On November 8, 1847, James Young Simpson administered the first chloroform anesthetic for childbirth (**D**) [13–15].
15. **D**. Small beer, with an ethanol content between 0.5 and 2.8%, was widely consumed from Medieval times to the present. The ethanol, along with the hops, inhibited bacterial growth and was likely safer to consume than water until modern times. It has not notably been prescribed for pain with childbirth (**A**). Medicinal alcohol has been widely used for a variety of ailments until the twentieth century. There was no advocacy in sixteenth-century CE Scotland for use as childbirth analgesia (**B**). White willow bark tea contains salicin, which has anti-inflammatory effects like acetylsalicylic acid. Salicin is not particularly

effective for childbirth analgesia. Opium was widely used therapeutically from prehistoric times until the present. Paracelsus introduced opium to Western Europe in the sixteenth century. In the 1660s, English physician Thomas Sydenham popularized the tincture of opium, a solution of opium in alcohol. In the sixteenth-century CE, it was not advocated for pain with childbirth (**C**). On June 15, 1591, Euphemia Maclean was burned alive on Castle Hill in Edinburgh by order of King James VI (later King James I of England). Along with other charges, she was accused of being offered and accepting pain relief during childbirth (**D**) [16, 17].

16. **D**. Wu Lien-teh was born in Penang and became the first medical student of Chinese descent to study at the University of Cambridge. He had a multifaceted career and was involved in many medical and social issues. During the Manchurian plague of 1910–1911, he ascertained the mode of spread of the plague. To prevent the spread of the plague, he developed the Wu mask, adding layers of gauze and cotton to the design of the surgical mask. The Wu mask is the forerunner of today's N95 respirator (**A**). Buwei Yang Chao was a Chinese American physician and writer. She attended Tokyo Women's Medical College and took up cooking after she found Japanese food to be inedible. She was one of the first women to practice Western medicine in China. She later became the author of an English-language Chinese cookbook, "How to Cook and Eat in Chinese," inventing the terms "stir fry" and "pot sticker" (**B**). Li Zhisui was Mao Zedong's personal physician and confidante. He was born in Beijing, China, in 1919. During the Great Proletarian Cultural Revolution, Mao's wife, Jiang Qing, accused him of trying to poison her, causing him to flee. After emigrating to the United States, he wrote a biography of Mao entitled "The Private Life of Chairman Mao" (**C**). Guang-Bo Zhang was the first anesthesiologist to administer and study the effects of labor epidural analgesia in China. Between September 1963 and March 1964, she conducted an observational study evaluating neuraxial analgesia for laboring women. She presented her research but was unable to publish due to the Great Proletarian Cultural Revolution, which began in 1966 (**D**) [18].
17. **C**. Ginko Ogino was Japan's first licensed female doctor. She was born into a wealthy family and had an arranged marriage at age 16. She soon divorced her husband, after contracting gonorrhea from him. Japanese society looked down on divorced women, and women affected by gonorrhea were considered prostitutes. After having to visit male doctors with a "shameful" disease, she resolved to become a doctor herself to help women in similar circumstances. In 1885, she became the first registered female doctor in Japan. Her life inspired the novel "Beyond the Blossoming Fields" (2009) by Jun'ichi Watanabe (**A**). At the age of 7, Tsuda Umeko became Japan's first female exchange student, traveling to the United States. Returning to Japan after 11 years, Tsuda was alarmed by the treatment of women in her home country and determined to improve the lot of her countrywomen. In 1900, she founded Joshi Eigaku Juku (now Tsuda University), one of the first private institutions offering higher education to women (**B**). Tsuda Umeko will be featured on new Japanese banknotes issued

in 2024 (**B**). Akiko Yosano, born Shō Hō, was the nom de plume of a Japanese author, poet, feminist, and pacifist. She had intravenous labor analgesia for her fifth son in 1916. She was given a mixture of an opioid alkaloid, Pantopon, and scopolamine and had a painless labor and delivery. Pantopon is a preparation of the hydrochloride salts of the opium alkaloids; it was sometimes called "Opium in a syringe" (**C**). Toshiko Tamura was the nom de plume of an early modern feminist novelist in the Shōwa period of Japan. Her birth name was Toshi Satō (**D**) [19].

18. **B**. Oskar Kreis (1872–1958) was a gynecologist and obstetrician who received his training at the Basle University Women's Hospital. In 1900, he pioneered the use of spinal anesthesia for labor analgesia, using spinal cocaine in six parturients [20].
19. **D**. Humphry Davy (1778–1829), a British chemist and inventor, noted the analgesic effect of nitrous oxide and considered the potential to be used for surgical operations but never translated his research into clinical practice. Davy coined the name "laughing gas" for nitrous oxide (**A**). Horace Wells, an American dentist, demonstrated insensitivity to pain from a dental extraction on December 11, 1844 (**B**). Arthur Ernest Guedel (1883–1956) developed the cuffed endotracheal tube and the oropharyngeal airway (also known as an oral airway, OPA, or Guedel pattern airway) (**C**). Stanislav Sigismund Klikovich (1853–1910) was the first clinician to use a mixture of nitrous oxide and oxygen to provide analgesia during labor. After studying medicine at the Academy of Medicine and Surgery in St Petersburg, he studied the use of mixtures of oxygen and nitrous oxide (**D**). Prior to Klikovich's research, nitrous oxide had become established as a useful anesthetic agent, with unconsciousness resulting primarily from the hypoxia which occurred because of asphyxia. He introduced the use of a mixture of nitrous oxide and oxygen to provide analgesia without loss of consciousness or risk of hypoxia, recommending a mix with oxygen 20% and nitrous oxide 80%. Klikovich published observations on 25 parturients to whom he had given the oxygen/nitrous oxide mixture [21].
20. **D**. Benjamin Ward Richardson was a British anesthetist who introduced 14 anesthetics (but not lidocaine) into clinical practice (**A**). Heinrich Friedrich Wilhelm Braun introduced the newly synthesized procaine (Novocaine) into clinical practice in 1905. It rapidly displaced the use of cocaine (**B**). Otto Eisleb, a chemist with IG Farben in Germany, synthesized tetracaine in 1928, which is still used at the present time. Eisleb went on to develop meperidine (pethidine) during World War II (**C**). Torsten Gordh, MD, Sweden's first anesthesiologist, participated in the toxicity testing and clinical testing of compound LL30 (lidocaine, lignocaine) starting in 1944. Procaine was the local anesthetic commonly in use prior to lidocaine, but it had significant limitations with toxicity, very short duration of action, and the need to reconstitute prior to use. Lidocaine was developed with a goal to avoid these limitations. Nils Löfgren, Ph.D., along with his assistant, Bengt Lundqvist (1922–1953), synthesized a series of compounds and found the characteristics that were desired in lidocaine. They, of course, initially tested it on themselves. After 3 years of toxicity testing and

trials in volunteers, Gordh tried the compound in a wide variety of settings: corneal anesthesia, ENT, infiltration anesthesia, peripheral nerve and plexus blocks, chronic pain conditions, and spinal anesthesia. Lidocaine was found to have a rapid onset, reduced toxicity, and longer duration (four times or longer than procaine) (**D**) [22].

References

1. Dunn PM. Sir James Young Simpson (1811-1870) and obstetric anesthesia. Arch Dis Child Fetal Neonatal Ed. 2002;86:F207. https://doi.org/10.1136/fn.86.3.f207.
2. Caton D. The history of obstetric anesthesia. In: Chestnut's obstetric anesthesia: principles and practice, 6th ed. Elsevier; 2020. p. 2–11.
3. Whitfield A. A short history of obstetric anesthesia. Res Medica. 1992;3(1):28–30. https://doi.org/10.2218/resmedica.v3i1.972.
4. Gibson ME. An early history of anesthesia in labor. J Obstet Gynecol Neonatal Nurs. 2017;46(4):619–27. https://doi.org/10.1016/j.jogn.2016.10.013.
5. Calthorpe N. The history of spinal needles: getting to the point. Anesthesia. 2004;59(12):1231–41. https://doi.org/10.1111/j.1365-2044.2004.03976.x.
6. Wulf HF. The centennial of spinal anesthesia. Anesthesiology. 1998;89(2):500–6. https://doi.org/10.1097/00000542-199808000-00028. PMID: 9710410.
7. Sicard A. Les injections medicamenteuses extra-durales par voie sacrococcygienne. Compt Rend Soc De Biol. 1901;53:396–8.
8. Frolich MA, Caton D. Pioneers in epidural needle design. Anesth Analg. 2001;93:215–20.
9. Calthorpe N. The history of spinal needles: getting to the point. Anaesthesia. 2004;59:1231–41.
10. Huber RL. Hypodermic needle. US patent 2409979. 1946.
11. Chua SM, Sia AT. Automated intermittent epidural boluses improve analgesia induced by intrathecal fentanyl during labour. Can J Anaesth. 2004;51(6):581–5. https://doi.org/10.1007/BF03018402. PMID: 15197122.
12. Gambling DR, Yu P, Cole C, McMorland GH, Palmer L. A comparative study of patient controlled epidural analgesia (PCEA) and continuous infusion epidural analgesia (CIEA) during labour. Can J Anaesth. 1988;35(3):249–54.
13. McKenzie AG. Historic timeline of obstetric anesthesia. In: Clark V, Van de Velde M, Fernando R, editors. Oxford textbook of obstetric anaesthesia, Oxford textbook in anaesthesia. Oxford: Oxford Academic, 2016. https://doi.org/10.1093/med/9780198713333.001.0001.
14. Pittinger CB. The anesthetization of Fanny Longfellow for childbirth on April 7, 1847. Anesth Analg. 1987;66(4):368–9. PMID: 3551691.
15. Goerig M, Streckfuss W. Adam Hammer (1818–1878)—Anmerkungen zu einem vergessenen Pionier der Atheranwendung in der Geburtshilfe [Adam hammer (1818–1878)—remarks on a forgotten pioneer of ether anaesthesia in obstetrics]. Anasthesiol Intensivmed Notfallmed Schmerzther. 2004;39(5):265–75. German. PMID: 15156417. https://doi.org/10.1055/s-2004-814542
16. Menz G, Aldred P, Vriesekoop F. Growth and survival of foodborne pathogens in beer. J Food Prot. 2011;74(10):1670–5. https://doi.org/10.4315/0362-028X.JFP-10-546. PMID: 22004814.
17. Lurie S. Euphemia Maclean, Agnes Sampson and pain relief during labour in 16th century Edinburgh. Anaesthesia. 2004;59:834–5. https://doi.org/10.1111/j.1365-2044.2004.03891.x.
18. Cai ZY, Hu LQ, Stellaccio FS, Wang DX. Recognizing the Chinese pioneer of neuraxial labor analgesia: Dr Guang-Bo Zhang and her unpublished manuscript from more than a half-century ago. Anesth Analg. 2019;128(1):119–22. https://doi.org/10.1213/ANE.0000000000003845. PMID: 30300175.

19. Okutomi T. [Akiko Yosano, the famous Japanese poet and writer, is the first lady who experienced labor analgesia in Japan?]. Masui. 2011;60(10):1214–20. Japanese. PMID: 22111370.
20. Schneider MC, Holzgreve W. 100 years ago: Oskar Kreis, a pioneer in spinal obstetric analgesia at the University Women's Clinic of Basel [in German]. Anaesthesist. 2001;50:525–528.
21. Richards W, Parbrook GD, Wilson J. Stanislav Klikovich (1853-1910). Pioneer of nitrous oxide and oxygen analgesia. Anaesthesia. 1976;31(7):933–40. https://doi.org/10.1111/j.1365-2044.1976.tb11906.x. PMID: 788546.
22. Gordh T. Lidocaine: the origin of a modern local anesthetic. 1949. Anesthesiology. 2010;113(6):1433–7. https://doi.org/10.1097/ALN.0b013e3181fcef48. PMID: 21068652.

Further Reading

Caton D. The history of obstetric anesthesia. In: Chestnut's obstetric anesthesia: principles and practice. Philadelphia: Elsevier; 2020.

Neurologic and Neuromuscular Pathophysiology of Pregnancy

Donald Lee and Mark Zakowski

Questions

1. **What is the normal opening CSF pressure for pregnant woman?**
   A. 6–15 cm H_2O
   B. 25–50 cm H_2O
   C. 50–75 mmHg
   D. 75–100 mmHg
2. **Which of the following neurologic changes occurs with pregnancy?**
   A. Decrease in cerebral blood flow
   B. Increase in epidural venous plexus blood volume
   C. Increase in spinal CSF volume
   D. Decrease in epidural pressure within the spinal canal
3. **Uterine enlargement in pregnant women contributes to all of the following, *except*:**
   A. Decrease in the lumbar lordotic curve
   B. Sciatica
   C. Brachial plexus neuropathy
   D. Meralgia paresthetica
4. **Gait changes during pregnancy are associated with which *one* of the following:**
   A. Increase in anterior tilt of the pelvis
   B. Decrease in anterior tilt of the pelvis
   C. Increase in hip flexion
   D. Decrease in width of gait

D. Lee · M. Zakowski (✉)
Department Anesthesiology, Cedars-Sinai Medical Center, Los Angeles, CA, USA
e-mail: donald.lee@cshs.org; mark.zakowski@cshs.org

A. C. Sinha, I. F. Pasca (eds.), *Peripartum Care of the Pregnant Patient*,
https://doi.org/10.1007/978-3-031-62756-9_2

5. **Which hormone contributes to the instability of the symphysis pubis and sacroiliac joints during gestation?**
   A. Human chorionic gonadotropin hormone (hCG)
   B. Relaxin
   C. Progesterone
   D. Estrogen
6. **Which of the following statements is *false*:**
   A. Disc herniation is a common cause of back pain during pregnancy
   B. Carpal tunnel syndrome is a common cause of hand and wrist pain during pregnancy
   C. Coccydynia often develops postpartum
   D. De Quervain's tenosynovitis may develop postpartum
7. **Which statement is *true* regarding patients with multiple sclerosis during the peripartum period?**
   A. Relapse rates are decreased during the postpartum period.
   B. General anesthesia has fewer relapses than epidural or spinal anesthesia.
   C. There is a positive association with worsening neurologic conditions with any form of neuraxial anesthesia.
   D. Neuraxial (epidural or intrathecal) opioids have no harmful effects in multiple sclerosis.
8. **Which of the following is *not* true regarding pregnant patients with autonomic dysreflexia (aka autonomic hyperreflexia)?**
   A. Neuraxial labor analgesia should be used to reduce the risk of autonomic dysreflexia.
   B. Continuous hemodynamic monitoring is recommended during labor.
   C. Spinal cord injury at or above the T10 level results in autonomic dysreflexia.
   D. Hypertension due to autonomic dysreflexia occurs during uterine contractions and resolves between contractions.
9. **Which statement is correct regarding pregnant patients with neurocutaneous syndromes?**
   A. Radiographic imaging is required prior to neuraxial anesthesia administration.
   B. Asymptomatic patients do not require radiographic imaging prior to neuraxial anesthesia administration.
   C. Neurofibromas decrease in size during pregnancy.
   D. There are no concerns about increased intracranial pressure (ICP) during labor and delivery.
10. **Which is *not true* regarding pregnant patients with increased intracranial pressure (ICP)?**
   A. Unintentional dural puncture during epidural anesthesia placement may increase the chances of brain herniation.
   B. Intra-arterial blood pressure monitoring is recommended prior to the induction of anesthesia.

C. High-dose mannitol given for the reduction of ICP does not affect the fetus.
D. Hyperventilation may cause uterine artery vasoconstriction and a leftward shift in the maternal oxyhemoglobin dissociation curve.

11. **What percentage of women report pelvic pain during pregnancy?**
A. 10%
B. 20%
C. 30%
D. 40%

12. **Which of the following occurs in patients with significant scoliosis during pregnancy?**
A. Diaphragmatic activity restriction
B. Increase in pulmonary residual and closing capacities
C. Lower ventilation-perfusion mismatch
D. Increase in arterial oxygen content

13. **Which antirheumatic medication may be continued throughout pregnancy?**
A. NSAIDs
B. Azathioprine
C. Methotrexate
D. Leflunomide

14. **Which of the following is the *most common* antenatal complication in patients with open spinal dysraphism?**
A. Recurrent urinary tract infection
B. Hydrocephalus
C. Kyphoscoliosis
D. Paraparesis

15. **Which of the following statements regarding lumbopelvic pain during pregnancy is *true*?**
A. Pregnancy-related lumbopelvic pain is a contraindication to neuraxial anesthesia.
B. Elective assisted vaginal delivery (vacuum or forceps) protects against postpartum pelvic girdle pain.
C. There is no significant relationship between the use of epidural analgesia and long-term backache.
D. Higher doses of local anesthetic with epidural analgesia are recommended.

16. **Which of the following statements are *true* regarding pregnant women with myasthenia gravis?**
A. Myasthenia gravis worsens during pregnancy.
B. Magnesium therapy may be given to myasthenic patients with preeclampsia or preterm labor.
C. Maternal IgG antibodies to the acetylcholine receptor do not transfer across the placenta.
D. Neuraxial anesthetic techniques for cesarean delivery may be relatively contraindicated with significant bulbar involvement or respiratory compromise.

17. **Meralgia paresthetica is caused by the compression of which nerve?**
    A. Femoral nerve
    B. Obturator nerve
    C. Lateral femoral cutaneous nerve
    D. Ilioinguinal nerve
18. **Which is the first-line analgesic for pregnant patients with tension headaches?**
    A. Caffeine
    B. Ergotamine
    C. Acetaminophen
    D. NSAIDs
19. **Which of the following statements regarding disorders of the vertebral column and spinal cord is *not true*?**
    A. Neuraxial anesthesia is contraindicated for patients with a spinal cord stimulator.
    B. Prior discectomies or microdiscectomies rarely compromise the epidural space.
    C. Closed spinal dysraphism lesions are typically safe for neuraxial anesthesia.
    D. Neuraxial anesthesia is generally considered safe in patients with degenerative disc disease.
20. **Which is *not true* regarding patients with epilepsy during pregnancy?**
    A. Pregnancy may increase the frequency of seizures in 33% of epileptics.
    B. Substituting new antiepileptic agents after conception is not usually recommended.
    C. Valproate is associated with significantly higher rates of major congenital malformations.
    D. Epilepsy is a contraindication to neuraxial analgesia.

Answers and Explanations

1. **A**. CSF pressure does not change during pregnancy and remains low. The lateral position for lumbar puncture or spinal anesthesia may have very slow CSF flow filling the hub of the needle due to low CSF pressure. Uterine contractions and Valsalva/pushing during the second stage of labor may increase epidural vein size, transiently increasing CSF pressure [1].
2. **B**. Maternal cerebral blood flow increases during pregnancy due to a decrease in cerebrovascular resistance and an increase in internal carotid artery diameter (**A**). Uterine enlargement and vena caval compression in the supine position causes increased abdominal pressure and engorgement of the epidural veins (**B**), thus ultimately increasing epidural pressure (**D**). The spinal CSF volume is reduced due to the volume of epidural fat and epidural venous plexus enlargement (engorgement) during pregnancy (**C**) [2].

3. **A**. Uterine enlargement shifts weight anterior/forward when standing, causing an increase in the lumbar lordotic curve (**A**) and an anterior tilt of the upper pelvis, which may stretch the lateral femoral cutaneous nerve, causing meralgia paresthetica and sensory loss over the anterolateral thigh (**C**). Late in pregnancy, these changes may also lead to sciatica (**B**). Subsequent anterior flexion of the neck and slumping of the shoulders can also cause brachial plexus neuropathy.
4. **A**. Gait changes during pregnancy. To help maintain stability, the anterior tilt of the pelvis increases with trimester progression, which may contribute to lower back pain. Hip flexion and extension decrease with reduced step length and wider stance (**C**, **D**). External rotation increases with a wider stance (**D**). Pregnant women have a greater risk of falling due to altered biomechanics [3, 4].
5. **B**. Relaxin is an insulin-like growth factor polypeptide hormone synthesized from the corpus luteum and placenta that is associated with remodeling of collagen fibers and pelvic connective tissue. Relaxin increases tenfold during gestation, which induces ligamentous softening and peripheral and pelvic joint laxity. Loosening of the pelvis allows easier passage of the fetus through the pelvis and vaginal canal. Loosening of other ligamentous structures has been attributed to greater joint instability and back pain.
6. **A**. Degenerative spondylolisthesis is aggravated by pregnancy; however, disc herniation rarely causes back pain during pregnancy (**A**). Coccydynia occurs at 4–15% postpartum and may be caused by pressure on the coccyx during childbirth or dislocation of the apex of the coccyx (**C**). Carpal tunnel syndrome is a common cause of hand and wrist pain during pregnancy due to swelling (**B**), while De Quervain's tenosynovitis often develops postpartum when repetitive lifting of the infant causes irritation to the wrist (**D**).
7. **D**. Regardless of the use of neuraxial analgesia or anesthesia, the incidence of relapse during the postpartum period is higher (**A**). Prospective studies show no evidence that neuraxial (spinal or epidural) anesthesia is associated with neurologic injury or relapse rates in multiple sclerosis (**B**, **C**) [5, 6].
8. **C**. Although decreased sensation to labor contractions occurs with spinal cord injury at the T10 level, spinal cord injury at or above the *T6* level leads to autonomic dysreflexia (AKA autonomic hyperreflexia) (**C**). The American College of Obstetrics and Gynecology (ACOG) recommends the use of neuraxial analgesia to reduce the risk of autonomic dysreflexia (**A**). ACOG also notes that continuous blood pressure monitoring (**B**) be used and that the timing of hypertension episodes can help distinguish autonomic dysreflexia (intermittent elevation of blood pressure with contractions) from preeclampsia, which would exhibit continued elevation of blood pressure [7].
9. **A**. With the presence of asymptomatic paraspinal and intracranial tumors, neuraxial anesthesia should be administered after careful clinical and radiographic evaluations (**A**, **B**). Pregnancy may exacerbate the disease by increasing tumor growth (**C**). Increased maternal intracranial pressure (ICP) occurs with pushing, creating a Valsalva maneuver during the second stage of labor (**D**).

10. **C**. In pregnant women with increased intracranial pressure (ICP) due to mass effect, an unintentional dural puncture associated with epidural anesthesia placement can result in a sudden loss of CSF in the spinal canal, decreasing spinal CSF pressure, resulting in a pressure differential between the spinal canal and intracranial space, potentially increasing brain herniation. Therefore, many anesthesia providers favor general anesthesia for cesarean delivery in patients with a significant brain neoplasm (**A**). To preserve cerebral and utero-placental perfusion, avoidance of aortocaval compression, prophylactic or early use of vasopressor medications, and intra-arterial blood pressure monitoring instituted before induction of anesthesia are generally recommended (**B**). Since mannitol may cause fetal hyperosmolality, reduced fetal lung fluid production, decreased fetal urine production, and increased fetal plasma sodium concentration, lower doses of 0.25–0.5 mg/kg are recommended (**C**). Normal maternal pCO_2 during the third trimester is approximately 4 kPa (30 mmHg), and further hyperventilation can cause decreased transfer of oxygen to the fetus due to maternal left shifting (higher affinity) of maternal hemoglobin (**D**) [1].
11. **B**. Approximately 20% of women report pelvic pain during pregnancy. Pelvic girdle pain is usually caused by the altered weight distribution of pregnancy in addition to pelvic laxity/joints moving unevenly. Among those who reported pelvic pain, 10% continued to have pelvic pain after delivery and during the postpartum period.
12. **A**. As the uterus enlarges, the maternal diaphragmatic activity is restricted (**A**), and the pulmonary residual and closing capacities decrease (**B**), which causes greater ventilation-perfusion mismatch (**C**) and decreased arterial oxygen content (**D**).
13. **B**. Azathioprine may be used during pregnancy at lower doses less than 2 mg/kg/day (**B**). NSAID use in early pregnancy has been associated with an increased incidence of early pregnancy loss. Premature closure of the ductus arteriosus and increased risk for neonatal bleeding may occur if NSAIDs are used later in pregnancy (**A**). Methotrexate and leflunomide are highly teratogenic (**C**, **D**). The American College of Obstetrics and Gynecology (ACOG) identifies acetaminophen as a safe pain reliever during pregnancy.
14. **A**. The most common maternal antenatal complication in patients with open spinal dysraphism is recurrent urinary tract infection. Cesarean delivery is performed only for obstetric indications [8].
15. **C**. During the second stage of labor, elective assisted vaginal delivery may be used to decrease maternal physical and cardiac work; however, it does not protect against postpartum pelvic girdle pain (**B**). Dilute solutions of local anesthetic used for epidural analgesia during labor will minimize motor block and help maintain muscle tone across the pelvis, potentially reducing stress across the relaxed sacroiliac joints (**D**). Lumbosacral or lower back pain are not contraindications to neuraxial anesthesia or analgesia (**A**). Careful positioning and checking during labor or cesarean section may be helpful to prevent exacerbating preexisting back pain.

16. **D**. Neuraxial techniques are preferred for labor analgesia to decrease maternal stress and preserve strength and reserve for second-stage labor; cesarean delivery requires a higher sensory/motor block; thus, significant respiratory compromise warrants caution (**D**). The course of myasthenia gravis during pregnancy is highly variable (**A**). Magnesium is a competitive calcium antagonist. Magnesium therapy (typically therapeutic range 4–6 mEq/L) for uterine tocolysis or for seizure prophylaxis in severe preeclampsia may increase muscle weakness, thereby precipitating a myasthenic crisis. Thus, anticonvulsants (e.g., phenytoin) are recommended for seizure prophylaxis in patients with myasthenia gravis and preeclampsia (**B**). Maternal IgG antibodies to the acetylcholine receptor are transferred across the placenta, and approximately 10–20% of newborns experience transient neonatal myasthenia gravis (**C**).
17. **C**. Obesity and the exaggerated lordosis of pregnancy can put pressure on or stretch the lateral femoral cutaneous nerve, causing lateral thigh sensory loss and paresthesias. Symptoms typically resolve within 3 months of delivery.
18. **C**. ACOG recommends caffeine be limited to less than 200 mg/day, and some evidence suggests an even lower amount (**A**). Ergotamine is relatively contraindicated due to possible increases in uterine tone (**B**). NSAIDs should be limited during the third trimester due to premature closure of the fetal ductus arteriosus, oligohydramnios, and prolongation of pregnancy (**D**).
19. **A**. It is typically safe to administer neuraxial anesthesia for patients with spinal cord stimulators if there is no expected mechanical interference with the device or wires. While any surgery can produce scarring, the overwhelming majority of patients with microdiscectomies achieve normal labor epidural pain relief and epidural spread of medication (**B**, **D**). Degenerative disc disease is not a contraindication to epidural anesthesia; many patients with radiculopathy receive epidural steroid injections.
20. **D**. Due to the increased risk for teratogenicity associated with polytherapy, substituting new antiepileptic agents after conception is not usually recommended (**B**). Epilepsy is not a contraindication to the administration of neuraxial analgesia despite the potential effect of antiepileptic drugs on the coagulation system and metabolism of other medications (**C**). Pregnancy has been associated with an increase in seizures, although this may in part be due to altered metabolism and pharmacokinetics (**A**). Antiseizure medications should be closely monitored and adjusted.

References

1. Godoy DA, Robba C, Paiva WS, Rabinstein AA. Acute intracranial hypertension during pregnancy: special considerations and management adjustments. Neurocrit Care. 2022;36(1):302–16. https://doi.org/10.1007/s12028-021-01333-x. Epub 2021 Sep 7. PMID: 34494211.

2. Kacmar RM, Gaiser R. Chapter 2. Physiologic changes pregnancy; Preston R. Chapter 47. Musculoskeletal disorders; Lim G, Bader AM. Chapter 48. Neurologic and neuromuscular disease. In: Chestnut DH, Wong CA, Tsen LC, et al., editors. Chestnut's obstetric anesthesia: principles and practice, 6th ed. Elsevier; 2020.
3. Branco MA, Santos-Rocha R, Vieira F, Aguiar L, Veloso AP. Three-dimensional kinematic adaptations of gait throughout pregnancy and postpartum. Acta Bioeng Biomech. 2016;18(2):153–62. PMID: 27406315.
4. Mei Q, Gu Y, Fernandez J. Alterations of pregnant gait during pregnancy and postpartum. Sci Rep. 2018;8(1):2217. https://doi.org/10.1038/s41598-018-20648-y. PMID: 29396468.
5. Hopkins AN, Alshaeri T, Akst SA, Berger JS. Neurologic disease with pregnancy and considerations for the obstetric anesthesiologist. Semin Perinatol. 2014;38:359–69. PMID: 25176638.
6. Kopp SL, Jacob AK, Hebl JR. Regional anesthesia in patients with preexisting neurologic disease. Reg Anesth Pain Med. 2015;40:467–78. PMID: 26115188.
7. Obstetric management of patients with spinal cord injuries: ACOG committee opinion, number 808. Obstet Gynecol. 2020;135(5):e230-e236. doi: https://doi.org/10.1097/AOG.0000000000003842. PMID: 32332418.
8. Jackson AB, Mott PK. Reproductive health care for women with spina bifida. ScientificWorldJournal. 2007;7:1875–83. PMID: 18060325.

Airway and Respiratory Challenges of Pregnancy

Avrodet Mourkus and Charles Schoepflin

Questions

1. **Functional respiratory changes during pregnancy include which of the following**:
   A. Increased functional residual capacity
   B. Increased tidal volume
   C. Decreased minute ventilation
   D. Increased total lung capacity
2. **Anatomical and physiological changes, specifically of the respiratory tract, of the parturient may be exacerbated by all the following, EXCEPT:**
   A. Upper respiratory tract infection
   B. Preeclampsia
   C. Gestational diabetes
   D. Fluid overload
3. **True or False: The symptoms and diagnostic procedures for the treatment of pneumonia are different for pregnant vs nonpregnant women.**
   A. True
   B. False
4. **Which of the following puts pregnant women at a higher risk of failed tracheal intubation?**
   A. Mucosal edema
   B. Difficulty visualizing oropharyngeal structures

A. Mourkus
University of California Riverside, Riverside, CA, USA
e-mail: Avrodet.Mourkus@medsch.ucr.edu

C. Schoepflin (✉)
Riverside University Health System, Moreno Valley, CA, USA

Loma Linda University, Loma Linda, CA, USA
e-mail: C.Schoepflin@ruhealth.org

A. C. Sinha, I. F. Pasca (eds.), *Peripartum Care of the Pregnant Patient*,
https://doi.org/10.1007/978-3-031-62756-9_3

C. Obesity
D. All the above

5. **The risk of pulmonary embolism is significantly increased in parturients due to which issues associated with pregnancy.**
   A. Hypercoagulability
   B. Decreased maternal age
   C. Cesarean delivery
   D. Both A and C
6. **Complications of difficult or failed intubation in the parturient include which of the following:**
   A. Preterm labor
   B. Postpartum hemorrhage
   C. Aspiration of gastric content
   D. Preeclampsia
7. **During pregnancy, upward diaphragm displacement can be as high as:**
   A. 10 cm
   B. 14 cm
   C. 7 cm
   D. 4 cm
8. **Asthma during pregnancy may be associated with which one of the following adverse effects:**
   A. High neonatal birth weight
   B. Preterm labor
   C. Hypotension
   D. Decreased perinatal mortality
9. **Failed intubation is eight times more common in pregnancy than in other populations due to which one of the following reasons:**
   A. Caudal uterine displacement
   B. Increased lung compliance
   C. Increased neck range of motion
   D. Increased mucosal edema
10. **Which of the following physiological changes during pregnancy shorten the time for airway manipulation before significant hypoxia?**
    A. Hypoventilation
    B. Reduced functional residual capacity
    C. Increased oxygen consumption
    D. B and C
11. **Which of the following can aid in the anesthetic management of an anticipated difficult airway during labor and delivery?**
    A. Elective cesarean section with planned neuraxial anesthesia
    B. Elective cesarean section with general anesthesia and laryngeal mask airway
    C. Elective cesarean section with general anesthesia and awake fiberoptic intubation
    D. Elective cesarean section with general anesthesia and video laryngoscopic-guided intubation

12. **Which of the following hormones stimulates respiratory alkalosis during pregnancy?**
    A. Human chorionic gonadotropin hormone (hCG)
    B. Luteinizing hormone
    C. Estrogen
    D. Progesterone
13. **A 19 y/o G1P0 female 40-week gestation presents for primary C-section secondary to fetal breach presentation. Neuraxial anesthesia is performed without complications, but prior to incision, the mother becomes increasingly agitated and tachypneic. Vital signs were BP, 120/80; RR:, 26; HR, 100 bpm; and O_2 saturation, 98%. Physical examination was unremarkable and demonstrated adequate anesthesia levels for surgery. Choose the next best course of action:**
    A. Sedation with midazolam
    B. Induction of general anesthesia and intubation for airway protection
    C. Patient reassurance and further monitoring
    D. Cancel the operation until the patient stabilizes
14. **Inhalational induction is more rapid in pregnant individuals than in non-pregnant populations due to the following:**
    A. Increased sensitivity to anesthetics
    B. Increased minute ventilation
    C. Decreased functional residual capacity
    D. All the above
15. **Which of the following is one of the most effective and popular rescue devices for failed intubation?**
    A. Laryngeal mask airway (LMA)
    B. Esophageal tracheal Combitube
    C. Laryngeal tube-S
    D. None of the above
16. **Preoxygenation before administration of general anesthesia of obese parturients should achieve end-tidal oxygen concentrations (etO_2) of:**
    A. 60%
    B. 80%
    C. >90%
    D. <90%
17. **Which of the following associated with pregnancy can hinder laryngoscopy?**
    A. Diaphragm elevation
    B. Breast engorgement
    C. Decreased mucosal edema
    D. Increased lung compliance
18. **Laryngeal edema can develop very rapidly in a preeclamptic patient without many warning signs.**
    A. True.
    B. False.
    C. There are always warning signs.

D. Change in phonation is not a warning sign.

19. **Increased progesterone during pregnancy causes an enlargement of the trachea, which contributes to:**
    A. Increased functional residual capacity
    B. Decreased tidal volume
    C. Increased alveolar ventilation
    D. Increased expiratory reserve volume
20. **The incidence of failed intubation is ____ times higher than that in the general population.**
    A. 8
    B. 12
    C. 20
    D. 30

Answers and Explanations

1. The correct answer is **B**. During pregnancy, the tidal volume increases to meet increased oxygenation demands of the parturient and the fetus. The minute ventilation also increases (**C**) due to the increased need for CO_2 elimination. The functional residual capacity decreases by as much as 20% due to the larger expiratory volume (**A**), and the total lung capacity slightly decreases (**D**) [1].
2. The correct answer is **C**. There are several anatomical changes during pregnancy such as mucosal edema and swelling of the respiratory tract. These changes can be exacerbated by a mild upper respiratory tract infection (**A**), preeclampsia (**B**) which is often associated with edema, and fluid overload (**D**) [2]. There is no direct evidence that gestational diabetes affects the respiratory tract of a pregnant person (**C**).
3. The correct answer is **B**. The treatment and diagnostic testing for pneumonia is the same for pregnant and nonpregnant individuals, but the rate of morbidity and mortality from influenza and pneumonia is significantly higher in pregnancy [1]. One-third of women with respiratory failure in pregnancy have had pneumonia during their pregnancy. The heightened susceptibility to complications from influenza and pneumonia is thought to stem from physiological changes during pregnancy, including reduced functional residual capacity and diminished cell-mediated immunity.
4. The correct answer is **D**. Mucosal edema associated with pregnancy puts the parturient at an eight times greater risk of failed intubation over the general population (**A**) [1]. During preoperative airway assessment, there is a strong correlation between difficulty visualizing oropharyngeal structures and difficulty with intubation (**B**). Obese parturients are at an increased risk of failed intubation and higher maternal mortality rates (**C**).
5. The correct answer is **D**. The parturient's hypercoagulable state, which is a physiological preparation for delivery, increases their risk of pulmonary embolism [3]. Increased patient age (>35 years old) is one of the patient

characteristics that has been shown to increase the risk of pulmonary embolism (**B**) [4]. Surgical procedures increase the risk of pulmonary embolism and when compared to vaginal delivery, platelet counts are increased in cesarean delivery (**C**) [4].

6. The correct answer is **C**. Several anatomical changes in the parturient including decreased esophageal sphincter tone, delayed gastric emptying, and increased gastric pressure increase the risk of aspiration of gastric contents (**C**) [1, 2]. While preterm labor (**A**), postpartum hemorrhage (**B**), and preeclampsia (**D**) are common obstetric complications, they are not directly related to intubation and its complications.
7. The correct answer is **D**. During pregnancy, the cephalad displacement of the diaphragm can be up to 4 cm (**D**) [1, 5, 6]. This displacement leads to a loss of lung volume and consequently, a decreased functional residual capacity.
8. The correct answer is **B**. Asthma during pregnancy can lead to adverse effects including preterm labor (**B**), chronic hypertension (**C**), and increased perinatal mortality rate (**D**) [7]. The parturient's history of asthma may be related to low birth weight [7, 8].
9. The correct answer is **D**. Increased mucosal edema can decrease visualization of the airway structures and therefore lead to difficult and, consequently, failed intubation (**D**). During pregnancy, there is cranial diaphragm and uterine displacement by up to 4 cm [6] (**A**), which causes decreased lung compliance (**B**). Increased weight during pregnancy can cause decreased neck range of motion and, consequently, difficult intubation (**A**).
10. The correct answer is **D**. The reduction in functional residual capacity in pregnancy due to increased respiratory demand, mechanical compression, and cephalad dislocation of the diaphragm plays a significant role in the shortened time for airway manipulation (**B, C**) [9]. There is associated hyperventilation during pregnancy due to the increased respiratory demand (**A**).
11. The correct answer is **A**. In some cases, an elective cesarean section can be performed due to the anticipation of difficult airway management [10]. The other options are not proven to be most effective in managing anticipated difficult airways in the setting of elective cesarean deliveries (**B, C, and D**).
12. The correct answer is **D**. Increased levels of progesterone during pregnancy stimulate respiratory alkalosis due to increased tidal volume and respiratory rate, with a metabolic correction of decreased bicarbonate levels (**D**) [11]. The other hormones are not known to play a role in the development of respiratory alkalosis (**A, B, and C**).
13. The correct answer is **C**. In the operating room during cesarean section, especially for first-time parturients and emergency procedures, the experience is extremely stressful. However, the patient should continue to be monitored for respiratory failure or cardiorespiratory collapse. Additionally, the use of amnestics should be avoided prior to delivery of the fetus (**A**).
14. The correct answer is **D**. Altered physiology during pregnancy affects drug metabolism which consequently increases sensitivity to anesthetics (**A**) [11–13]. Common respiratory changes in pregnancy that contribute to rapid inhalational

induction include increased minute ventilation (**B**) and decreased functional residual capacity (**C**).

15. The correct answer is **A**. The laryngeal mask airway has been shown to be 99% effective on the first attempt (**A**) [14]. While the other choices are also effective (**B and C**), the LMA is the most effective due to its accommodation to the altered anatomy seen in pregnant women.
16. The correct answer is **C**. Airway management guidelines of obstetric patients recommend preoxygenation prior to general anesthesia, with goals to achieve end-tidal oxygen concentrations (etO_2) of >90% (**C**) [15].
17. The correct answer is **B**. Breast engorgement during pregnancy can hinder laryngoscopy, therefore requiring proper positioning of the parturient (**B**) [16]. There is increased mucosal edema (**C**) and decreased lung compliance (**D**) associated with pregnancy.
18. The correct answer is **B**. Laryngeal edema can occur very rapidly in a pre-eclamptic patient without any warning signs (**B**) [17]. Warning signs can include facial edema, voice change, or enlargement of the tongue; therefore, caution should be exercised during extubation.
19. The correct answer is **C**. The ventilatory stimulating effect of progesterone causes the hyperventilation observed in pregnant women (**C**) [17, 18]. Consequently, there will be decreased functional residual capacity (**A**), increased tidal volume (**B**), and decreased expiratory reserve volume (**D**).
20. The correct answer is **A**. Airway management in the obstetric population is more difficult due to many factors including anatomical and physiological changes including edema, metabolic changes, and obesity. These changes lead to a higher incidence of failed intubation [19].

References

1. Mighty HE. Acute respiratory failure in pregnancy. Clin Obstet Gynecol. 2010;53:360.
2. Munnur U, de Boisblanc B, Suresh MS. Airway problems in pregnancy. Crit Care Med. 2005;33:S259.
3. Pulmonary embolism in pregnancy. Lancet. 2010;375:500–512.
4. Pulmonary embolism and stroke in relation to pregnancy: how can high-risk women be identified? Am J Obstet Gynecol. 2002;186:198–203.
5. Lapinsky SE. Acute respiratory failure in pregnancy. Sage J. 2015;8:126.
6. MRI evaluation of maternal cardiac displacement in pregnancy: implications for cardiopulmonary resuscitation. Am J Obstet Gynecol. 2015;213:401.e1–401.e5.
7. Maternal asthma and risk of preterm delivery. Ann Epidemiol. 2003;13:267–272.
8. Pregnancy related treatment disparities of acute asthma exacerbations in the emergency department. Respir Med. 2011;105:1434–1440.
9. Izakson A, Cohen Y, Landau R. Physiologic changes in the airway and the respiratory system affecting management in pregnancy. In: Principles and practice of maternal critical care. 2020. pp 271–283. https://doi.org/10.1007/978-3-030-43477-9_20.
10. Mushambi MC, Athanassoglou V, Kinsella SM. Anticipated difficult airway during obstetric general anaesthesia: narrative literature review and management recommendations. Anaesthesia. 2020;75:945–61.

11. Kidney physiology in pregnancy. Adv Chronic Kidney Dis. 2020;27:449–454.
12. Jeong H. Altered drug metabolism during pregnancy: hormonal regulation of drug-metabolizing enzymes. Expert Opin Drug Metab Toxicol. 2010;6:689. https://doi.org/10.1517/17425251003677755.
13. Anesthesia in pregnant patients for nonobstetric surgery. J Clin Anesth. 2006;18:60–66.
14. Principles and practices of obstetric airway management. Anesthesiol Clin. 2008;26:109–125.
15. High-flow humidified nasal preoxygenation in pregnant women: a prospective observational study. Br J Anaesth. 2019;122:86–91.
16. Munnur U, Bandi VD, Gropper MA. Airway management and mechanical ventilation in pregnancy. In: Pulmonary problems in pregnancy. 2009. pp. 385–403. https://doi.org/10.1007/978-1-59745-445-2_23.
17. Rocke DA, Scoones GP. Rapidly progressive laryngeal oedema associated with pregnancy-aggravated hypertension. Anaesthesia. 1992;47:141–3.
18. Hirnle L, et al. Respiratory function in pregnant women. In: Neurobiology of respiration. 2013. pp. 153–160. https://doi.org/10.1007/978-94-007-6627-3_23.
19. Teoh WH. Airway management during pregnancy and the peripartum period. In: Principles and practice of maternal critical care. 2020. pp. 285–304. https://doi.org/10.1007/978-3-030-43477-9_21.

Endocrinologic Disorders of Pregnancy

Ashley Almajan and Ioana F. Pasca

Questions

1. **A physiological drop in which hormone can be expected during the first trimester of pregnancy?**
   A. TSH
   B. HCG
   C. FT4
   D. ACTH
2. **How often will hypothyroid patients require TSH levels to be drawn during the first half of pregnancy?**
   A. Every 4 weeks
   B. Every 6 weeks
   C. Every 8 weeks
   D. Every 12 weeks
3. **Failure to treat maternal hypothyroidism during pregnancy can lead to which of the following:**
   A. Decreased risk of miscarriage
   B. Higher birth weight

A. Almajan
Riverside University Health System, Moreno Valley, CA, USA
e-mail: Ashley.Almajan@ruhealth.org

I. F. Pasca (✉)
Riverside University Health System, Moreno Valley, CA, USA

Department of Anesthesiology, Critical Care, and Neurocritical Care, Loma Linda University at Riverside University Health System, Loma Linda, CA, USA

University of California San Diego, San Diego, CA, USA

University of California Riverside, Riverside, CA, USA
e-mail: i.pasca@ruhealth.org

A. C. Sinha, I. F. Pasca (eds.), *Peripartum Care of the Pregnant Patient*,
https://doi.org/10.1007/978-3-031-62756-9_4

C. Increased intellectual functioning in offspring
D. Low birth weight

4. **Subclinical hypothyroidism should be treated with T4 replacement if serum TSH is between 2.5–10 mU/L *except* in patients who:**
A. Are pregnant
B. Attempting pregnancy
C. Have a large goiter
D. Have no symptoms and are not pregnant or attempting pregnancy

5. **Postpartum thyroiditis will present with which of the following characteristics?**
A. Hyper- or hypothyroid symptoms and a painless goiter
B. Hyper- or hypothyroid symptoms and a painful goiter
C. Painful and tender goiter
D. Nonthyroidal illness syndrome

6. **Which antithyroid drug is recommended for Graves' disease in pregnant patients during the first trimester?**
A. Methimazole
B. Propylthiouracil
C. Radioiodine
D. Methadone

7. **Which are the most serious side effects of propylthiouracil?**
A. Hepatic toxicity and agranulocytosis
B. Kidney toxicity and thrombocytopenia
C. Graves ophthalmopathy and periorbital edema
D. Pretibial myxedema and adrenal insufficiency

8. **Which of the following is the most appropriate diagnostic test for a pregnant patient with a 3-week history of palpitations, heat intolerance, tremulousness, and evidence of goiter on exam?**
A. Thyroid ultrasound
B. Total triiodothyronine measurement
C. Thyroid-stimulating immunoglobulin measurement
D. Thyroid scintigraphy with radioactive iodine uptake

9. **Which of the following is the preferred agent for the management of both type 1 and type 2 diabetes during pregnancy?**
A. Insulin
B. Chlorpropamide
C. Nateglinide
D. Rosiglitazone

10. **Which of the following blood sugar values are diagnostic of gestational diabetes mellitus when using the two-step approach?**
A. 126 mg/dL followed by 1 h GTT 160 mg/dL
B. 140 mg/dL followed by 1 h GTT 190 mg/dL
C. 136 mg/dL followed by 3 h GTT 135 mg/dL
D. 140 mg/dL followed by 3 h GTT 139 mg/dL

11. **Which of the following is the optimal HgbA1c goal level that should be achieved during pregnancy without causing significant hypoglycemia?**
    A. <6%
    B. <7%
    C. <7.5%
    D. <8%
12. **How will the insulin requirements of a pregnant patient with previously diagnosed diabetes mellitus be expected to change during the second trimester?**
    A. Insulin requirements will decrease
    B. Insulin requirements will remain the same
    C. Insulin requirements will increase
    D. Patient will no longer require insulin during pregnancy
13. **When should screening for gestational diabetes occur?**
    A. Between 16 and 20 weeks gestation
    B. Between 21 and 23 weeks gestation
    C. Between 24 and 28 weeks gestation
    D. Between 29 and 32 weeks gestation
14. **Immediately after delivery, a previously healthy patient is noted to have severe hypotension along with massive hemorrhage. Following delivery, the patient is unable to lactate her newborn, experiencing genital and axillary hair loss, dry skin, and generalized weakness. Which of the following is the most likely explanation?**
    A. Ischemic stroke
    B. Brain neoplasm
    C. Postpartum psychosis
    D. Sheehan's syndrome
15. **Which of the following medications is considered safe in pregnancy?**
    A. Levothyroxine
    B. Lisinopril
    C. Ibuprofen
    D. Atorvastatin
    E. Lithium

Answers and Explanations

1. **A**: Increase in hCG (**B**) will stimulate the TSH receptor causing increased thyroid hormone production free T4 (**C**). Increased thyroid hormone production stimulates the negative feedback loop, resulting in decreased TSH (**A**). ACTH (**D**) rises in proportion to increasing cortisol in pregnancy [1].
2. **A**: Due to increasing requirements, TSH will need to be checked every 4 weeks, and the dosing may be adjusted 25–50% more than prepregnancy requirements [2].

3. **D**: Untreated hypothyroidism in pregnancy can lead to low birth weight, increased risk of miscarriage and stillbirth, and increased risk of pre-eclampsia [3].
4. **D**: The American Thyroid Association guidelines recommend that subclinical hypothyroidism should be treated in pregnancy (**A**), those attempting pregnancy (**B**), the presence of a large goiter (**C**), and symptomatic patients with anti-TPO antibodies [2].
5. **A**: Postpartum thyroiditis will present with hyper- or hypothyroid symptoms and a painless goiter. Patients will follow a typical pattern starting with the hyperthyroid phase followed by the euthyroid phase, followed by the hypothyroid phase and eventually ending in the euthyroid phase, with 20% remaining in the hypothyroid phase. Hyper- or hypothyroid with a painful goiter includes subacute, infectious, and radiation thyroiditis (**B**, **C**). Nonthyroidal illness syndrome (euthyroid sick syndrome) is seen in critically ill (hospitalized patients) or starving patients characterized by low to low-normal TSH and free T4 and very low free T3 (**D**) [4].
6. **B**: The American Thyroid Association recommends propylthiouracil (**B**), as it is associated with a lower frequency of birth defects than methimazole (**A**). Radioiodine is not recommended during pregnancy, as it can lead to fetal hypothyroidism, intellectual disability, and increased risk of malignancy in the infant (**C**). Methadone is not used to treat thyroid disfunction (**D**).
7. **A**: The most serious potential side effects of propylthiouracil include hepatic toxicity and agranulocytosis [3].
8. **C**: The patient presented with symptoms of hyperthyroidism. Autoantibodies are usually not measured unless a thyroid uptake and scan cannot be performed (e.g., in pregnancy, patient received recent contrast) (**C**). A thyroid ultrasound (**A**) is usually performed if there is a palpable nodule accompanied by TSH level suggestive of hypothyroid or euthyroid. The majority of thyroid hormone produced is thyroxine (T4). Free thyroxine (FT4) and TSH are generally measured when testing thyroid disorders. The total triiodothyronine level (T3) (**B**) is seldom obtained; it is the product of deiodination of T4 in peripheral tissues. Thyroid scintigraphy with radioactive iodine uptake will show an enlarged gland with diffusely increased uptake, but it is not recommended in pregnancy [2].
9. **A**: Insulin is the first-choice agent in pregnancy because it does not cross the placenta. (**B**) Chlorpropamide is a first-generation sulfonylurea that can lead to fetal hypoglycemia and congenital anomalies. There is no data regarding the use of nateglinide during pregnancy and is therefore not recommended (**C**). Rosiglitazone (**D**) crosses the placenta and may lead to delayed growth and insulin resistance [5].
10. **B**: The two-step approach for screening and diagnosis of diabetes in pregnancy is recommended by the American College of Obstetricians and Gynecologists (ACOG). In step one, give 50 g oral glucose solution and following 1 h measure venous plasma or serum glucose concentration with glucose >135 mg/dL or >140 mg/dL requiring the administration of a 100 g oral glucose tolerance test. In step two, administer 100 g of oral glucose solution and measure plasma or

serum glucose during fasting. Proposed cutoffs for diagnosing gestational diabetes mellitus include fasting blood glucose >95 mg/dL, 1-h blood glucose >180 mg/dL, 2-h glucose >155 mg/dL, and 3-h glucose >140 mg/dL post administration [6].

11. **A**: The HbA1C target in pregnancy is 6–6.5% (42–48 mmol/mol); <6% (42 mmol/mol) may be optimal if this can be achieved without significant hypoglycemia, but the target may be relaxed to <7% (53 mmol/mol) if necessary to prevent hypoglycemia. The HbA1C goal is lower in pregnancy due to increased red cell turnover [7].
12. **C**: During the second trimester, there is a rapid increase in insulin resistance, necessitating an increase in insulin dose, usually approximately 50% more, to achieve the recommended glycemic target. In the first trimester, insulin requirements may be lower (**A**), as contra-insulin hormones produced by the placenta are usually not produced until the 24th week of gestation [7].
13. **C**: Screening for gestational diabetes should occur between 24 and 28 weeks gestation. Earlier testing has not been shown to be beneficial. In a randomized trial, early pregnancy diabetes screening (14–20 weeks) because of obesity alone (BMI ≥30 kg/m^2) did not demonstrate a reduction in a composite of adverse outcomes, including macrosomia, primary cesarean delivery, hypertensive disease of pregnancy, shoulder dystocia, neonatal hyperbilirubinemia, or hypoglycemia [8].
14. **D**: Sheehan's syndrome is characterized by postpartum hypopituitarism due to necrosis of pituitary gland. Often seen following massive hemorrhage during delivery or the immediate postpartum period and is associated with severe hypotension or shock. Ischemic stroke (**A**) and brain neoplasm (**B**) do not typically present with hair loss or dry skin. Postpartum psychosis (**C**) will present with insomnia, anxiety, irritability, mood fluctuations, and abnormal thought content [9].
15. **A**: Levothyroxine is considered safe in pregnancy. ACE inhibitors (**B**) are known to cause intrauterine growth restriction, still birth, and oligohydramnios. Ibuprofen (**C**) may cause premature closure of the ductus arteriosus and oligohydramnios. Atorvastatin (**D**) may cause congenital anomalies and delayed fetal development. Lithium (**E**) is known to cause Ebstein anomaly [10].

References

1. Pregnancy and thyroid disease—National Institute of Diabetes and Digestive and Kidney Diseases. https://www.niddk.nih.gov/-/media/Files/Endocrine-Diseases/Pregnancy_Thyroid_Disease_508.pdf?la=en. Accessed 11 Feb 2023.
2. Hypothyroidism in pregnancy. American Thyroid Association. n.d. https://www.thyroid.org/hypothyroidism-in-pregnancy/. Accessed 17 Dec 2022.
3. Alexander EK, Pearce EN, Brent GA, et al. 2017 guidelines of the American Thyroid Association for the diagnosis and management of thyroid disease during pregnancy and the postpartum. Thyroid. 2017;27(3):315–89.

4. Postpartum thyroiditis. American Thyroid Association. n.d. https://www.thyroid.org/postpartum-thyroiditis/. Accessed 17 Dec 2022.
5. Kavitha N, De S, Kanagasabai S. Oral hypoglycemic agents in pregnancy: an update. J Obstet Gynecol India. 2013. https://www.ncbi.nlm.nih.gov/pmc/articles/PMC3664692/. Accessed 17 Dec 2022.
6. ACOG practice bulletin no. 190: gestational diabetes mellitus. Obstet Gynecol. 2018;131(2):e49–e64. https://doi.org/10.1097/AOG.0000000000002501.
7. Management of diabetes in pregnancy: standards of medical care in diabetes—2018. Diabetes Care. 2017;41(Supplement 1):S137–S143. https://doi.org/10.2337/dc18-s013.
8. Harper LM, Jauk V, Longo S, Biggio JR, Szychowski JM, Tita AT. Early gestational diabetes screening in obese women: a randomized controlled trial. Am J Obstet Gynecol. 2020;222(5):495.e1–8. https://doi.org/10.1016/j.ajog.2019.12.021.
9. Shivaprasad C. Sheehan's syndrome: newer advances. Indian J Endocrinol Metab. 2011;15 Suppl 3(Suppl3):S203–7. https://doi.org/10.4103/2230-8210.84869.
10. Hannaman RA, Hatchell CA. Women's and men's health-obstetrics. In: Internal medicine review core curriculum, 2021-2022. MedStudy; 2020.

Peripartum Hypertensive Disease

PJ McGuire

Questions

1. **In 2017, the American College of Cardiology/American Heart Association (ACC/AHA) proposed new blood pressure guidelines and updated recommendations for antihypertensive medication initiation and intensification. Which of the following is MOST consistent with the new ACC/AHA recommendations?**
   A. A diastolic blood pressure treatment target goal of <90 mmHg.
   B. A systolic blood pressure treatment target goal of <130 mmHg.
   C. Blood pressure treatment goals only apply to adults with other comorbidities.
   D. Blood pressure treatment goals only apply to adults >65 years old.
2. **A 23-year-old G2P1 at 34 weeks presents to Labor and Delivery Triage complaining of foamy urine. Her blood pressure is 152/95, and she is diagnosed with preeclampsia. Which of the following is the MOST common cause of morbidity in women with preeclampsia?**
   A. Myocardial infarction
   B. Stroke
   C. Postpartum hemorrhage
   D. Suicide
3. **A 25-year-old G1P0 with a protein to creatinine ratio of 0.5 is diagnosed with preeclampsia. All of the following are risk factors for preeclampsia, EXCEPT:**
   A. A history of chronic hypertension
   B. Multiparity

P. J. McGuire (✉)
Yale New Haven Hospital, New Haven, CT, USA
e-mail: pj.mcguire@yale.edu

A. C. Sinha, I. F. Pasca (eds.), *Peripartum Care of the Pregnant Patient*,
https://doi.org/10.1007/978-3-031-62756-9_5

C. Assisted reproductive technology
D. A history of chronic renal disease

4. **A 30-year-old G2P2 who is postpartum day two from a cesarean delivery for preeclampsia collapses unexpectedly while getting out of bed. All of the following are within the top five causes of pregnancy-related maternal mortality in the United States, EXCEPT:**
   A. Hemorrhage
   B. Cardiovascular conditions
   C. Anesthetic complications
   D. Mental health conditions (includes deaths by suicide or overdose/poisoning related to substance use disorder)
5. **A 32-year-old G1P0 presents to Labor and Delivery Triage complaining of a frontal headache, blurry vision, and photophobia with a blood pressure of 148/95. Preeclampsia is confirmed by labs. While the RN is preparing a magnesium sulfate infusion, the patient experiences an acute onset tonic-clonic seizure. Which of the following is the MOST appropriate first-line treatment?**
   A. Benzodiazepines
   B. Levetiracetam
   C. Magnesium sulfate
   D. Phenytoin
6. **A 36-year-old G4P1 who suffered from severe preeclampsia necessitating cesarean delivery at 37 weeks in her last pregnancy comes in for a postpartum visit. She complains of chronic fatigue, shortness of breath with exertion, and swelling in her ankles. Her BNP is elevated. Which of the following is the MOST appropriate next step in her management?**
   A. Start a beta-blocker and ACE inhibitor
   B. Albuterol, as needed
   C. Start midodrine
   D. Start a potassium-channel blocker
7. **A magnesium infusion for a 29-year-old G2P1 with preeclampsia has been running for over 12 hours. The patient's blood pressure is 85/58. She is somnolent, flushed, and complaining of shortness of breath. Her serum magnesium level results and it is 12 mg/dL. Which of the following is the MOST appropriate first line of treatment?**
   A. Calcium gluconate
   B. Diphenhydramine
   C. Epinephrine
   D. Intralipid emulsion
8. **A 33-year-old G1P0 comes in for a high-risk obstetric anesthesia consult for a BMI 55. Her BP is 155/90, and her SpO2 is 95%. As an early recognition tool for preeclampsia, providers should be alerted by all the following signs or symptoms of preeclampsia EXCEPT:**
   A. Maternal heart rate 115 bpm
   B. Category I fetal heart tracing

C. Urine output <40 mL/h
D. Shortness of breath at rest

9. **A 28-year-old G2P1 at 18 weeks comes in for a routine obstetrical visit. Her blood pressure is 145/90. All her laboratory results, including a urine test, are within normal limits. Which of the following is the MOST appropriate diagnosis?**
   A. Gestational hypertension
   B. Ongoing/chronic hypertension
   C. Preeclampsia
   D. HELLP
10. **A 28-year-old G2P1 at 25 weeks comes in for a routine obstetrical visit. Her blood pressure is 145/90, and she complains of a headache. She is sent to Triage at the Labor and Delivery suite, where her labs show a serum creatinine concentration of 1.2 mg/dL. She has no history or risk factors for renal disease. Which of the following is the MOST appropriate diagnosis?**
   A. Gestational hypertension
   B. Ongoing/chronic hypertension
   C. Preeclampsia
   D. HELLP
11. **A 28-year-old G2P1 at 25 weeks comes in for a routine obstetrical visit. Her blood pressure is 125/80, and she complains of a headache. Her last pregnancy was complicated by preeclampsia necessitating an urgent cesarean delivery at 34-weeks gestation. For this pregnancy, she is prescribed low-dose aspirin to prevent or delay the onset of preeclampsia. Which of the following is the MOST likely mechanism of action of aspirin in this scenario?**
   A. Enhancement of descending serotoninergic pathway inhibition
   B. Inhibition of the reuptake of norepinephrine and serotonin
   C. Inhibition of spinal nociceptive transmission
   D. Decreased thromboxane A2 production
12. **A 28-year-old G2P1 at 25-weeks comes in for a routine obstetrical visit. Her blood pressure is 165/115, and she complains of right upper quadrant pain. She is sent to Triage at the Labor and Delivery suite where her labs show an alanine transaminase level of 155 U/L and aspartate aminotransferase level of 146 U/L, but platelets are within normal limits. She has no history or risk factors for liver disease. Which of the following is the MOST appropriate diagnosis?**
   A. Gestational hypertension
   B. Preeclampsia
   C. Preeclampsia with severe features
   D. HELLP
13. **A 25-year-old G1P0 at 40-weeks is diagnosed with preeclampsia and admitted to the Labor and Delivery suite. During your anesthetic evaluation, she complains of a headache and blurry vision. Suddenly, she has a tonic-clonic seizure. Her vitals are within normal limits, including her SpO_2which is**

99%. What is the MOST appropriate next step of care after you call for help?

A. Emergent intubation
B. Administer midazolam
C. Open airway and give supplemental oxygen by a nonrebreather mask
D. Emergent CT head imaging

14. **A 36-year-old G4P1 who suffered from severe preeclampsia necessitating early cesarean delivery at 37-weeks in her last delivery comes in for a postpartum visit. She complains of chronic fatigue, shortness of breath with exertion and swelling in her ankles. Her BNP is elevated. Which of the following is the MOST likely diagnosis?**
    A. HELLP
    B. Preeclampsia
    C. Peripartum cardiomyopathy
    D. Normal postpartum physiological changes
15. **A 28-year-old G4P1 at 36-weeks who is ruptured and in active labor is admitted to the Labor and Delivery suite. Her blood pressure is 150/100, and she complains of frothy urine. An hour ago, she took aspirin 81 mg and is now requesting an epidural. Which of the following is the MOST appropriate next step?**
    A. She cannot have an epidural due to her aspirin use.
    B. Wait 4–6 h, then place an epidural.
    C. Obtain a CBC.
    D. Nothing is needed; you can place the epidural now.
16. **A 32-year-old G2P1 at 36 -weeks is taking aspirin 81 mg for preeclampsia prevention. Which of the following BEST describes the pathophysiology of preeclampsia?**
    A. Upregulation of factor X levels
    B. sFLT1-mediated systemic endothelial dysfunction
    C. Upregulation of the renin-angiotensin-aldosterone system (RAAS)
    D. Progesterone-mediated upregulation of bradykinin
17. **A 32-year-old G2P1 at 38 weeks with a BMI of 62 presents to Triage complaining of a headache that is refractory to analgesics. Her BP is 165/115. LDH is normal, but her platelets are 60 K. She is diagnosed with preeclampsia with severe features. Shortly thereafter, she goes into labor, making fast cervical change, and asks for an epidural. Which of the following is MOST consistent with current society for obstetric anesthesia and perinatology (SOAP) guidelines for safe neuraxial placement in patients with thrombocytopenia?**
    A. Platelet count $\geq$70 K.
    B. Platelet count $\geq$100 K.
    C. There is no current guideline for optimal platelet count.
    D. You can place an epidural now since this is a new finding.
18. **You're a medical student on your obstetric anesthesia rotation. You've just learned that maternal mortality in pregnancy has been steadily rising in**

the USA and is associated with the widest and most persistent inequality in all US public health, according to the CDC. Which of the following ethnic groups is associated with the GREATEST risk of dying in pregnancy?
   A. Ashkenazi Jewish descendants
   B. Non-Hispanic Caucasians
   C. Non-Hispanic African Americans
   D. Hispanic descendants

19. **A 32 yo G1P0 at 35 weeks presents to Triage complaining of colicky epigastric abdominal pain with nausea and vomiting. Her blood pressure is 165/115, her platelet count is 55 K, and a peripheral blood smear shows schistocytes and burr cells. She is diagnosed with HELLP syndrome, and you proceed to the OR for urgent cesarean delivery under general anesthesia. You prepare propofol and succinylcholine for RSI and a 6.5 cm endotracheal tube for intubation. Which of the following is the MOST appropriate next step in management?**
   A. Aggressively coload the patient with IV fluids.
   B. Start a third IV.
   C. Administer dexamethasone.
   D. Take precautions to blunt the hemodynamic response to laryngoscopy and intubation.
20. **A 28 yo G2P1 at 33 weeks comes in for a routine obstetrical visit. She has a history of chronic hypertension. Which of the following is the MOST common fetal complication associated with women with chronic hypertension in pregnancy?**
   A. Cerebral palsy
   B. Omphalocele
   C. Fetal growth restriction
   D. Hypoglycemia

Answers and Explanations

1. **B**. The 2017 ACC/AHA guidelines recommend an SBP treatment target goal of <130 mmHg and a DBP treatment target goal of <80 mmHg for adults <65 years of age and those ≥65 years of age with diabetes, CKD, a history of CVD, or a 10-year predicted CVD risk ≥10% [1].
2. **B**. Complications of preeclampsia include multi-end-organ failure, but the most common and dreaded complication is hemorrhagic stroke [2].
3. **B**. Nulliparity is a risk factor for preeclampsia, not multiparity. Other risk factors for preeclampsia include age > 35, multiple gestation, BMI > 30, diabetes (includes gestational), OSA, autoimmune disorders like systemic lupus erythematosus and antiphospholipid syndrome, and thrombophilia [3].
4. **C**. According to the CDC, the top five underlying causes of pregnancy-related deaths from 2017 to 2019 were (1) mental health conditions, (2) hemorrhage, (3) cardiac and coronary conditions, (4) infection, and (5) thrombotic embolism [4].

5. **C**. This patient is having an eclamptic seizure and the first line medication therapy is magnesium sulfate. If the seizure is nonterminating, you may consider giving a benzodiazepine such as midazolam or small doses of propofol [5].
6. **A**. This patient presents with heart failure symptoms and most likely has peripartum cardiomyopathy. Treatment is supportive and usually directed at treating the heart failure symptoms. Postpartum, selective Beta 1 blockers and ACE inhibitors have been known to reduce mortality [6].
7. **A**. This patient has signs and symptoms of magnesium toxicity for which the treatment is calcium gluconate (or calcium chloride) [7].
8. **B**. A category I fetal heart tracing is normal and therefore should not alert you to a diagnosis of preeclampsia. A high heart rate, low urine output, and shortness of breath at rest are alarms for preeclampsia and warrant further screening [8].
9. **B**. This patient presents with chronic hypertension which occurs before pregnancy or before 20 weeks gestation. Gestational hypertension is used to describe cases in which elevated blood pressure without proteinuria develops in a woman after 20 weeks gestation and blood pressure levels return to normal postpartum. As many as one quarter of women with gestational hypertension will develop proteinuria, i.e., preeclampsia [9].
10. **C**. The combination of blood pressure of 140 mmHg or more or diastolic blood pressure of 90 mmHg or more and the presence of renal insufficiency as seen by a serum creatinine concentration greater than 1.1 mg/dL in the absence of other renal disease is a diagnosis of preeclampsia [8].
11. **D**. Aspirin at low doses (below 300 mg) irreversibly inactivates the COX-1 enzyme, decreasing the production of prostaglandins and thromboxane and inhibiting inflammation and platelet aggregation. It has been postulated that this can help prevent preeclampsia [10].
12. **C**. The combination of blood pressure greater than 160 mmHg and a diastolic blood pressure of greater than 110 mmHg coupled with impaired liver function resulting in test results that are more than twice the upper limit of normal is a diagnosis of preeclampsia with severe features [8].
13. **C**. This patient presented with eclampsia. After you have called for help, the initial steps are to secure the airway and give supplemental oxygen ensuring a normal SpO_2. You must also position the patient with a left lateral tilt. If the patient becomes hypoxic or the seizure is nonterminating, intubation should be considered. Magnesium sulfate is the initial treatment for an eclamptic seizure. A benzodiazepine can be administered if a bolus of magnesium fails or if the seizure is nonterminating [11].
14. **C**. This patient has many risk factors for and is showing signs of peripartum cardiomyopathy including shortness of breath, pretibial edema, and fatigue [6].
15. **C**. This patient shows signs and symptoms of preeclampsia. Low-dose aspirin is not a contraindication for epidural placement, and there is no need to wait for any time period. However, obtaining a platelet level from a CBC is necessary to ensure an appropriate level, as this patient could be progressing to HELLP.

16. **B**. The pathophysiology of preeclampsia is caused by abnormal remodeling of the spiral arteries of the placenta. It is thought that this is caused by increased circulating sFlt1, which helps to decrease circulating levels of free vascular endothelial growth factor (VEGF) and placental growth factor (PlGF), resulting in systemic endothelial dysfunction [12].
17. **A**. This patient has a high risk of bleeding due to her thrombocytopenia. Currently, there is a consensus statement based on class IIa and level C-LD evidence that if the platelet count is ≥70 K, then there is likely to be a low risk of spinal epidural hematoma, and it is reasonable to proceed with a neuraxial procedure if clinically indicated. For platelet counts between 50 and 70 K, a risk-benefit ratio may justify proceeding with neuraxial placement [13].
18. **C**. In 2020, the maternal mortality rate for non-Hispanic Black women was 55.3 deaths per 100,000 live births, 2.9 times the rate for non-Hispanic White women. Data from the CDC show that there is a statistically significant increase in mortality rate ($p < 0.05$) for non-Hispanic Black women compared to rates for non-Hispanic White and Hispanic women [14].
19. **D**. Care must *always* be taken to minimize the hypertensive response to laryngoscopy and intubation to prevent complications such as intracranial hemorrhage or pulmonary edema. (Cantwell R, et al. Saving Mothers' Lives: Reviewing maternal deaths to make motherhood safer: 2006–2008. The Eighth Report of the Confidential Enquiries into Maternal Deaths in the United Kingdom. BJOG. 2011 Mar;118 Suppl 1:1–203.) Medications that may be used include the following: labetalol titrated with 10 mg IV boluses up to 1 mg/kg prior to induction; esmolol 2 mg/kg IV during induction, or 1 mg/kg IV with lidocaine; nitroglycerin 1.5–2.5 mcg/kg IV; nicardipine 15–30 mcg/kg IV, or 100–200 mcg bolus during induction; remifentanil 1 mcg/kg IV during induction, which crosses the placenta and may cause transient neonatal respiratory depression; or fentanyl 1–3 mcg/kg IV [15].
20. **C**. Common fetal/neonatal complications in women with chronic hypertension who are now pregnant include fetal growth restriction/small for gestational age infant, preterm delivery, congenital anomalies, stillbirth, and neonatal death [16].

References

1. Colantonio LD, et al. 2017 ACC/AHA blood pressure treatment guideline recommendations and cardiovascular risk. J Am Coll Cardiol. 2018;72(11):1187–97.
2. Bushnell C, Chireau M. Preeclampsia and stroke: risks during and after pregnancy. Stroke Res Treat. 2011;2011:858134.
3. Rana S, et al. Preeclampsia. Circ Res. 2019;124(7):1094–112.
4. Trost SL, Beauregard J, Njie F, et al. Pregnancy-related deaths: data from maternal mortality review committees in 36 US states, 2017–2019. Atlanta: Centers for Disease Control and Prevention, US Department of Health and Human Services; 2022.
5. Magley M, Hinson MR. Eclampsia. [Updated 2022 Feb 16]. In: StatPearls [Internet]. Treasure Island: StatPearls Publishing; 2022

6. Behrens I, Basit S, Lykke JA, et al. Association between hypertensive disorders of pregnancy and later risk of cardiomyopathy. JAMA. 2016;315(10):1026–33. https://doi.org/10.1001/jama.2016.1869.
7. Ajib FA, Childress JM. Magnesium toxicity. [Updated 2022 Nov 7]. In: StatPearls [Internet]. Treasure Island: StatPearls Publishing; 2022.
8. Gestational hypertension and preeclampsia: ACOG practice bulletin, number 222. Obstet Gynecol. 2020;135(6):e237-e260. PMID: 32443079. https://doi.org/10.1097/AOG.0000000000003891
9. Sibai B, Ramadan M, Chari R, Friedman S. Pregnancies complicated by HELLP syndrome (hemolysis, elevated liver enzymes, and low platelets): subsequent pregnancy outcome and long-term prognosis. Am J Obstet Gynecol. 1995;172:125–9.
10. Rolnik DL, Nicolaides KH, Poon LC. Prevention of preeclampsia with aspirin. Am J Obstet Gynecol. 2022;226(2S):S1108–19.
11. Parthasarathy S, Kumar VR, Sripriya R, Ravishankar M. Anesthetic management of a patient presenting with eclampsia. Anesth Essays Res. 2013;7(3):307–12. CMQCC PREECLAMPSIA TOOLKIT PREECLAMPSIA CARE GUIDELINES CDPH-MCAH Approved: 12/20/13.
12. Maynard SE, et al. Excess placental soluble fms-like tyrosine kinase 1 (sFlt1) may contribute to endothelial dysfunction, hypertension, and proteinuria in preeclampsia. J Clin Invest. 2003;111(5):649–58.
13. Bauer ME, Arendt K, Beilin Y, Gernsheimer T, Perez Botero J, James AH, Yaghmour E, Toledano RD, Turrentine M, Houle T, MacEachern M, Madden H, Rajasekhar A, Segal S, Wu C, Cooper JP, Landau R, Leffert L. The Society for Obstetric Anesthesia and Perinatology interdisciplinary consensus statement on neuraxial procedures in obstetric patients with thrombocytopenia. Anesth Analg. 2021;132(6):1531–44. https://doi.org/10.1213/ANE.0000000000005355. PMID: 33861047.
14. Hoyert DL. Maternal mortality rates in the United States, 2020. NCHS Health E-Stats; 2022.
15. Cantwell R, et al. Saving Mothers' Lives: Reviewing maternal deaths to make motherhood safer: 2006–2008. The Eighth Report of the Confidential Enquiries into Maternal Deaths in the United Kingdom. BJOG. 2011;118(Suppl 1):1–203.
16. ACOG practice bulletin no. 203 summary: chronic hypertension in pregnancy. Obstet Gynecol. 2019; 133:215.

Further Reading

ACOG: pregnancy and heart disease. Obstet Gynecol. 2019.

Creanga AA, et al. Pregnancy-related mortality in the United States, 2006-2010. Obstet Gynecol. 2015;125:5–12.

Melchiorre K, et al. Hypertensive disorders of pregnancy and future cardiovascular health. Front Cardiovasc Med. 2020;7:59.

Cardiac Disease in Pregnancy

Jonathan Molina Cifuentes and Kristen L. Fardelmann

Questions

1. **During a physical exam on a 35-year-old female at 28 weeks gestation, you may find all the following changes, *except*:**
   A. A systolic murmur
   B. The presence of a third heart sound (S3)
   C. Accentuation of the first heart sound (S1)
   D. Rightward displacement of the point of maximal cardiac impulse
2. **At term, what is the overall increase of the left ventricular (LV) mass?**
   A. 25%
   B. 50%
   C. 75%
   D. 95%
3. **Which of the following statements is true:**
   A. Intraosseous, vertebral, paravertebral, epidural veins and the azygos system contribute to venous return, especially when a pregnant patient is in supine position.
   B. There is no difference in inferior vena cava (IVC) volume when laterally tilting a pregnant patient at term 15° or 30°.
   C. Femoral arterial blood pressure and brachial arterial blood pressure remain the same when a pregnant patient at term is positioned supine.
   D. Supine hypotension syndrome occurs a few seconds after placing a patient at term in supine position.

J. M. Cifuentes (✉) · K. L. Fardelmann
Yale School of Medicine, New Haven, CT, USA
e-mail: Jonathan.molinacifuentes@yale.edu; kristen.fardelmann@yale.edu

A. C. Sinha, I. F. Pasca (eds.), *Peripartum Care of the Pregnant Patient*,
https://doi.org/10.1007/978-3-031-62756-9_6

4. **A healthy 22-year-old female G1P0 at 39 weeks gestation presents in active labor. A successful labor epidural was placed for analgesia and an uncomplicated vaginal and placental delivery followed. Which statement best represents the hemodynamic changes immediately after delivery?**
   A. Decrease of LV wall mass due to the changes in LV wall stress and reduction of hormonal concentrations in the plasma
   B. Increase in stroke volume caused by an increase in venous return and the displacement of blood from the intervillous space to the systemic circulation
   C. Return of systolic and diastolic blood pressure to prepregnancy levels
   D. No change in left ventricular end-diastolic volume
5. **Which of the following electrocardiogram (ECG) changes is an *abnormal* finding during third trimester and delivery?**
   A. ST-segment depression
   B. Changes of T-wave morphology
   C. Left-axis deviation up to 15–20°
   D. ST-segment elevation
6. **Which of the following statements is true regarding brain natriuretic peptide (BNP):**
   A. BNP levels do not increase during an uncomplicated pregnancy.
   B. BNP levels should not be measured in patients with congenital heart disease given the high variability and the lack of correlation with cardiovascular complications.
   C. Patients with known cardiac disease and severe chronic hypertension should have a baseline BNP.
   D. BNP may increase in patients with congenital heart disease, but not in patients with preeclampsia.
7. **A 42-year-old female with a 36-week breech pregnancy comes to the preop clinic. She is complaining of new-onset chest discomfort for 5 weeks noted when climbing stairs, and resting on her bed, that does not increase with physical activity. After obtaining a normal ECG, you decide to obtain cardiac enzymes. The following statements are true, *except*:**
   A. Cardiac troponin levels are not elevated during uncomplicated pregnancy.
   B. CK-MB levels are normal during uncomplicated pregnancy.
   C. Troponin levels in patients with preeclampsia and a concurrent myocardial infarction are higher compared to stable patients with underlying preeclampsia.
   D. Heterophil antibodies may interfere with the troponin assay and produce falsely elevated levels.
8. **Which of the following is *not* a risk score system used to predict adverse cardiac events in pregnancy?**
   A. CARPREG I and II Risk Index
   B. ZAHARA (Zwangerschap bij Aangeboren HARtAfwijking) risk score
   C. ASCVD Risk Estimator
   D. mWHO (modified World Health Organization) risk score

9. **A 25-year-old female, with a 30-week gestation pregnancy, a history of scoliosis and dural ectasia, presents to the emergency department with acute thoracoabdominal pain of 10/10 intensity. On physical exam, you noticed her height is 6′1″, she has arachnodactyly and a mid-systolic click on auscultation. Which of the following acute aortic syndromes is the most prevalent in this population?**
   A. Type B aortic dissection
   B. Type A aortic dissection
   C. Abdominal aortic pseudoaneurysm
   D. Intramural hematoma
10. **A 41-year-old female with a 27-week pregnancy, chronic hypertension, type 2 non-insulin-dependent diabetes mellitus, and smoking presents with acute chest pain. After performing a percutaneous coronary intervention for circumflex artery severe stenosis and placement of a drug-eluting stent, she was placed on medical therapy. The patient may receive the following medications, *except*:**
   A. Aspirin
   B. Clopidogrel
   C. Atorvastatin
   D. Nitroglycerin
11. **According to The American College of Obstetricians and Gynecologists, which of the following patients is recommended for antibiotic endocarditis prophylaxis during labor at the time of membrane rupture:**
   A. A 22-year-old female with active opioid use disorder
   B. A 29-year-old with a history of rheumatic mitral stenosis
   C. An 18-year-old with a repaired transposition of the great vessels without prosthesis
   D. A 42-year-old with a previous history of infective endocarditis
12. **A 32-year-old female with a history of recurrent syncope and Lyme disease complicated by a complete heart block is coming for an urgent cesarean section due to placenta previa. She underwent pacemaker implantation 2 years ago without complication. On the last interrogation 6 months ago, it was noted that she is pacer-dependent, with a DDD mode and an HR of 80. Which of the following statements is correct?**
   A. The pacemaker needs to be reprogrammed to a synchronous mode given that the electromagnetic interference during the cesarean section is significant.
   B. If central access is needed, femoral vein central lines should be used given the concern for damage to the pacemaker leads.
   C. There is no need to reprogram the pacemaker. However, a magnet and external pacing pads should be readily available.
   D. Placing a magnet on her device will inactivate the implantable cardioverter defibrillator (ICD) function.

13. **According to the CDC's Pregnancy Mortality Surveillance System, what percentage of pregnancy-related deaths were caused by cardiovascular conditions and cardiomyopathy in the United States between 2016 and 2018:**
    A. 1–10%
    B. 11–20%
    C. 21–30%
    D. 31–40%
14. **Recommendations for the administration of cardiopulmonary resuscitation (CPR) in pregnancy include all of the following, *except*:**
    A. Supine positioning with manual left uterine displacement during CPR.
    B. Hand positioning for chest compressions should be placed 2–3 cm higher on the sternum than in nonpregnant patients.
    C. Stop magnesium sulfate and administer IV/IO calcium chloride 10 mL in 10% solution.
    D. Perimortem cesarean delivery aims for delivery of the fetus by 5 min after onset of resuscitation.
15. **Patients with a history of preeclampsia have an increased lifelong risk of all the following, *except*:**
    A. Heart failure
    B. Myocardial infarction
    C. Diabetes mellitus
    D. Stroke
16. **Pregnant patients with congenital heart disease are at increased risk for all the following, *except*:**
    A. Fetal distress during labor
    B. Preeclampsia
    C. Arrhythmia
    D. Heart failure
17. **A 36-year-old G3P2 with a history of hypertrophic obstructive cardiomyopathy presents in labor with anticipated vaginal delivery. Anesthetic management considerations include:**
    A. Avoidance of increased systemic vascular resistance
    B. Maintaining tachycardia
    C. Allowance of hypovolemia
    D. Maintaining afterload
18. **In patients with cardiovascular disease in pregnancy, independent prepregnancy predictors for the occurrence of death or heart failure include all of the following, *except*:**
    A. New York Heart Association (NYHA) Class > II
    B. Systemic ventricular ejection fraction (EF) <30%
    C. mWHO IV
    D. Anticoagulation use

19. **Cardio-obstetric experts recommend all of the following antihypertensive medications in pregnancy, *except*:**
    A. β-blockers
    B. Calcium channel blockers
    C. Angiotensin-converting enzyme inhibitors
    D. Hydralazine
20. **A 43-year-old G3P2 at 38 weeks gestation with preeclampsia develops symptoms of shortness of breath on exertion, fatigue, chest tightness, and peripheral edema. Which of the following tests is required for diagnosis?**
    A. Echocardiogram
    B. Duplex ultrasonography
    C. Chest X-ray
    D. Electrocardiogram
21. **All the following are associated with worse outcomes in patients with peripartum cardiomyopathy, *except*:**
    A. Left ventricular dilation
    B. African-American ethnicity
    C. Concomitant preeclampsia
    D. Left ventricular ejection fraction of 35%
22. **According to the CARPREG II Risk Prediction Index, the predicted risk for primary cardiac events in a patient with coronary artery disease and a history of arrhythmia and mild left ventricular systolic dysfunction with baseline NYHA functional class II is:**
    A. 10%
    B. 15%
    C. 20%
    D. 40%
23. **Anesthetic management considerations for patients with Eisenmenger syndrome include:**
    A. Administration of β-blockade
    B. Maintenance of afterload
    C. Permissive hypercarbia
    D. Epidural loss of resistance technique with air

Answers and Explanations

1. **D**. The point of maximal impulse is shifted superiorly and laterally due to the elevation of the diaphragm with the enlarging uterus. In addition, pregnancy causes an increase in blood volume and, thus, an increase in stretch and force of contraction [6]. Due to early closure of the mitral valve in pregnancy, the first heart sound (S1) is accentuated. In quiet settings, you may appreciate the presence of third (S3) and fourth (S4) heart sounds. More than 90% of patients exhibit new murmurs in pregnancy. A grade II systolic murmur is commonly heard at the left sternal border, and it is commonly attributed to mild tricuspid regurgitation in the setting of dilation of the tricuspid annulus secondary to increased intravascular volume. All these findings are considered benign [7].

2. **B**. At term, echocardiographic studies have shown an increase in LV mass up to 50% at term. This is caused by an increase in the size of the preexisting cardiomyocytes, resulting in an eccentric hypertrophy. Cardiac output is increased by about 50% by the end of the second trimester secondary to increased stroke volume and heart rate and remains increased throughout the third trimester. LV end-diastolic volume increases while the LV end-systolic volume is unchanged, leading to an increase in ejection fraction. Other changes include increased annular diameters of the mitral, tricuspid, and pulmonic valves. However, the aortic annulus is not affected [6, 7].
3. **A**. Compression of the IVC occurs as early as 13 weeks of gestation. Angiographic studies have shown an increase of up to 75% in femoral and IVC pressures at term in the supine position. When tilting a patient laterally by 30°, compression of the IVC improves compared to the supine position. However, a lateral tilt of 15° has not shown any difference in IVC volume. At term, a decrease in venous return can be significant and may decrease the stroke volume and cardiac output by up to 20%. However, not all patients experience symptoms from this phenomenon, as blood return can be maintained via intraosseous, vertebral, paravertebral, and epidural veins and the azygos system [6]. Supine hypotension syndrome of pregnancy is a decrease in blood pressure in the supine position associated with clinical symptoms that may include: chest discomfort, nausea, vomiting, lightheadedness, dizziness, visual disturbances, dyspnea, restlessness, and an urge to change position. It usually occurs within 3–10 min after laying supine. In addition to differences in the collateral venous system between symptomatic versus asymptomatic patients, differences in baroreflex sensitivity have also been proposed [8]. Risks factors include the size/shape of the uterus, multiple pregnancies, and obesity. Aortic compression, originally described in angiographic studies, occurs at the level of the lumbar lordosis and is supported by a difference in arterial blood pressure between the upper and lower extremities. However, recent MRI studies have failed to demonstrate a significant decrease in aortic cross-sectional areas from a gravid uterus in a supine position [8].
4. **B**. During labor, uterine contractions displace blood from the intervillous space through the ovarian venous outflow system and into the systemic circulation leading to increased venous return. This phenomenon is called autotransfusion. In addition, decreased IVC compression, lower extremity venous pressure, and elimination of the low resistance vascular placental bed at the time of delivery contributes to an increase in cardiac output and stroke volume up to 150% of prepregnancy values. All other answer choices do not occur in the immediate postdelivery period. Blood pressure may remain lower compared to prepregnancy levels, and these effects may persist due to possible long-lasting vascular changes [6, 9].
5. **D**. The ECG of pregnant patients may show left-axis deviation given the rotation and upward and left-shifting of the heart. ST-segment depression, especially in patients undergoing cesarean section regardless of the type of anesthesia, T wave changes, and the presence of Q waves are also normal

findings. All these findings are related to the changes of chamber volumes and stretching of the conduction pathway. The use of oxytocin has been associated with ST-segment depression and is not associated with myocardial damage. ST-segment elevation is an abnormal finding in pregnancy and should always be considered pathologic [6, 7].

6. **C**. BNP is a hormone mainly produced by the heart ventricles, and its levels may increase in response to increased filling pressures, heart failure, myocardial trauma, arrhythmias, acute pulmonary embolism, infection/sepsis, pulmonary hypertension, renal insufficiency, burns, cirrhosis, and many other conditions. However, in uncomplicated pregnancies, BNP levels may increase up to two-fold compared to nonpregnant patients and return to normal values within the first week after delivery [10]. BNP levels have been known to be increased in pregnant patients with preeclampsia, severe chronic hypertension, congenital heart disease, and known cardiovascular disease [6]. In a prospective study of patients with structural heart disease, a BNP $\leq$ 100 pg/mL had a negative predictive value of 100% for identifying cardiac events during pregnancy [11]. In patients with congenital heart disease, a N-terminal pro-BNP >128 pg/mL at 20 weeks of gestation is an independent predictor of adverse cardiovascular events defined as heart failure, need for invasive cardiac procedure, myocardial infarction (MI), new arrhythmias, cardiac arrest, death, and thromboembolic complications [12]. Individual and careful assessment of BNP levels is necessary, as increases in BNP may suggest decompensation in the setting of change in clinical status.
7. **B**. CK-MB levels are elevated up to two to four times the upper limit of normal due to its production by the uterus and placental tissue. Thus, CK-MB is not a specific marker for the diagnosis of MI during pregnancy; however, it is sensitive for MI in pregnancy. Troponins are not elevated during an uncomplicated pregnancy, but they may be increased in patients with gestational hypertension and preeclampsia. However, in patients with MI and underlying preeclampsia, troponin levels are higher than expected for the underlying preeclampsia alone [6]. Troponins can be falsely elevated due to multiple conditions including high fibrin, presence of heterophil antibodies, hemolysis, and renal failure [13].
8. **C**. The most applied score systems to assess for cardiovascular events in pregnancy are ZAHARA, CARPREG (CARdiac disease in PREGnancy study), CARPREG II, and mWHO [6]. Many studies have evaluated the performance of these tests with CARPREG II, the most recently evaluated. The CARPREG risk score consists of four predictors: previous cardiac events, baseline NYHA functional class, LV obstruction, and reduced LV ejection fraction. Each risk represents a point with increasing total points correlating with increased risk of adverse events [14]. ZAHARA is a weighted risk score with eight predictors that incorporate cardiac diagnosis, severity of disease, use of cardiac medications, history of arrythmia, and baseline cardiac function [15]. The mWHO considers pregnancy risk based on cardiac condition [16]. The CARPREG II score incorporates ten predictors for maternal cardiac complications that include cardiac history, baseline functional status, cardiac diagnoses, and

severity of disease [1, 17]. The Task Force for the Management of Cardiovascular Diseases during Pregnancy of the European Society of Cardiology (ESC) recommends the mWHO classification due to its accuracy for risk assessment [17].

9. **B**. Marfan syndrome is one of the most common inherited connective tissue disorders. It is an autosomal dominant condition associated with mutations of the FBN1 gene that encodes for the connective tissue protein fibrillin-1. Sporadic mutations are seen in up to 25% of the patients. It leads to multiple disorders such as aortic root disease, mitral valve prolapse, musculoskeletal disorders (including excessive linear growth of long bones, arachnodactyly, joint laxity, pectus deformity, abnormal arm span/height, scoliosis, etc.), ocular abnormalities (including ectopia lentis and myopia), dural ectasia (usually lumbosacral on up to 63–92% of patients), and pulmonary disease (emphysema and bullae) [18]. In particular, dilation of the aorta is seen in up to 80% of adult patients, which most commonly occurs in the aortic root and is often accompanied by aortic regurgitation [6, 19]. The mWHO risk classification categorizes Marfan syndrome without aortic dilatation as Class II–III with moderate risk of maternal morbidity or mortality, Marfan syndrome with aorta 40–45 mm Class III with significantly increased risk of maternal mortality or severe morbidity, and Marfan syndrome >45 mm Class IV with pregnancy highly discouraged [20]. Pregnancy and the postpartum period are the highestrisk periods for aortic dissection and rupture in these patients, likely due to increased intimal shear forces in the setting of the hyperdynamic circulatory state and the possible estrogen-induced effects on the aortic wall composition. The most common type of dissections in pregnancy is Stanford type A (with an average of 4.8 cm at the time of dissection) [6]. Traditionally, pregnant patients with Marfan syndrome with or without aortic disease are placed on β-blocker therapy (labetalol or extended-release metoprolol). However, there is limited evidence regarding the efficacy of β-blockers preventing aortic dissection in pregnant patients with Marfan syndrome [21]. In this patient with a viable pregnancy, who presents with type A dissection during the third trimester, it is recommended to proceed with urgent cesarean delivery followed by aortic surgery. In the event of dissection during the first or second trimester, surgical repair should be performed, anticipating the fetal risk during hypothermic circulatory arrest [6]. For type B dissections, medical therapy or TEVAR is preferred unless an intervention is needed (percutaneous or surgical) to treat rupture, subacute aortic leaking or malperfusion [22].

10. **C**. Acute coronary syndrome is uncommon in young women. However, as pregnancies increase in older women, its prevalence has increased. Some of the common risk factors in this population include age > 35 years, lower socioeconomic status, African American, preexistent hypertension, diabetes mellitus, obesity, smoking, cocaine/amphetamine use, dyslipidemia, and treatment for infertility [23]. Up to 40% of patients with MI have evidence of atherosclerosis, but spontaneous coronary artery dissection can be observed in up to 27% and is more frequently observed in the peripartum and postpartum periods [6]. Diagnosis follows the same approach as the general population and includes

symptoms, ECG changes, and elevation in cardiac biomarkers. When managing these patients, it is important to individualize their treatment. Treatment includes revascularization with percutaneous coronary intervention and possible stenting, coronary artery bypass graft surgery, or conservative medical therapy (in the case of coronary dissection). When the mechanism of infarction is related to atherosclerosis, there are multiple approaches that include the use of drug-eluting stents or bare metal stents and balloon angioplasty. If stents are chosen, dual antiplatelet therapy is recommended for 12 months [6]. However, in patients with a high risk of bleeding, dual antiplatelet therapy can be used for at least one month and can be extended up to 3 months if there is a risk of recurrent ischemia. If delivery occurs during that time, the teams involved should be prepared to manage the increased bleeding. Patients with stents should continue with aspirin indefinitely. For delivery, the goal is to minimize the cardiac workload by using early epidural analgesia, left lateral position, assisted vaginal delivery, or cesarean section if unstable or for obstetric indications [20, 24]. Clopidogrel may be used in pregnancy and should be stopped for at least 7 days prior to placement of neuraxial anesthesia [6]. Other medications that can be used in this population include nitrates, β-blockers, and heparin. However, statins, angiotensin-converting enzyme inhibitors and angiotensin II receptor blockers are contraindicated due to the associated teratogenicity with their use [4, 5].

11. **D**. Infective endocarditis in pregnancy is rare. However, it carries a high maternal and fetal mortality of up to 15% and 22%, respectively [6]. Most commonly, infective endocarditis is associated with intravenous drug use or preexisting structural heart disease (congenital or rheumatic heart disease) in pregnancy. High-risk patients that may benefit from antibiotic prophylaxis after rupture of membranes are patients with prosthetic cardiac valve or a valve repaired with prosthetic material, an unrepaired or palliated cyanotic CHD, repaired CHD with prosthetic material within 6 months of procedure or with residual defects near prosthetic material and history of bacterial endocarditis [25].
12. **C**. Pregnant patients with pacemakers or ICDs follow the same recommendations as their nonpregnant counterparts. For operative obstetric procedures (including cesarean section), there is no significant electromagnetic interference given the distance to the implanted device. A magnet and pacing/defibrillation pads should be immediately available. Continuous cardiac monitoring during labor and following delivery is recommended. Central lines can be placed carefully [6].
13. **C**. According to the CDC's Pregnancy Mortality Surveillance System (PMSS), cardiomyopathy (12.5%) and other cardiovascular conditions (16.2) contribute to almost 30% of all pregnancy-related deaths in the United States between 2016 and 2018. Hypertensive disorders of pregnancy contribute to an additional 6.8% of pregnancy-related deaths over the same period [3].
14. **B**. High-quality chest compressions at a rate of at least 100 per minute and a depth of at least 2 inches with full recoil and minimal interruptions of less than 10 s are essential to optimize cardiopulmonary resuscitation and survival. The

patient should be placed supine on a hard surface with manual left uterine displacement. It is no longer recommended to adjust hand placement in the pregnant patient compared to the nonpregnant patient. During cardiac arrest, magnesium sulfate should be discontinued and reversal with IV/IO calcium chloride 10 mL in 10% solution or calcium gluconate 30 mL in 10% solution should be administered. If return of spontaneous circulation (ROSC) does not occur by 4 min of resuscitative efforts, perimortem cesarean delivery is recommended to improve the chance of ROSC and maternal and fetal survival [26, 27].

15. **C**. After adjusting for age, body mass index, and diabetes mellitus, preeclampsia is associated with a fourfold increased future incidence of heart failure and a twofold increased future risk of coronary artery disease, stroke, and death secondary to cardiovascular disease. Diabetes mellitus is both a risk factor for preeclampsia and cardiovascular disease [28].
16. **A**. When compared to patients without CHD, patients with CHD have greater risk for adverse events during delivery including heart failure (aOR 22.6), arrhythmias (aOR 12.4), thromboembolic events (aOR 2.4), preeclampsia (aOR 1.5), and placental previa (aOR 1.5). Infants of patients with CHD were more likely to experience preterm delivery and fetal growth restriction and less likely to have fetal distress. Compared to women without CHD, women with CHD are more likely to deliver via cesarean section or operative vaginal delivery and experience hemorrhage. Patients with CHD experienced longer lengths of stay and higher total charges [29, 30].
17. **D**. Anesthetic hemodynamic management goals for patients with hypertrophic obstructive cardiomyopathy and aortic stenosis include maintenance of normal heart rate and rhythm with avoidance of tachycardia, maintenance of afterload, and avoidance of hypovolemia. It is essential to maintain coronary perfusion pressure to the hypertrophied LV myocardium. Early and effective neuraxial analgesia with slow titration of local anesthetics minimizes hemodynamic alterations and limits the sympathetic catecholamine response to the stress and pain of labor. Consideration should be given to continuous telemetry, strict monitoring of fluid balance, early recognition of hemorrhage and resuscitation, treatment of hypotension with phenylephrine infusion, and invasive arterial blood pressure monitoring [20].
18. **B**. In patients with cardiovascular disease in pregnancy, independent risk factors for heart failure and/or maternal death include prepregnancy NYHA>II, systemic ventricular ejection fraction of <40%, signs of heart failure, mWHO IV, and anticoagulation use [2].
19. **C**. Angiotensin-converting enzyme inhibitors and angiotensin receptor blockers are contraindicated in pregnancy secondary to risk for fetal malformations such as renal dysgenesis and calvarial hypoplasia and fetal growth restriction. Labetalol, nifedipine, and hydralazine are first-line antihypertensive medications in pregnancy [4, 5].
20. **A**. Peripartum cardiomyopathy (PPCM) is defined as new-onset nonischemic cardiomyopathy with systolic dysfunction (LV ejection fraction <45%) without

a reversible cause presenting near the end of pregnancy or in the postpartum period in a woman without known heart disease [4]. PPCM is a diagnosis of exclusion in patients with new-onset LV systolic dysfunction. The incidence is higher in black women, older maternal age, hypertensive disorders of pregnancy, and multiple gestation pregnancies. Echocardiogram is required for diagnosis to assess LV systolic dysfunction. Echocardiogram may also reveal left and/or right ventricular dilation or dysfunction, mitral and/or tricuspid regurgitation, atrial enlargement, pulmonary hypertension, and intracardiac thrombus (10–17% of initial echocardiograms). Electrocardiogram may reveal nonspecific abnormalities and may be normal. Chest X-ray reveals pulmonary edema and is not diagnostic of cardiomyopathy [31].

21. **D**. LV ejection fraction less than 30% is the most reliable predictor of adverse outcomes and is associated with lower rates of recovery. Other predictors of adverse outcomes include LV dilation, LV thrombus, right ventricular systolic dysfunction, obesity, concomitant preeclampsia, and African-American ethnicity [31].
22. **D**. According to the CARPREG II Risk Index, the patient described has a 41% risk of primary cardiac events. The patient receives 2 points for coronary artery disease, 3 points for prior arrhythmia, and 2 points for mild LV systolic dysfunction for a total of >4 points. Primary cardiac events may include arrhythmias, heart failure, and cardiac arrest among other events [1].
23. **B**. Patients with Eisenmenger syndrome require maintenance of afterload to minimize right-to-left shunting and cyanosis. Cyanosis should be treated with phenylephrine. Hypercarbia, hypoxia, and acidemia may increase pulmonary vascular resistance and worsen right-to-left shunting. Avoidance of β-blockade is appropriate as it may act as a myocardial depressant and decrease right ventricular contractility. Monitoring techniques include continuous telemetry, pulse oximetry with consideration of invasive blood pressure monitoring, central line placement, and pulmonary artery catheterization. Multidisciplinary management with a cardiovascular anesthesiologist should be considered. Neuraxial anesthesia may be used with slow titration. Placement of neuraxial anesthesia should be performed with loss of resistance to saline technique to limit paradoxical embolism. Filters should also be placed on intravenous lines [20].

References

1. Silversides CK, Grewal J, Mason J, et al. Pregnancy outcomes in women with heart disease the CARPREG II study. J Am Coll Cardiol. 2018;71:2419–30. https://doi.org/10.1016/j.jacc.2018.02.076.
2. Roos-Hesselink J, Baris L, Johnson M, et al. Pregnancy outcomes in women with cardiovascular disease: evolving trends over 10 years in the ESC registry of pregnancy and cardiac disease (ROPAC). Eur Heart J. 2019;40:3848. https://doi.org/10.1093/eurheartj/ehz136.
3. CDC. Pregnancy mortality surveillance system. 2022. https://www.cdc.gov/reproductivehealth/maternal-mortality/pregnancy-mortality-surveillance-system.htm. Accessed 22 Feb 2023.

4. Mehta LS, Warnes CA, Bradley E, et al. Cardiovascular considerations in caring for pregnant patients: a scientific statement from the American Heart Association. Circulation. 2020;141:e884–903. https://doi.org/10.1161/cir.0000000000000772.
5. American College of Obstetricians and Gynecologists' Presidential Task Force on Pregnancy and Heart Disease and Committee on Practice Bulletins—Obstetrics. ACOG practice bulletin no. 212: pregnancy and heart disease. Obstet Gynecol. 2019;133:e320–56. https://doi.org/10.1097/aog.0000000000003243.
6. Vidovich MI. Cardiovascular disease. In: Elsevier Inc. (ed) Chestnut's obstetric anesthesia: principles and practice, 6th ed. Elsevier Inc.; 2020
7. Kacmar RM, Gaiser R. Physiologic changes in pregnancy. In: Chestnut's obstetric anesthesia: principles and practice. 2020
8. Massoth C, Chappell D, Kranke P, Wenk M. Supine hypotensive syndrome of pregnancy: a review of current knowledge. Eur J Anaesthesiol. 2021;39:236–43. https://doi.org/10.1097/eja.0000000000001554.
9. Meah VL, Cockcroft JR, Backx K, et al. Cardiac output and related haemodynamics during pregnancy: a series of meta-analyses. Heart. 2016;102:518. https://doi.org/10.1136/heartjnl-2015-308476.
10. Hameed AB, Chan K, Ghamsary M, Elkayam U. Longitudinal changes in the B-type natriuretic peptide levels in normal pregnancy and postpartum. Clin Cardiol. 2009;32:E60–2. https://doi.org/10.1002/clc.20391.
11. Tanous D, Siu SC, Mason J, et al. B-type natriuretic peptide in pregnant women with heart disease. J Am Coll Cardiol. 2010;56:1247–53. https://doi.org/10.1016/j.jacc.2010.02.076.
12. Kampman MAM, Balci A, van Veldhuisen DJ, et al. N-terminal pro-B-type natriuretic peptide predicts cardiovascular complications in pregnant women with congenital heart disease. Eur Heart J. 2014;35:708–15. https://doi.org/10.1093/eurheartj/eht526.
13. Zaidi A, Cowell R. False positive cardiac troponin elevation due to heterophile antibodies: more common than we recognise? BMJ Case Rep. 2010;2010:bcr1120092477. https://doi.org/10.1136/bcr.11.2009.2477.
14. Siu SC, Sermer M, Colman JM, et al. Prospective multicenter study of pregnancy outcomes in women with heart disease. Circulation. 2001;104:515–21. https://doi.org/10.1161/hc3001.093437.
15. Drenthen W, Boersma E, Balci A, et al. Predictors of pregnancy complications in women with congenital heart disease. Eur Heart J. 2010;31:2124–32. https://doi.org/10.1093/eurheartj/ehq200.
16. Thorne S, MacGregor A, Nelson-Piercy C. Risks of contraception and pregnancy in heart disease. Heart. 2006;92:1520. https://doi.org/10.1136/hrt.2006.095240.
17. Regitz-Zagrosek V, Roos-Hesselink JW, Bauersachs J, et al. 2018 ESC guidelines for the management of cardiovascular diseases during pregnancy. The task force for the management of cardiovascular diseases during pregnancy of the European Society of Cardiology (ESC). Eur Heart J. 2018;39:3165–241. https://doi.org/10.1093/eurheartj/ehy340.
18. Loeys BL, Dietz HC, Braverman AC, et al. The revised Ghent nosology for the Marfan syndrome. J Med Genet. 2010;47:476. https://doi.org/10.1136/jmg.2009.072785.
19. Bruno L, Tredici S, Mangiavacchi M, et al. Cardiac, skeletal, and ocular abnormalities in patients with Marfan's syndrome and in their relatives. Comparison with the cardiac abnormalities in patients with kyphoscoliosis. Br Heart J. 1984;51:220. https://doi.org/10.1136/hrt.51.2.220.
20. Meng M-L, Arendt KW. Obstetric anesthesia and heart disease: practical clinical considerations. Anesthesiology. 2021;135:164–83. https://doi.org/10.1097/aln.0000000000003833.
21. Smith K, Gros B. Pregnancy-related acute aortic dissection in Marfan syndrome: a review of the literature. Congenit Heart Dis. 2017;12:251–60. https://doi.org/10.1111/chd.12465.
22. Zhu J-M, Ma W-G, Peterss S, et al. Aortic dissection in pregnancy: management strategy and outcomes. Ann Thorac Surg. 2017;103:1199–206. https://doi.org/10.1016/j.athoracsur.2016.08.089.

23. Jalnapurkar S, Xu KH, Zhang Z, et al. Changing incidence and mechanism of pregnancy-associated myocardial infarction in the state of California. J Am Heart Assoc. 2021;10:e021056. https://doi.org/10.1161/jaha.121.021056.
24. Roth A, Elkayam U. Acute myocardial infarction associated with pregnancy. Ann Intern Med. 1996;125:751. https://doi.org/10.7326/0003-4819-125-9-199611010-00009.
25. Committee on Practice Bulletins-Obstetrics. ACOG practice bulletin no. 199: use of prophylactic antibiotics in labor and delivery. Obstet Gynecol. 2018;132:e103–19. https://doi.org/10.1097/aog.0000000000002833.
26. Lipman S, Cohen S, Einav S, et al. The Society for Obstetric Anesthesia and Perinatology consensus statement on the management of cardiac arrest in pregnancy. Anesth Analg. 2014;118:1003–16. https://doi.org/10.1213/ane.0000000000000171.
27. Jeejeebhoy FM, Zelop CM, Lipman S, et al. Cardiac arrest in pregnancy. Circulation. 2015;132:1747–73. https://doi.org/10.1161/cir.0000000000000300.
28. Wu P, Haththotuwa R, Kwok CS, et al. Preeclampsia and future cardiovascular health: a systematic review and meta-analysis. Circ Cardiovasc Qual Outcomes. 2017;10:e003497. https://doi.org/10.1161/circoutcomes.116.003497.
29. Schlichting LE, Insaf TZ, Zaidi AN, et al. Maternal comorbidities and complications of delivery in pregnant women with congenital heart disease. J Am Coll Cardiol. 2019;73:2181–91. https://doi.org/10.1016/j.jacc.2019.01.069.
30. Thompson JL, Kuklina EV, Bateman BT, et al. Medical and obstetric outcomes among pregnant women with congenital heart disease. Obstet Gynecol. 2015;126:346–54. https://doi.org/10.1097/aog.0000000000000973.
31. Davis MB, Arany Z, McNamara DM, et al. Peripartum cardiomyopathy JACC state-of-the-art review. J Am Coll Cardiol. 2020;75:207–21. https://doi.org/10.1016/j.jacc.2019.11.014.

Anesthesia for the Parturient with Cardiovascular Disease

John Bouz and Peter Cheng

Questions

1. **A 36-year-old parturient with severe eclampsia on magnesium sulfate presents for cesarean delivery. What is the antihypertensive drug of choice prior to induction?**
   A. Labetalol
   B. Hydralazine
   C. Nitroglycerin
   D. Nitroprusside
2. **A 29-year-old postpartum presents with dyspnea, cough, postural hypotension, and hemoptysis. Echocardiogram demonstrates left ventricular ejection fraction <0.45, M-mode fractional shortening <30%, and left-end diastolic dimensions >2.7 cm/m^2. Which diagnosis is correct?**
   A. Diastolic dysfunction
   B. Pulmonary embolus
   C. Amniotic fluid embolus
   D. Peripartum cardiomyopathy
   E. Pericardial effusion
3. **For parturients with Eisenmenger syndrome presenting in labor, which statement is true?**
   A. Uterine contraction increases pulmonary arterial hypertension.
   B. General anesthesia reduces the right-to-left shunt.
   C. Reduction of systemic vascular resistance increases pulmonary perfusion.

J. Bouz (✉)
Riverside University Health System, Moreno Valley, CA, USA
e-mail: J.Bouz@ruhealth.org

P. Cheng
Riverside University Health System, Moreno Valley, CA, USA

Loma Linda University, Loma Linda, CA, USA

A. C. Sinha, I. F. Pasca (eds.), *Peripartum Care of the Pregnant Patient*,
https://doi.org/10.1007/978-3-031-62756-9_7

   D. Oxygen increases the blood flow across the right-to-left shunt.

4. **Which physiologic change of pregnancy occurs?**
   A. Myocardial contractility increases.
   B. Diastolic blood pressure decreases more than systolic blood pressure.
   C. Systemic vascular resistance increases.
   D. The renin-angiotensin-aldosterone system is diminished.
5. **A parturient with severe mitral stenosis suddenly develops hypotension and tachycardia after a labor epidural anesthetic. Which choice is best?**
   A. Fluid administration
   B. Ephedrine
   C. Epinephrine
   D. Phenylephrine
6. **For a parturient presenting with stable ventricular arrhythmia and a history of arrhythmogenic right ventricle cardiomyopathy, which drug is the best choice?**
   A. Beta-blockers
   B. Sodium channel blockers
   C. Amiodarone
   D. Verapamil
7. **Which statement about ECG changes is true during the third trimester of normal pregnancy?**
   A. Tall T waves
   B. Q waves in lead II
   C. Right axis deviation
   D. Increased QTc interval
8. **For parturients with pulmonary artery hypertension, which uterotonic is the drug of choice?**
   A. Methergine
   B. Carboprost
   C. Oxytocin
   D. Hemabate
9. **A parturient with critical aortic valvular stenosis develops severe hypotension after a labor epidural anesthetic. What is the best management option listed?**
   A. Fluid challenge
   B. Epinephrine
   C. Phenylephrine
   D. Beta-agonist
10. **Which statement about parturients with severe mitral stenosis is true?**
   A. Uterine contractions are well-tolerated.
   B. Pulmonary capillary wedge pressure decreases.
   C. Tachycardia is poorly tolerated.
   D. Immediately after delivery, the central volume decreases and is well-tolerated.

11. **Which is NOT a common potential complication in parturients with mechanical heart valve?**
    A. Thromboembolism
    B. Endocarditis
    C. Valvular outflow obstruction
    D. Dysrhythmia
12. **Which cardiovascular complication is uncommon with COVID-19 Infection during pregnancy?**
    A. Hypertensive disorders
    B. Thromboembolism
    C. HELLP Syndrome
    D. Myocardial infraction
13. **For the management of hypertension during pregnancy, which statement is true?**
    A. Esmolol is the safest beta-blocker.
    B. Intravenous nitroglycerine is the drug of choice for preeclampsia and seizure.
    C. For severe hypertension (over 160/110 mmHg), intravenous labetalol and magnesium are the drugs of choice.
    D. For eclampsia associated with seizure, labetalol is the first-line antihypertensive drug.
14. **For the treatment for peripartum cardiomyopathy, which statement is true?**
    A. Levosimendan reduces pulmonary capillary wedge pressure, improves cardiac output, and is effective.
    B. Calcium channel blockers are safe and effective.
    C. β-1 blockers are preferred over β-2 blockers.
    D. Diuretic preload reduction is recommended.
15. **Regarding venous thromboembolism (VTE) during pregnancy, which statement is true?**
    A. D-dimer testing to rule out pulmonary embolus is accurate.
    B. Warfarin is safe and effective during pregnancy.
    C. For acute small pulmonary embolus and small deep vein thrombosis, unfractionated heparin is recommended.
    D. For stable pulmonary embolus, low-molecular-weight heparin is preferred.
16. **Which of the following drugs, if used during pregnancy, is associated with an increased risk of fetal cardiovascular and central nervous system malformations as well as oligohydramnios due to fetal kidney malfunction?**
    A. Beta-blockers
    B. Hydralazine
    C. ACE inhibitors
    D. Verapamil
17. **Per AHA guidelines, all the following are recommended for pregnant women with chronic aortic dilation, EXCEPT:**
    A. Strict blood pressure control

B. Yearly echocardiograms
C. Cesarean delivery in women with significant aortic enlargement, dissection, or severe aortic valve regurgitation
D. Prophylactic surgery in the setting of progressive aortic dilation and/or advancing aortic valve regurgitation

18. **It is reasonable to administer antibiotic prophylaxis against infective endocarditis for vaginal delivery at the time of membrane rupture in all of the following, EXCEPT:**
A. Prosthetic heart valve
B. Unrepaired cyanotic congenital heart disease
C. Surgically constructed palliative shunts and/or conduits
D. Mitral valve prolapse

Answers and Explanations

1. **A**. Labetalol will decrease maternal blood pressure without comprising fetal circulation [1]. In contrast, the slow onset time for hydralazine precludes its use in an emergent situation. Nitroglycerin-induced hypotension may be unpredictable. Nitroprusside has the risk of fetal cyanide toxicity.
2. **D**. The criteria for the diagnosis of peripartum cardiomyopathy follows: (1) development of heart failure in last month of pregnancy or 5 months postpartum, (2) absence of preexisting heart disease, and (3) echocardiographic findings with left ventricular end-diastolic dimension >2.7 cm/m^2 and M-mode fractional shortening <30% or left ventricular ejection fraction <45% [2].
3. **A**. Uterine contractions cause autotransfusion and increase pulmonary artery hypertension, risking heart failure and arrhythmia. General anesthesia reduces systemic vascular resistance and increases the right-to-left shunt. The right-to-left shunt reduces pulmonary perfusion and increases hypoxia. Oxygen is a pulmonary vasodilator and decreases the blood flow across the right-to-left shunt [3].
4. **B**. Myocardial contractility and ejection fraction remain unchanged. The mean and diastolic blood pressure decreases more than the systolic blood pressure. Systemic vascular resistance decreases. The renin-angiotensin-aldosterone system is activated [4].
5. **D**. Fluid challenge may cause pulmonary edema and heart failure. Ephedrine and epinephrine cause tachycardia. Phenylephrine supports blood pressure without inducing tachycardia given that it targets alpha-1 receptors which could cause reflex bradycardia.
6. **A**. Beta-blockers are the first drugs of choice, while sodium channels blockers are the second drugs of choice. Amiodarone causes adverse effects on the thyroid, lung, liver, and eyes, and verapamil is ineffective in this context [5].
7. **D**. During the third trimester, T waves will be inverted or flattened with an increase in the QTc interval, left axis deviation, and Q wave in lead III [6].

8. **C**. Methergine causes generalized smooth muscle contractions and can elevate pulmonary artery hypertension. Carboprost can cause bronchospasm and worsen right heart failure. Oxytocin has minimal effects on pulmonary vascular resistance and is safe and effective. Hemabate may cause bronchoconstriction and pulmonary artery hypertension [7].
9. **C**. Phenylephrine will increase systemic vascular resistance and blood pressure. Fluid challenge risks pulmonary edema and heart failure. Epinephrine will cause tachycardia. Beta-agonists will also cause tachycardia [8].
10. **C**. Uterine contraction increases preload which is poorly tolerated in mitral stenosis. Pulmonary artery capillary wedge pressure increases and risks pulmonary hypertension. Tachycardia decreases left ventricular filling and must be avoided. Central blood volume increases after delivery and may decompensate the heart [8].
11. **D**. Complications of mechanical heart valves include thromboembolism, hemolysis, and outflow obstruction [8]. Dysrhythmia has not been reported as a common complication.
12. **C**. Hypertensive disorders, thromboembolism, and myocardial infarction have all been reported in parturients after being infected with COVID-19. HELLP Syndrome has not been reported in this patient population [9].
13. **C**. Esmolol causes fetal bradycardia. Intravenous magnesium and labetalol are the drugs of choice for preeclampsia and seizure. For severe hypertension (over 160/110 mmHg), intravenous labetalol is the antihypertensive drug of choice. For eclampsia associated with seizure, magnesium is the first-line antihypertensive drug [10].
14. **C**. While levosimendan reduces pulmonary capillary wedge pressure and improves cardiac output, it has not been shown to be effective. Calcium channel blockers are safe and effective but cause uterine hypoperfusion. β-1 blockers are preferred over β-2 blockers to avoid the anti-tocolytic activity of the latter. Diuretics reduce preload and pulmonary edema but can cause dehydration, uterine hypoperfusion, and maternal metabolic acidosis [2].
15. **D**. D-dimer testing increases with each trimester and has no specificity. Warfarin is teratogenic. For acute small pulmonary embolism and small deep vein thrombosis, unfractionated heparin is recommended. For stable pulmonary embolism, low-molecular-weight heparin is preferred [10].
16. **C**. Beta-blockers are safe in pregnancy although prolonged, and high-dose use is associated with fetal growth restriction. Hydralazine is safe to use during pregnancy. ACE inhibitors have been associated with fetal cardiovascular and neural tube defects. They have also been associated with adverse outcomes due to their effect on fetal renal vascular tone causing fetal kidney malfunction and decreased fetal urine output, resulting in oligohydramnios. Verapamil is likely not teratogenic in the first trimester, and its use in the second and third trimesters is safe and effective for cardiac arrhythmias [11].
17. **B**. Strict blood pressure control is recommended. Monthly or bimonthly echocardiograms are recommended to measure aortic dimensions. Cesarean delivery in women with significant aortic enlargement, dissection, or severe aortic

valve regurgitation is recommended. Prophylactic surgery in the setting of progressive aortic dilation and/or advancing aortic valve regurgitation is recommended [11].

18. **D**. Per the guidelines from AHA, ACC, and ACOG, infective endocarditis (IE) antibiotic prophylaxis is not recommended during vaginal or cesarean section in the absence of structural heart disease. Based on limited evidence for choice B, the high-risk cardiac conditions for which it is reasonable to give IE antibiotic prophylaxis for vaginal delivery at time of membrane rupture include prosthetic heart valve, prosthetic material used for heart valve repair, history of IE, unrepaired cyanotic congenital heart disease, repaired congenital heart disease (palliative shunts and/or conduits, prosthetic material or percutaneously inserted devices/material during the first 6 months after the procedure, residual defects in proximity to prosthetic material or percutaneously inserted device), and cardiac transplantation recipient with valvulopathy [11]. Mitral valve prolapse is not an indication for antibiotic prophylaxis.

References

1. Datta S, Kodali BS, Segal S, Datta S, Kodali BS, Segal S. Anesthesia for cesarean delivery. In: Obstetric anesthesia handbook, 5th ed. 2010. pp. 179–230.
2. Bhattacharyya A, Basra SS, Sen P, Kar B. Peripartum cardiomyopathy: a review. Tex Heart Inst J. 2012;39(1):8–16.
3. Yuan SM. Eisenmenger syndrome in pregnancy. Braz J Cardiovasc Surg. 2016;31(4):325–9. https://doi.org/10.5935/1678-9741.20160062.
4. Sanghavi M, Rutherford JD. Cardiovascular physiology of pregnancy. Circulation. 2014;130(12):1003–8. https://doi.org/10.1161/CIRCULATIONAHA.114.009029.
5. Wichter T, Milberg P, Wichter HD, Dechering DG. Pregnancy in arrhythmogenic cardiomyopathy. Herzschrittmacherther Elektrophysiol. 2021;32(2):186–98. https://doi.org/10.1007/s00399-021-00770-7.
6. Sumalatha B, Jyotsna M, Indrani G. Electrocardiographic changes during Normal pregnancy. Indian J Cardiovasc Dis Women WINCARS. 2017;2(3):35–8.
7. McNeil A, Chen J, Meng ML. Pulmonary hypertension in pregnancy—the Anesthesiologist's perspective. Int J Cardiol Congenit Heart Dis. 2021;5:100234.
8. Kuczkowski KM, van Zundert A. Anesthesia for pregnant women with valvular heart disease: the state-of-the-art. J Anesth. 2007;21(2):252–7. https://doi.org/10.1007/s00540-007-0504-3.
9. Briller JE, Aggarwal NR, Davis MB, et al. Cardiovascular complications of pregnancy-associated COVID-19 infections. JACC Adv. 2022;1(3):100057. https://doi.org/10.1016/j.jacadv.2022.100057.
10. Mehta LS, Warnes CA, Bradley E, et al. Cardiovascular considerations in caring for pregnant patients: a scientific statement from the American Heart Association [published correction appears in Circulation. 2020 Jun 9;141(23):e904] [published correction appears in Circulation. 2021 Mar 23;143(12):e792-e793]. Circulation. 2020;141(23):e884–903. https://doi.org/10.1161/CIR.0000000000000772.
11. Chestnut DH, Nathan N. Chapter 41. Chestnut's obstetric anesthesia: principles and practice. Elsevier; 2020.

Uteroplacental Physiology

Ronald B. Johnson

Questions

1. **Hormone production unique to the placenta includes the following:**
   A. Human placental lactogen
   B. Progesterone
   C. Placental growth hormone
   D. Human chorionic gonadotropin
   E. All of the above
2. **The fetus is dependent on the placenta for the following:**
   A. Hepatic function
   B. Pulmonary function
   C. Renal function
   D. All of the above
3. **Progesterone production in pregnancy:**
   A. Is produced entirely by the ovary
   B. Is produced entirely by the placenta
   C. Is unimportant for the continuation of pregnancy
   D. Is produced by the corpus luteum in the first 8 weeks of pregnancy
4. **The main site of exchange for nutrients and gases between the maternal bloodstream and the fetus is as follows:**
   A. Embryonic mesoderm
   B. Maternal decidua
   C. Syncytiotrophoblast
   D. Amnion

R. B. Johnson (✉)
Department of Gynecology and Obstetrics, Loma Linda University School of Medicine, Loma Linda, CA, USA

Riverside University Health System—Medical Center, Moreno Valley, CA, USA
e-mail: ronald.johnson@ruhealth.org

A. C. Sinha, I. F. Pasca (eds.), *Peripartum Care of the Pregnant Patient*,
https://doi.org/10.1007/978-3-031-62756-9_8

5. **Mechanisms of transfer of nutrients and gases between mother and fetus include the following:**
   A. Solvent drag
   B. Simple diffusion
   C. Transcellular transfer
   D. Endo- and exocytosis
   E. All of the above
6. **Amniotic fluid in the second half of pregnancy is produced primarily by the following:**
   A. Transmembranous flow across the amniotic membrane
   B. Fetal lung secretion
   C. Fetal urination
   D. Fetal swallowing
7. **Respiratory gas exchange crosses the placenta by:**
   A. Simple diffusion
   B. Bulk flow
   C. Facilitated diffusion
   D. Protein channels
8. **True or false: Oxygen and carbon dioxide are lipophilic molecules.**
9. **The low level of fetal oxygenation is compensated by:**
   A. High oxygen extraction by fetal organs
   B. Fetal cardiac output
   C. Fetal shunting of blood to critical anatomy
   D. Small fetus
10. **Chronic fetal hypoxia results in:**
    A. Increase in fetal plasma norepinephrine
    B. Decrease in fetal placental insulin
    C. Decrease in fetal growth
    D. All of the above
11. **The fetal response to acute hypoxia includes the following:**
    A. Increased cardiac output
    B. Increased umbilical blood flow
    C. Increased flow to the CNS and heart
    D. All of the above
12. **Respiratory disturbances of acid–base balance in the mother cause analogous disturbances in the fetus:**
    A. Seconds
    B. Minutes
    C. Hours
    D. Days
13. **The majority of uteroplacental oxygen consumption is by the:**
    A. Myometrium
    B. Decidual membranes
    C. Intervillous space
    D. Placental villous tree

14. **Inhalation of oxygen by a pregnant patient:**
    A. Can dramatically increase fetal PaO_2
    B. Is safe at 100% concentration for long periods if at atmospheric pressure
    C. Influences the shape of the maternal and fetal oxygen dissociation curves
    D. Can cause fetal pulmonary toxicity
15. **The CO_2 affinity of fetal blood compared to maternal blood is:**
    A. Higher
    B. Lower
    C. Equal
    D. Not relevant

Answers and Explanations

1. **E**. The placenta is an endocrine organ releasing humoral agents that are responsible for paracrine and autocrine signaling. It can produce peptide hormones and steroid hormones. The trophoblasts of the chorionic villi uniquely produce human chorionic gonadotropin, human placental lactogen, parathyroid hormone-related protein, and insulin-regulating ligands. Other hormones produced are corticotropin-releasing hormone, estrogen, progesterone, glucocorticoids, and vascular endothelial growth factor [1–3].
2. **D**. The placenta is responsible for the diffusion of gases and transport of nutrients across its membranes and regulates the growth of the fetus and the placenta itself.
3. **D**. Progesterone is vital for maintenance of pregnancy and is produced solely by the corpus luteum, a temporary organ in the ovary which dissolves after the first 8–12 weeks of pregnancy. After this time, there is sufficient placental tissue to take over production and is responsible, along with relaxin, which is an insulin-like hormone, for maintaining a quiescent uterus for the remainder of pregnancy.
4. **C**. The syncytiotrophoblast layer is responsible for most of the exchange of nutrients and gases responsible for normal fetal growth and development [3, 4].
5. **E**. Drug transfer across the placenta occurs by pinocytosis, passive diffusion, active transport, and facilitated diffusion [5].
6. **C**. Fetal urination is the primary source of amniotic fluid production after 18 weeks of pregnancy. Prior to that, transmembranous and intermembranous flow across fetal vessels on the placental surface are responsible. Defects in fetal pulmonary and renal or GI function will affect amniotic fluid volume in late pregnancy.
7. **A**. Transport of oxygen from the atmosphere to the fetal tissues is a sequence of six steps that alternate bulk and diffusional transport [6].
    Step 1. Transport from atmosphere to alveoli
    Step 2. Diffusion across alveolar membrane
    Step 3. Transport from lungs to placenta
    Step 4. Diffusion across the placenta
    Step 5. Transport from placenta to fetus

Step 6. Diffusion into fetal tissues

8. **True**. Oxygen and carbon dioxide are lipophilic molecules that cross the placenta by simple diffusion. Blood flow is the rate limiting step for exchange. The partial pressure and the difference between maternal and fetal hemoglobin affinity for oxygen are important factors that regulate the rate of exchange [7].
9. **B**. The blood that carries oxygen to the fetus in the third trimester via the umbilical vein has mean normal O_2 saturation and PO_2 values significantly lower than maternal arterial blood. The fetal cardiac output is significantly higher than the adult resting cardiac output, creating a high ratio of blood flow to oxygen compensation [8].
10. **C**. The lowering of oxygen available to the fetus during gestation is compensated by a decrease in growth factors resulting in fetal growth restriction.
11. **C**. Although the cardiac output and umbilical flow remain the same, the blood flow to the CNS and heart increases.
12. **B**. The high diffusibility of CO_2 across the placenta causes analogous disturbances in the fetus in a matter of minutes. A low maternal $PaCO_2$ will cause fetal respiratory alkalosis, and a high maternal $PaCO_2$ will be reflected in fetal respiratory acidosis when a well-perfused placenta is present.
13. **D**. Approximately 70–80% of uteroplacental oxygen consumption is by the placental villous tree. The major mechanism that allows the umbilical circulation to extract oxygen from such an organ is uterine hyperemia.
14. **C**. The shape of the maternal and fetal oxygen dissociation curves dictates that a dramatic increase in maternal PaO_2 causes only a small increase in fetal PaO_2. Oxygen (100%) at atmospheric pressure can cause lung toxicity if given for extended periods of time. Breathing 50% is considered safe.
15. **B**. Fetal blood affinity for CO_2 is lower than that of maternal blood, thereby favoring CO_2 transfer from the fetus to the mother. Mild maternal hyperventilation results in a fall in $PaCO_2$ levels favoring a transfer of CO_2 from the fetal compartment to maternal blood.

References

1. Cunningham F et al. Implantation and placental development. In: Williams obstetrics. McGraw Hill; 2014.
2. Randhawa R, Cohen P. The role of the insulin-like growth factor system in prenatal growth. Mol Genet Metab. 2005;86:84.
3. Settle P, Mynett K, Speake P, et al. Polarized lactate transporter activity and expression in the syncytiotrophoblast of the term human placenta. Placenta. 2004;25:496.
4. Brownhill P, Mahendran D, Owen D, et al. Denudations as paracellular routes for alphafetoprotein and creatinine across the human syncytiotrophoblast. Am J Physiol Regul Integr Comp Physiol. 2000;278:R677.
5. Griffiths SK, Campbell JP. Placental structure, function and drug transfer. Contin Educ Anaesth Crit Care Pain. 2015;15(2):84–9. https://doi.org/10.1093/bjaceaccp/mku013.
6. Meschia G. Supply of oxygen to the fetus. J Reprod Med. 1979;23:160.

7. Herrera E, Amusquivar E, Lopez-Soldado I, Ortega H. Maternal lipid metabolism and placental lipid transfer. Horm Res. 2006;65(Suppl 3):59.
8. Carter AM. Factors affecting gas transfer across the placenta and the oxygen supply to the fetus. J Dev Physiol. 1989;12:305.

Renal and Hepatic Pathophysiology of Pregnancy

Bowei Su, Jae Woong Lee, Aymen Alian, and Justin Calvert

Questions

1. **How is glomerular filtration rate (GFR) affected by pregnancy?**
   A. Decreased by 30%
   B. Maintained
   C. Increased by 25%
   D. Increased by 50%
2. **All of the following are expected with a normal pregnancy, EXCEPT:**
   A. Glucosuria
   B. Hydronephrosis
   C. Unchanged BUN and Cr
   D. Anemia
3. **Physiologic proteinuria in pregnant women over 24 hours is defined as:**
   A. <100 mg
   B. <300 mg
   C. <500 mg
   D. <1000 mg
4. **What is the most accurate method of estimating GFR during pregnancy?**
   A. Creatinine clearance
   B. Cystatin C clearance
   C. 24-h urine collection
   D. Renal ultrasound

B. Su · J. Calvert (✉)
Department of Anaesthesiology, Riverside University Health System Medical Center, Moreno Valley, CA, USA
e-mail: B.su@ruhealth.org; a.calvert@ruhealth.org

J. W. Lee · A. Alian
Department of Anaesthesiology, Yale University, New Haven, CT, USA
e-mail: Jaewoong.lee@yale.edu; aymen.alian@yale.edu

A. C. Sinha, I. F. Pasca (eds.), *Peripartum Care of the Pregnant Patient*,
https://doi.org/10.1007/978-3-031-62756-9_9

5. **Preeclampsia may present with:**
   A. Hypoalbuminemia
   B. Hyperalbuminemia
   C. Thrombocytosis
   D. Hypouricemia
6. **Which antihypertensive medication should be discontinued during pregnancy?**
   A. Methyldopa
   B. Labetalol
   C. Nifedipine
   D. Lisinopril
7. **During pregnancy, free drug concentrations are generally:**
   A. No effect
   B. Decreased
   C. Maintained
   D. Increased
8. **Alpha-1 acid glycoprotein preferentially binds:**
   A. Acidic drugs
   B. Neutral drugs
   C. Basic drugs
   D. None of the above
9. **Which is *not* a mechanism of decreased systemic vascular resistance during pregnancy?**
   A. Reduced responsiveness to vasopressors such as angiotensin II, norepinephrine, and vasopressin
   B. Increased vascular expression of angiotensin II type 1 receptor
   C. Increased nitric oxide synthesis
   D. Production of relaxin by the placenta and decidua
10. **During the first trimester, the most common reason for the elevation of LFTs is as follows:**
    A. Hepatitis B
    B. Hyperemesis gravidarum
    C. HELLP syndrome
    D. Hepatorenal syndrome
11. **If an abdominal ultrasound of cholestasis during a second trimester pregnancy is indeterminate, what follow-up imaging should be ordered?**
    A. MRI without gadolinium contrast
    B. MRI with gadolinium contrast
    C. CT
    D. KUB radiograph
12. **What is NOT a common cause of elevation of liver transaminases in the third trimester?**
    A. Eclampsia
    B. HELLP syndrome
    C. Acute fatty liver disease

D. All of the above

13. **What is the lower normal limit of serum albumin (g/dL) at the third trimester during normal pregnancy?**
    A. 4.1
    B. 3.1
    C. 2.6
    D. 2.3
14. **What is the most common cause of nonobstetric abdominal surgery during pregnancy?**
    A. Diverticulitis
    B. Cholelithiasis
    C. Appendicitis
    D. Pyelonephritis
15. **What is NOT a risk factor for the development of intrahepatic cholestasis of pregnancy (ICP)?**
    A. Younger maternal age
    B. Multiparity
    C. Prior history of ICP
    D. Hepatitis C infection
16. **A third trimester G5P4 parturient presents with nausea, vomiting, jaundice, and labs show hyperbilirubinemia, LFT elevations, profound hypoglycemia, and thrombocytopenia, which may be indicative of the following:**
    A. Eclampsia
    B. HELLP syndrome
    C. Acute fatty liver of pregnancy
    D. None of the above
17. **Which P450 enzyme is the most abundant and involved in the metabolism of more than half of all approved drugs?**
    A. CYP 2D6
    B. CYP 3A4
    C. CYP 2C9
    D. CYP 2E1
18. **What is the recommended dosing of ursodeoxycholic acid for treatment of intrahepatic cholestasis of pregnancy (ICP) gvb?**
    A. 10–15 mg/kg
    B. 20–25 mg/kg
    C. 30–35 mg/kg
    D. None of the above
19. **In the third trimester, alkaline phosphatase (ALP) will most likely:**
    A. Decrease to half of prepregnancy levels
    B. No change with prepregnancy levels
    C. Increase to twice that of prepregnancy levels
    D. Increase tenfold from prepregnancy levels

Answers and Explanations

1. **D**. GFR will increase 40–50% by the end of the first trimester to a peak rate of 180 mL/min and is maintained until approximately 36 weeks gestation. This is due to an expansion of plasma volume of 30–50%, leading to a decrease in oncotic pressure. **A–C** are incorrect [1–3].
2. **C**. BUN and Cr will decrease with pregnancy due to hyperactive kidney function with increased GFR. Glucosuria (**A**) is expected at physiological plasma glucose levels, as there is less effective glucose reabsorption and variability with excretion. Kidneys will also increase in length and volume during pregnancy, leading to hydronephrosis (**B**) in 63% of pregnant women with a peak incidence at 28 weeks. Erythropoietin secretion is upregulated with pregnancy, leading to an 18–25% increase in red blood cells; however, plasma volume exceeds this increase and results in net dilutional anemia (**D**) [1, 2].
3. **B**. Physiologic proteinuria is twice the limit of nonpregnant women; however, proteinuria over 300 mg/24-h period must be examined for any evidence of preeclampsia. **A**, **C**, and **D** are incorrect [1, 3].
4. **C**. Calculators based on creatinine and cystatin C clearance tend to underestimate GFR, so the preferred method is 24-h urine collection to calculate creatinine clearance [1].
5. **A**. Due to abnormal proteinuria, preeclampsia may also present with low serum albumin. The patient also presented with low platelet levels <100,000 (**C**) and elevated levels of serum uric acid (**D**) [1–3].
6. **D**. ACE inhibitors and ARBs are associated with teratogenicity and should be discontinued prior to pregnancy. **A–C** are safe to use during pregnancy [3].
7. **D**. Due to lower serum albumin levels during pregnancy, there is reduced protein binding with free drug. As a result, a higher fraction of intravascular free drug is able to diffuse to target tissues [4].
8. **C**. Alpha-1 acid glycoprotein preferentially binds to basic drugs, whereas albumin binds preferentially to acidic (**A**) and neutral (**B**) drugs [4].
9. **B**. Angiotensin II levels are elevated by the second trimester. At late gestation, its levels reach approximately 50% above nonpregnant levels. Despite angiotensin II type 1 receptor having a vasoconstrictive effect, during pregnancy, there is elevated vascular angiotensin II type 2 receptor expression mediated by estrogen, which causes net vasodilation rather than vasoconstriction [1–3].
10. **B**. Hyperemesis gravidarum accounts for the main cause of hypertransaminasemia, occurring in 0.3–2% of pregnancies with elevation up to 20 times the normal limit. **A**, **C**, and **D** are incorrect [2, 5].
11. **A**. Ultrasound is the preferred imaging modality that is safe for pregnancy, allowing for differentiation between intra- and extrahepatic causes of cholestasis. If imaging remains inconclusive, an MRI during the second/third trimester can be used without gadolinium contrast. The contrast crosses the placenta and is excreted by fetal kidneys into amniotic fluid, where it remains for prolonged periods and increases the risk of GI/pulmonary harm [5].

12. **D**. HELLP syndrome, acute fatty liver disease, preeclampsia/eclampsia, and intrahepatic cholestasis of pregnancy are all common reasons for acute hypertransaminasemia in the third trimester [2, 5].
13. **D**. In the third trimester, the expected serum albumin concentration is 2.3–4.2 g/dL. This is thought to be related to the dilutional effect of the increased plasma volume and increased excretion through the kidney. The reference for the first trimester is 3.1–5.1, and that for the second trimester is 2.6–4.5 g/dL [1, 5].
14. **C**. Appendicitis is the most common cause of nonobstetric abdominal surgery in pregnancy. Appendicitis occurs in up to 1/500 pregnancies. Cholelithiasis is common in pregnancy and occurs due to elevated estrogen causing cholesterol saturation and increased gallstone formation; however, surgical intervention is less commonly needed [5].
15. **A**. ICP is one of the most common liver diseases during pregnancy and has a multifactorial etiology. Risk factors for the development of ICP include multiparity, IVF fertilization, advanced maternal age, history of ICP with prior pregnancy, hepatitis C infection, and family history [5].
16. **C**. Acute fatty liver of pregnancy most commonly occurs during the third trimester during weeks 28–40 gestation. It is an obstetric emergency and presents with jaundice, hepatic encephalopathy, and lab values consistent with acute liver failure. Treatment involves early recognition and prompt delivery, followed by intensive supportive therapy [3, 5].
17. **B**. CYP3A4 is the most abundant P450 enzyme and has increased activity during pregnancy. CYP2D6 (**A**) is involved in 25% of all medications, many of which are prescribed to pregnant women. CYP 2E1 (**D**) is notably involved in the metabolism of volatile anesthetics [4, 6].
18. **A**. ICP presents in the third trimester with pruritus on the palms and soles in the setting of increasing serum LFTs and bile acid levels. Ursodeoxycholic acid at a 10–15 mg/kg/day dosing is appropriate for managing pruritus and improving LFTs and fetal outcomes [5].
19. **C**. Due to an influx from placental isoenzyme production, ALP levels may increase two- to fourfold from regular adult values during the third trimester of pregnancy and require no further investigation in this range [5].

References

1. Cheung KL, Lafayette RA. Renal physiology of pregnancy. Adv Chronic Kidney Dis. 2013;20(3):209–14. https://doi.org/10.1053/j.ackd.2013.01.012. PMID: 23928384; PMCID: PMC4089195.
2. Tan EK, Tan EL. Alterations in physiology and anatomy during pregnancy. Best Pract Res Clin Obstet Gynecol. 2013;27(6):791–802. https://doi.org/10.1016/j.bpobgyn.2013.08.001. Epub 2013 Sep 4. PMID: 24012425.
3. Gonzalez Suarez ML, Kattah A, Grande JP, Garovic V. Renal disorders in pregnancy: core curriculum 2019. Am J Kidney Dis. 2019;73(1):119–30. https://doi.org/10.1053/j.ajkd.2018.06.006.

Epub 2018 Aug 16. Erratum in: Am J Kidney Dis 2019 Jun;73(6):897. PMID: 30122546; PMCID: PMC6309641.

4. Pinheiro EA, Stika CS. Drugs in pregnancy: pharmacologic and physiologic changes that affect clinical care. Semin Perinatol. 2020;44(3):151221. https://doi.org/10.1016/j.semperi.2020.151221. Epub 2020 Jan 25. PMID: 32115202; PMCID: PMC8195457.
5. Guarino M, Cossiga V, Morisco F. The interpretation of liver function tests in pregnancy. Best Pract Res Clin Gastroenterol. 2020;44–45:101667. https://doi.org/10.1016/j.bpg.2020.101667. Epub 2020 Feb 18. PMID: 32359686.
6. Betcher HK, George AL Jr. Pharmacogenomics in pregnancy. Semin Perinatol. 2020;44(3):151222. https://doi.org/10.1016/j.semperi.2020.151222. Epub 2020 Jan 25. PMID: 32081407; PMCID: PMC7214196.

Obesity and Pregnancy

Ioana F. Pasca and Ashish C. Sinha

Questions

1. **What is the prevalence of obesity (BMI >30 kg/m^2) among childbearing women, 20–39 years of age in the United States?**
   A. 10%
   B. 25%
   C. 40%
   D. 50%
2. **What is the frequency of >1 miscarriage after spontaneous conception in females with BMI >30 kg/m^2.**
   A. 11%
   B. 16%
   C. 24%
   D. 33%

I. F. Pasca (✉)
Riverside University Health System, Moreno Valley, CA, USA

Department of Anesthesiology, Critical Care, and Neurocritical Care, Loma Linda University at Riverside University Health System, Loma Linda, CA, USA

University of California San Diego, San Diego, CA, USA

University of California Riverside, Riverside, CA, USA
e-mail: i.pasca@ruhealth.org

A. C. Sinha
Riverside University Health System, Moreno Valley, CA, USA

Loma Linda University, Loma Linda, CA, USA

University of California Riverside, Riverside, CA, USA

Kaweah Health Medical Center, Visalia, CA, USA
e-mail: a.sinha@ruhealth.org

A. C. Sinha, I. F. Pasca (eds.), *Peripartum Care of the Pregnant Patient*,
https://doi.org/10.1007/978-3-031-62756-9_10

3. **Obesity in pregnancy increases all of the following, *except*:**
   A. Cesarean delivery
   B. Infection
   C. Accuracy of monitoring vital signs
   D. Fetal macrosomia
4. **Obesity is not an independent risk factor for which of the following:**
   A. Pulmonary aspiration
   B. Gallbladder disease
   C. Chronic back pain
   D. Pulmonary embolism
5. **Which of the following pulmonary changes occurs in the obese parturient?**
   A. Decreased expiratory reserve volume
   B. Increased forced vital capacity
   C. Increased ratio of FEV1 to FVC
   D. Increased total lung capacity (TLC)
6. **Which of the following describes supine hypotension syndrome in the morbidly obese parturient?**
   A. Increased
   B. No change
   C. Increase in venous return from the panniculus
   D. Decreased
7. **With every 100 g of fat increased during pregnancy, cardiac output increases by how many mL/min?**
   A. 3–5 mL/min
   B. 10–20 mL/min
   C. 30–50 mL/min
   D. 50–100 mL/min
8. **Which intravenous drug used during induction is dosed based on total body weight (TBW)?**
   A. Fentanyl
   B. Dexmedetomidine
   C. Succinylcholine
   D. Rocuronium
9. **Obese parturients may require less local anesthetic in epidurals due to the following:**
   A. Lower volumes of CSF
   B. Increased abdominal pressure
   C. Fatty infiltration of the epidural space
   D. All of the above
10. **All of the following are disadvantages of general anesthesia for delivery of obese parturients:**
    A. Increased risk of difficult airway
    B. Increased risk of peripartum hemorrhage
    C. Increased exposure of the fetus to medications
    D. Increased onset of action

11. **Select the recommended weight gain during pregnancy for the parturient with prepregnancy BMI >30 kg/m^2.**
    A. 12.5–18 kg
    B. 11.5–16 kg
    C. 7–11.5 kg
    D. 5–9 kg
12. **Which of the following factors increases the risk of difficult ventilation and intubation during general anesthesia for the delivery of obese parturients?**
    A. Friable mucous membranes
    B. Breast enlargement
    C. Airway edema
    D. Narrowing of the airway passages
    E. All of the above
13. **Increases in which procoagulant factor is associated with increased venous thromboembolism during obesity and pregnancy?**
    A. Protein S
    B. Fibrinogen
    C. Protein C
    D. Factor II
14. **Which of the following does not contribute to rapid desaturation during the induction of general anesthesia in obese parturients?**
    A. Decreased closing capacity
    B. Increase in oxygen consumption by the fetus
    C. Decreased FRC in pregnancy
    D. Increased work of breathing in obesity
15. **Compared to the normal weight parturient, the obese parturient is at increased risk for all of the following, *except*:**
    A. Faster cervical dilation
    B. Ineffective uterine contractions
    C. Failed induction of labor
    D. Fetal intolerance of labor
16. **The double catheter technique has been described when surgeons perform a supraumbilical vertical midline incision in superobese parturients with a large pannus for which of the following:**
    A. A lumbar CSE for intraoperative pain and a continuous local anesthetic catheter placed at the surgical incision
    B. A lumbar CSE for intraoperative anesthesia and a transversus abdominus plane block (TAP) continuous catheter for postoperative pain
    C. A lumbar CSE for intraoperative anesthesia and bilateral paravertebral catheters for postoperative pain
    D. A lumbar CSE for intraoperative anesthesia and a low thoracic epidural catheter for postoperative pain management
17. **Common obstetric complications in obese compared to nonobese parturients include the following:**
    A. Obstructive sleep apnea
    B. Gestational diabetes

C. Hypertensive disorders
D. Venous thromboembolism
E. All of the above

18. **Which of the following has not been shown in the use of ultrasound for neuraxial anesthetic placement for obese parturients undergoing C-section?**
    A. Reduce the number of attempts to successfully place a spinal anesthetic
    B. Reduce the risk of a failed epidural catheter
    C. Overdetermine the depth of the epidural space
    D. Reduce epidural needle redirection
19. **When administering propofol for emergency C-section of obese parturients, should dosing be based on LBW or TBW?**
    A. Induction: TBW and maintenance: TBW
    B. Induction: LBW and maintenance: TBW
    C. Induction: LBW and maintenance: LBW
    D. Induction: TBW and maintenance: LBW
20. **Obese parturients may require less local anesthetic with neuraxial techniques due to which of the following?**
    A. Higher volumes of CSF
    B. Lower abdominal pressure
    C. Fatty infiltration compressing the epidural space
    D. Decreased elimination half-life of local anesthetic

Answers and Explanations

1. **C**. In the current obesity epidemic, nearly 40% of women of childbearing age have a BMI of >30 kg/m^2. Predictive models anticipate that nearly 50% of the population will meet the criteria for obesity by 2030 [1, 2].
2. **B**. Women with obesity have increased rates of infertility and early miscarriages. The frequency of >1 miscarriage after spontaneous conception by BMI classification is 16.6% for obese and 11.8% for overweight compared to 10.7% in normal BMI [3].
3. **C**. Morbidly obese parturient patients have prolonged labor with an increased likelihood of cesarean delivery, increased risk of initial epidural failure, higher fetal birth weights, and increased risk of infection. Obesity presents increased challenges to tocolytic fetal monitoring as well as increased difficulty with hemodynamic monitoring [4].
4. **A**. Obesity is not an independent risk factor for aspiration. Aspiration occurs because of incorrect preoperative assessment and failure to modify the anesthetic technique to compensate for the increased aspiration risk. Wong et al. showed no difference in the gastric emptying of water in obese and nonobese pregnant patients [5, 6].
5. **A**. Obesity decreases expiratory reserve volume in proportion to increasing BMI. FEV1 to FVC remains unchanged. Forced vital capacity decreases as does FEV1 and TLC [7].

6. **A**. Supine hypotension syndrome is exaggerated in the obese parturient due to increased aortocaval compression and a significant decrease in venous return from the panniculus even leading to case reports of sudden death in morbidly obese patients in the supine position [8].
7. **C**. Every 100 g of fat increases cardiac output by 30–50 mL/min, increasing blood volume independently by 20–25%, which can increase pulmonary blood flow, pulmonary pressure, and even right heart strain [8].
8. **C**. Succinylcholine should be dosed using TBW. Pseudocholinesterase activity is closely associated with TBW. Fentanyl and dexmedetomidine dosing should use lean body weight (LBW). Rocuronium should be dosed using ideal body weight (IBW) [9].

Term	Equation
BMI (kg/m^2)	TBW (kg)/height (m^2)
IBW (kg)	Men = 50 kg + 2.3 kg/inch above 5 feet Women = 45.5 kg + 2.3 kg/inch above 5 feet
BSA (m^2)	$([\text{Height (cm)} \times \text{weight (kg)}]/3600)^{1/2}$
ABW (kg)	IBW + correction factor × (TBW − IBW)
FFM (kg)	Men: (0.285 × TBW) + (12.1 × height (m^2)) Women: (0.287 × TBW) + (9.74 × height (m^2))
LBW (kg)	Men: (1.1 × TBW) − (0.0128 × BMI × TBW) Women: (1.07 × TBW) − (0.0148 × BMI × TBW)

9. **D**. The elimination half-life of lidocaine is prolonged in obese patients. However, when the volume of distribution is corrected for TBW, the elimination half-life is comparable. Obese patients may require less local anesthetic for neuraxial blocks due to lower volumes of CSF, increased abdominal pressure, and fatty infiltration. Blocks extending above T5 should be avoided due to possible respiratory and autonomic blockade [9].
10. **D**. Because general anesthesia has a faster onset than neuraxial blockade, it is considered the standard of care for emergency cesarean delivery. However, there are several disadvantages of neuraxial blockade, including an increased risk of difficult ventilation and intubation, peripartum hemorrhage, thromboembolism, and increased fetal exposure to medications [8].
11. **D**. In 2009, the Institute of Medicine set the recommended allowable gestational weight gain for parturients to prevent inadequate weight gain, which is associated with small-for-gestational-age infants. In a parturient with a prepregnancy BMI >30 kg/m^2, the recommended weight gain is 5–9 kg. Gestational weight gain above the recommendations was associated with macrosomia and an increased risk of cesarean delivery [10].
12. **E**. The incidence of difficult intubation in morbidly obese parturients can be up to 33%. In normal pregnancy, increased airway vascularity results in interstitial airway edema, increased membrane friability, and narrowing of the airway passages. Increased adipose tissue deposition in the airway and engorgement of breast tissue also increases difficulty in mask ventilation and intubation [8].

13. **B**. The risk for venous thromboembolism is increased at least fourfold in pregnancy. Fibrinogen is a procoagulant that is increased in both normal pregnancy and obesity. Protein C and S are anticoagulant factors that are decreased in normal pregnancy. Obesity further increases hypercoagulability by increasing factor VII, factor VIII, and von Willebrand factor [8].
14. **A**. Obesity and pregnancy both result in increased oxygen consumption and CO_2 production. While pregnancy does not increase closing capacity, FRC may be decreased below closing capacity, resulting in airway closure during tidal respiration. On the other hand, obesity increases closing capacity through the collapse of the distal airways [8, 11].
15. **A**. Obese parturients have increased difficulties in all stages of labor, including slower cervical dilation, ineffective uterine contractions, failed induction of labor, fetal intolerance of labor, need for instrumental delivery, and progression to emergency cesarean delivery. Increased vigilance is required in placing and maintaining epidural catheters in obese parturients so that they can be used effectively in the event of an intrapartum complication [8].
16. **D**. A large pannus adds extra difficulty in performing a Pfannenstiel incision in obese parturients. Surgeons may perform a supraumbilical vertical midline incision, which can increase the risk of postoperative pain and respiratory complications. The use of a lumbar CSE allows for rapid onset of labor analgesia and the ability to augment medication if more time and analgesia is needed. A low thoracic epidural catheter may also be placed for postoperative analgesia and was described in a case series in 2015 in three superobese parturients (BMI: 73–95 kg/m^2) [4].

17. **E**. The increased odds ratio of obstetric complications in obese compared to nonobese parturients includes gestational diabetes, hypertensive heart disease, venous thromboembolism, induction of labor, cesarean delivery, postpartum hemorrhage, wound infection macrosomia, shoulder dystocia, prematurity, stillbirth, and obstructive sleep apnea [4].
18. **C**. Although there is a strong correlation between the predicted depth of the epidural space with ultrasound and the depth measured by the Tuohy needle, determining the depth of the epidural space may be underestimated as the distance from the probe increases. The ultrasound probe may compress the subcutaneous tissues, and the angle of the probe and needle may vary. Using ultrasound to identify the midline spinous processes as well as the transverse processes and ligamentum flavum has been shown to reduce the number of attempts to successfully place a spinal anesthetic for obese parturients (**A**),

reduce the risk of a failed epidural catheter (**B**), and reduce epidural needle redirection (**D**) [4].

19. **B**. Propofol can be given as a bolus for the induction of anesthesia or as a continuous infusion for the maintenance of anesthesia. Bolus dosing for nonobese patients is based on TBW; however, blood flow to fat is much less than that to lean tissue. Obese patients who are induced with LBW vs TBW propofol dosing had similar times of loss of consciousness, so LBW should be used for bolus dosing. There is no difference in the elimination half-time of propofol, so maintenance infusion should be based on TBW [9].
20. **C**. Obesity makes neuraxial anesthesia more challenging due to increased difficulty identifying anatomical structures. The elimination half-life of lidocaine is prolonged in obese patients; however, TBW dosing is recommended because the volume of distribution is also increased (**D**). Obese patients may require less local anesthetic with neuraxial techniques than nonobese parturients due to increased abdominal pressure (**B**), fatty infiltration compressing the epidural space (**C**), and lower volumes of CSF (**A**) [9].

References

1. Hales CM, Carroll MD, Fryar CD, Ogden CL. Prevalence of obesity and severe obesity among adults: United States, 2017–2018. NCHS Data Brief. 2020;1.
2. Ward ZJ, et al. Projected U.S. state-level prevalence of adult obesity and severe obesity. N Engl J Med. 2019;381:2440–50.
3. Boots C, Stephenson MD. Does obesity increase the risk of miscarriage in spontaneous conception: a systematic review. Semin Reprod Med. 2011;29(6):507–13. Epub 2011 Dec 8.
4. Taylor CR, Dominguez JE, Habib AS. Obesity and obstetric anesthesia: current insights. Local Reg Anesth. 2019;12:111–24.
5. Moon TS, Van de Putte P, De Baerdemaeker L, Schumann R. The obese patient: facts, fables, and best practices. Anesth Analg. 2021;132:53–64.
6. Wong CA, McCarthy RJ, Fitzgerald PC, et al. Gastric emptying of water in obese pregnant women at term. Anesth Analg. 2007;105:751–5.
7. Porhomayon J, Papadakos P, Singh A, Nader ND. Alteration in respiratory physiology in obesity for anesthesia-critical care physician. HSR Proc Intensive Care Cardiovasc Anesth. 2011;3(2):109–18.
8. Onuoha OC. Obesity in pregnancy. In: Sinha A, editor. Anesthesia for the obese patient. Oxford: Oxford University Press; 2021. p. 285–93.
9. Moon TS, Ogunnaike B. Pharmacokinetics and pharmacodynamics in obesity. In: Sinha A, editor. Anesthesia for the obese patient. Oxford: Oxford University Press; 2021. p. 39–48.
10. Goldstein RF, Abell SK, Ranashinha S, et al. Association of gestational weight gain with maternal and infant outcomes: a systematic review and meta-analysis. JAMA. 2017;317:2207.
11. Russell IF, Chambers WA. Closing capacity during pregnancy. BJA. 1981;53:1043.

Further Reading

Sinha A, editor. Anaesthesia for the obese patient. Oxford: Oxford University Press; 2021.

Blood Dyscrasias in Pregnancy

Thomas Cho and Ayman Ads

Questions

1. **What is the absolute platelet threshold for epidural placement during pregnancy?**
   A. 70,000
   B. 50,000
   C. 25,000
   D. No absolute threshold
2. **A 24 y/o G1P0 patient currently 38 weeks presents to the hospital for induction of labor. Past medical history is significant for protein C deficiency, with a known family history of venous thromboembolism in the past. Should this patient be started on VTE prophylaxis postpartum?**
   A. Yes: Due to the patient's family history of VTE, the patient is a candidate for postpartum VTE prophylaxis
   B. Yes: The patient's known history of protein C deficiency alone makes her a candidate for postpartum VTE prophylaxis
   C. No: Although the patient has a known history of inherited thrombophilia, the increased risk of major bleeding precludes her from starting postpartum prophylaxis
   D. No: Prophylaxis should never be offered to a pregnant patient, regardless of family history
3. **A 24 y/o G3P2 patient arrived at the ED with left calf pain. Duplex ultrasound shows acute VTE in the distal popliteal vein. She had no known**

T. Cho (✉)
Riverside University Health System, Moreno Valley, CA, USA
e-mail: T.Cho@ruhealth.org

A. Ads
Los Angeles General Medical Center, Los Angeles, CA, USA
e-mail: a.ayman@ruhealth.org

A. C. Sinha, I. F. Pasca (eds.), *Peripartum Care of the Pregnant Patient*,
https://doi.org/10.1007/978-3-031-62756-9_11

medical or family history of blood disorders. Renal function is normal, and the patient is otherwise healthy. Which of the following is recommended for VTE treatment in this patient?

A. Patient should be treated for an acute VTE with unfractionated heparin
B. Patient should be treated for an acute VTE with low molecular weight heparin (LMWH)
C. Patient should not be treated for an acute VTE, as no antithrombotic therapy is recommended over treatment
D. The patient should not be treated for acute VTE, as the clot is in the distal popliteal vein

4. **A 58 F with no PMH is scheduled for venous bypass graft surgery. Intraoperatively, the surgeon requests 5000 units of heparin to be injected subcutaneously, which you do. The rest of the surgery went well with no complications, and the patient was successfully extubated and eventually transferred to the floor. The next morning during the postoperative check, you notice that the patient has a superficial, painless hematoma on the forearm. CBC is notable for a platelet count of 30,000; preoperatively, it was 150,000. Which one of the following is NOT considered when calculating a 4T score of heparin induced thrombocytopenia?**
   A. Presence of thrombocytopenia
   B. Timing of platelet count drop
   C. New thrombosis
   D. PT and PTT prolongation
5. **A 28 y/o G5P4 presents to the OR for cesarean delivery. She has a history of multiple C-sections, and her most recent ultrasound is concerning for placenta accreta. After successful delivery of a baby boy at term, the surgery was complicated by uncontrolled blood loss, and the patient was converted to GA. The surgical team continues to have difficulty controlling blood loss, and after the patient has lost an estimated 2 L of blood, it is decided to start blood transfusion immediately. No coagulation results are available. Which of the following transfusion protocols is recommended for postpartum hemorrhage?**
   A. Start massive transfusion protocol at 1:1:3 RBC/FFP/platelets until bleeding is controlled
   B. Start with transfusion of 4 units PRBC, followed by 4 units FFP, followed by 1:1 RBC/FFP transfusion until bleeding is controlled
   C. Start massive transfusion protocol at 1:1:1 RBC/FFP/platelets
   D. Delay administering any products until all coagulation results are available
6. **According to the International Society on Thrombosis and Hemostasis (ISTH), what is the minimum blood fibrinogen concentration that should be maintained in postpartum hemorrhage?**
   A. 1 g/L
   B. 2 g/L
   C. 4 g/L
   D. Dependent on coagulation test results

7. **A 29 y/o G1P0 patient comes into the hospital for induction of labor. She wishes to have an epidural placed early in labor. Her only medication is daily aspirin. Her last dose was this morning prior to arriving at the hospital. Can she immediately proceed with an epidural?**
   A. Yes, there are no immediate contraindications
   B. Yes, but only after a 24-h washout period
   C. Yes, but she is at risk of developing a spinal/epidural hematoma
   D. No, she is on an anticoagulant
8. **A 31 y/o G4P3 patient presented to labor and delivery for induction of labor. The patient had a mechanical mitral valve and was previously on warfarin. After finding out she was pregnant, she was switched to therapeutic doses of low-molecular-weight heparin, which she had been taking as directed. She is currently in labor and is requesting an epidural. Her last injection of LMWH was over 12 h prior. Can she immediately proceed with an epidural?**
   A. Yes, there are no immediate contraindications
   B. Yes, as it has been over 12 h since last administration
   C. No, there needs to be a 24-h washout period
   D. No, as stopping anticoagulation for a mechanical heart valve is an absolute contraindication
9. **Which of the following factors has elevated concentrations during pregnancy?**
   A. Factor VIII
   B. Factor II
   C. Factor XIII
   D. Protein C
10. **What lab test is considered the best predictor of bleeding risk in pregnant patients with von Willebrand disease?**
    A. Platelet aggregation study
    B. Platelet count
    C. PT/PTT
    D. Factor VIII
11. **What is the most common true platelet dysfunction seen in pregnancy?**
    A. Bernard Soulier
    B. Thrombotic thrombocytopenic purpura
    C. Immune thrombocytopenia
    D. Thrombocytopenia 2/2 preeclampsia
12. **A 21-year-old G3P2 patient was diagnosed with immune thrombocytopenia. Platelet count is 25,000. What is the first-line therapy?**
    A. IVIG and corticosteroids
    B. Rituximab
    C. Cyclosporine
    D. Supportive care only
13. **A 19 y/o G2P0010 patient came into labor and delivered for induction of labor at 38 weeks gestation. The patient's history is notable for HbSS sickle**

cell disease. She has multiple sickle cell crises annually, and her last crisis required hospitalization for severe acute chest syndrome. The patient's current pregnancy has been uncomplicated, and she has been receiving good prenatal care. Which of the following prophylactic treatments should NOT be started?

A. Aspirin after the first trimester to prevent preeclampsia
B. Blood transfusion to prevent sickling during stage 3 of labor
C. Early fluid resuscitation through peripheral IVs
D. Tight O_2 saturation goals >94%

14. **A 28 y/o G1P0 at 31 weeks gestation presents to triage with abdominal pain. Initial CBC is notable for platelets of <20,000/μL. The patient had no history of blood disorders and was otherwise stable. The patient was diagnosed with immune thrombocytopenic purpura. She was started on IVIG and corticosteroids, but the thrombocytopenia did not improve. Given her presentation, what is the next best step?**

A. Platelet transfusion
B. Splenectomy
C. Rituximab
D. Azathioprine

15. **A 23 y/o G4P2 patient at 10 weeks gestation presented with abnormal uterine bleeding and fatigue for 2 weeks. She is admitted after CBC shows that she is pancytopenic. Bone marrow biopsy completed the next day showed hypocellular bone marrow, and she was diagnosed with aplastic anemia. What is the next best step for this patient?**

A. 1:1:1 transfusion
B. Stem cell transplantation
C. Pregnancy termination
D. Immunosuppression

16. **Two hours after delivering a healthy full-term baby, the mother started to have severe shortness of breath followed by collapse and a seizure. On exam, the patient had a blood pressure of 60/40 mmHg with a heart rate of 140 bps and crackles on lung auscultation. Shortly thereafter, the patient started to have profuse uterine bleeding as well as bleeding from all IV sites. What's the most likely cause of the patient collapse.**

A. Anaphylactic reaction
B. Venous thromboembolism
C. Amniotic fluid embolism
D. Air embolism

Answers and Explanations

1. **D**. Epidural-induced hematoma is a concern when placing an epidural in a patient with thrombocytopenia. It has been found that the risk of an epidural hematoma was low (less than 0.2%) in patients whose platelet count was greater

than 70,000 × 10^6/L. In parturients with platelet counts of <50,000 × 10^6/L, the upper bound risk was 11%, and there was a 3% risk of hematoma in those with platelet counts between 50,000 and 69,000 × 10^6/L. Different institutions have different thresholds, but there is no evidence to suggest that there is an absolute threshold [1].

2. **A**. Per the 2018 Clinical Practice Guidelines for Venous Thromboembolism in the Context of Pregnancy established by the American Society of Hematology, postpartum VTE prophylaxis should only be offered to patients with a select number of thrombophilic conditions and with a family history of VTEs [2]. These conditions include protein C deficiency, protein S deficiency, and anti-thrombin deficiency. Postpartum VTE prophylaxis is not recommended in those with a thrombophilic condition with no family history of VTEs.
3. **B**. The American Society of Hematology strongly recommends antithrombotic therapy over no antithrombotic therapy [2]. In addition, they specifically recommend LMWH over UFH.
4. **D**. The 4T score for heparin-induced thrombocytopenia (HIT) considers (A) the presence and magnitude of thrombocytopenia, (B) the timing of thrombocytopenia after heparin exposure, (C) the presence of new/worsening thrombosis, and (D) whether another cause can be identified as a cause of thrombocytopenia [3]. Lab values outside of platelet count are not considered in a 4T score. In one study, a low probability 4T score (≤ 3) was associated with a negative predictive value (NPV) of 0.998, while the PPV of a 4T score was limited. This suggests that the 4T score may be more useful in ruling out HIT if the 4T score is low.
5. **B**. Postpartum hemorrhage remains one of the leading causes of maternal mortality worldwide, and its pathophysiology is complex and includes both dilutional and consumption characteristics. According to the International Society on Thrombosis and Hemostasis (ISTH), there is no definitive protocol for PPH management, but care needs to be taken to monitor and adequately replete fibrinogen. Protocols such as 1:1:1 without monitoring current platelet levels may cause fluid overload without adequate repletion of fibrinogen. Likewise, focusing primarily on fibrinogen repletion may increase morbidity if the acute loss of RBCs may not be addressed in a timely manner. Therefore, given no/limited coagulation results, the ISTH recommends transfusing an initial 4 units of PRBCs, followed by 4 units of FPP, then 1:1 PRBC/FFP until hemostasis is achieved or coagulation tests are available [4]. If 8 units of PRBCs and 8 units of FFPs total are given and there are still no coagulation data available, then they recommend two pools of cryoprecipitate and one pool of platelets. Management of blood product transfusion can be guided by thromboelastogram (TEG) analysis, which can help the use of selective transfusion of blood products and coagulation factors.
6. **B**. The ISTH recommends a blood fibrinogen concentration of at least 2 g/L during any ongoing obstetric bleeding, regardless of PT/aPTT [4]. Either cryoprecipitate or fibrinogen concentrate may be used. However, they do recommend against the use of fibrinogen concentrate in an unmonitored or preemptive manner.

7. **A**. Women with sickle cell disease can be started on ASA daily from the end of the first trimester to reduce the risk of preeclampsia. Aspirin alone does not increase the risk for the development of a hematoma [5]. There is no washout period necessary. Additionally, there is no need to wait after aspirin discontinuation for catheter removal.
8. **C**. For patients on a therapeutic dose of LMWH, a 24-h interval between the last dose and epidural placement is required [5]. This is because of an increased risk of developing a spinal/epidural hematoma. Patients previously on warfarin for a mechanical heart valve are frequently transitioned to starting LMWH for anticoagulation in pregnancy due to the elevated risk of fetal abnormalities on warfarin. However, the timing and necessity of switching is controversial and has not been fully studied [5]. Regardless, those who have been on therapeutic doses of LMWH need a 24-h washout period before receiving neuraxial anesthesia.
9. **A**. Factors VII, VIII, and X and fibrinogen levels are elevated in pregnancy while protein S is decreased. Interestingly, those with von Willebrand disease type I, which is a quantitative disorder of insufficient vWF/factor VIII, see the deficiency corrected in pregnancy due to the increase in factor VIII concentrations [6].
10. **D**. von Willebrand disease is a bleeding disorder associated with deficiencies in von Willebrand factor and its associated factor, factor VIII. There are three types of vWF disease: type 1, which is a quantitative deficiency of vWF; type 2, which is a qualitative defect; and type 3, which is the absence of vWF. Factors VII, VIII, and X and fibrinogen levels are elevated in pregnancy. Women with von Willebrand disease may have lower levels of factor VIII, as vWF prevents factor 8 degradation, as such factor 8 levels are the best predictor of bleed risk [6].
11. **C**. Although gestational thrombocytopenia accounts for 70–80% of isolated thrombocytopenia, its pathophysiology appears to be from hemodilution or accelerated clearance and is thus not true thrombocytopenia [6]. Immune thrombocytopenic purpura (ITP) is therefore the most common true acquired thrombocytopenia.
12. **A**. IVIG and corticosteroids are first-line therapies, with a combination of the two being second-line [6]. The goal is to keep a platelet count of approximately 30,000 in the first trimester. However, the platelet count should be monitored frequently, especially in the third trimester. Rituximab and cyclosporine are reserved if IVIG and steroids have failed but have not been fully studied in pregnancy [6].
13. **B**. Sickle cell disease carriers (HbSA) have a lower risk of acute sickle crises compared to those with the homozygous mutation (HbSS) [7]. Prophylactic blood transfusions are no longer recommended in patients with sickle cell disease regardless of genotype [8]. Prophylactic transfusion has been shown to reduce the incidence of painful crises during the third trimester, but it does not affect fetal outcome and carries significant risks of acute transfusion reactions, alloimmunization, and DHTR [7]. Prophylactic transfusion can be considered

if the patient's sickle cell disease is not well controlled, if she has a history of having sickle cell crises during prior pregnancies, or if she has had other hematologic complications in the past due to sickle cell disease. Aspirin is routinely started after the first trimester to prevent preeclampsia.

14. **B**. ITP treatment with IVIG and/or steroids can be initiated in any of the trimesters if the platelet counts fall below 20–30,000/μL, there is bleeding, or the patient requires a procedure [9]. In the second or third trimester, a splenectomy is recommended if the thrombocytopenia remains refractory to IVIG/corticosteroids. Rituximab and azathioprine are treatments for ITP in nonpregnant patients but have not been studied in pregnancy.
15. **C**. Aplastic anemia is a potentially life-threatening pregnancy complication, increasing the risk of cerebral hemorrhage and sepsis. In nonpregnant patients, the first-line therapy for aplastic therapy is stem cell transplantation. However, transplantation is contraindicated in pregnancy due to the teratogenic effects of the necessary immunotherapy and radiotherapy [10].
16. **C**. Amniotic fluid embolism (AFE) incidence is 1:40,000 pregnancies and usually presents with severe shortness of breath, confusion that can progress to loss of consciousness. Severe hypotension, acute respiratory failure, and disseminated intravascular coagulation (DIC) are characteristic and can help direct the diagnosis toward AFE by exclusion when the cause of hemodynamic compromise is not clear. Prompt diagnosis and treatment of cardiopulmonary resuscitation with blood product transfusion is critical for survival [10].

References

1. Lee LO, Bateman BT, Kheterpal S, Klumpner TT, Housey M, Aziz MF, Hand KW, MacEachern M, Goodier CG, Bernstein J, Bauer ME, Multicenter Perioperative Outcomes Group Investigators. Risk of epidural hematoma after neuraxial techniques in thrombocytopenic parturients: a report from the Multicenter Perioperative Outcomes Group. Anesthesiology. 2017;126(6):1053–63. https://doi.org/10.1097/ALN.0000000000001630.
2. Bates SM, Rajasekhar A, Middeldorp S, McLintock C, Rodger MA, James AH, Vazquez SR, Greer IA, Riva JJ, Bhatt M, Schwab N, Barrett D, LaHaye A, Rochwerg B. American Society of Hematology 2018 guidelines for management of venous thromboembolism: venous thromboembolism in the context of pregnancy. Blood Adv. 2018;2(22):3317–59. https://doi.org/10.1182/bloodadvances.2018024802.
3. Cuker A, Gimotty PA, Crowther MA, Warkentin TE. Predictive value of the 4Ts scoring system for heparin-induced thrombocytopenia: a systematic review and meta-analysis. Blood. 2012;120(20):4160–7. https://doi.org/10.1182/blood-2012-07-443051. Epub 2012 Sep 18.
4. Collins P, Abdul-Kadir R, Thachil J, Subcommittees on Women's Health Issues in Thrombosis and Hemostasias and on Disseminated Intravascular Coagulation. Management of coagulopathy associated with postpartum hemorrhage: guidance from the SSC of the ISTH. J Thromb Hemost. 2016;14(1):205–10.
5. Fonseca NM, Pontes JPJ, Perez MV, Alves RR, Fonseca GG. SBA 2020: Atualização na diretriz da anestesia regional em uso de anticoagulants [SBA 2020: Regional anesthesia guideline for using anticoagulants update]. Braz J Anesthesiol. 2020;70(4):364–87. https://doi.org/10.1016/j.bjan.2020.02.006. Epub 2020 May 12.

6. Gernsheimer TB. Congenital and acquired bleeding disorders in pregnancy. Hematology Am Soc Hematol Educ Program. 2016;2016(1):232–5. https://doi.org/10.1182/asheducation-2016.1.232.
7. da Guarda CC, Yahouédéhou SCMA, Santiago RP, Neres JSDS, Fernandes CFL, Aleluia MM, Figueiredo CVB, Fiuza LM, Carvalho SP, Oliveira RM, Fonseca CA, Ndidi US, Nascimento VML, Rocha LC, Goncalves MS. Sickle cell disease: a distinction of two most frequent genotypes (HbSS and HbSC). PLoS One. 2020;15(1):e0228399. https://doi.org/10.1371/journal.pone.0228399.
8. Stoddard K, Sohal M, Bedson R. Anesthetic management of patients with sickle cell disease in obstetrics. BJA Educ. 2022;22(3):87–93. https://doi.org/10.1016/j.bjae.2021.11.005. Epub 2022 Jan 19.
9. Townsley DM. Hematologic complications of pregnancy. Semin Hematol. 2013;50(3):222–31. https://doi.org/10.1053/j.seminhematol.2013.06.004.
10. Stibbe KJ, Wildschut HI, Lugtenburg PJ. Management of aplastic anemia in a woman during pregnancy: a case report. J Med Case Rep. 2011;5:66. https://doi.org/10.1186/1752-1947-5-66.

Further Reading

Park YH. Diagnosis and management of thrombocytopenia in pregnancy. Blood Res. 2022;57(S1):79–85. https://doi.org/10.5045/br.2022.2022068.

Fetal Monitoring

Allen Wang and Erin I. Martin

Questions

1. **A parturient underwent an emergent cesarean delivery for velamentous cord prolapse under general anesthesia. Upon delivery, the neonate was unresponsive, cyanotic, and flaccid. Neonatal resuscitation was initiated, and at the 1-min mark, the neonate had no muscle tone, a pulse of 96 bpm, unresponsiveness to stimulation, peripheral cyanosis, and a weak cry. Resuscitation efforts continued, and at the 5-min mark, the neonate was grimacing to stimulation, a pulse of 125 bpm, peripheral cyanosis, extremities flexed with minimal muscle tone, and irregular breathing. Continued resuscitation efforts occurred, and at the 10-min mark, the neonate was highly reactive to stimulation, a pulse of 139 bpm, peripheral cyanosis, actively moving all extremities, and crying vigorously. What is the Apgar score at the 1-, 5- and 10-min mark?**
   A. 1 min, 2; 5 min, 3; and 10 min, 10
   B. 1 min, 3; 5 min, 6; and 10 min, 9
   C. 1 min, 3; 5 min, 6; and 10 min, 10
   D. 1 min, 0; 5 min, 5; and 10 min, 9

A. Wang (✉)
University of California, Davis, Sacramento, CA, USA

E. I. Martin
University of California, San Diego, La Jolla, CA, USA
e-mail: eim002@health.ucsd.edu

A. C. Sinha, I. F. Pasca (eds.), *Peripartum Care of the Pregnant Patient*,
https://doi.org/10.1007/978-3-031-62756-9_12

2. **A parturient at 39 weeks and 5 days presents for the onset of labor. Her pregnancy was complicated by gestational diabetes. She was 2 cm dilated, and external fetal heart rate monitoring (FHR) was performed. What is the FHR pattern?**

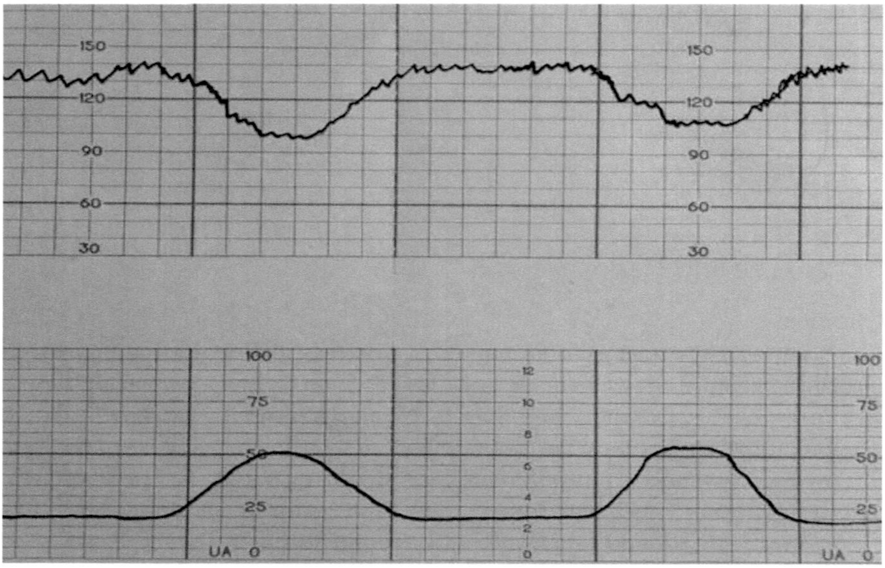

A. Early decelerations
B. Variable decelerations
C. Late decelerations
D. Sinusoidal

3. **A G1P0 parturient at 34 weeks and 3 days presents to the obstetric unit for feeling unwell. Her pregnancy was complicated with severe preeclampsia with a blood pressure measuring 220/110 mmHg. The patient was started on an antihypertensive cascade and magnesium therapy. Fetal heart rate (FHR) tracing is demonstrated below. What is the FHR pattern?**

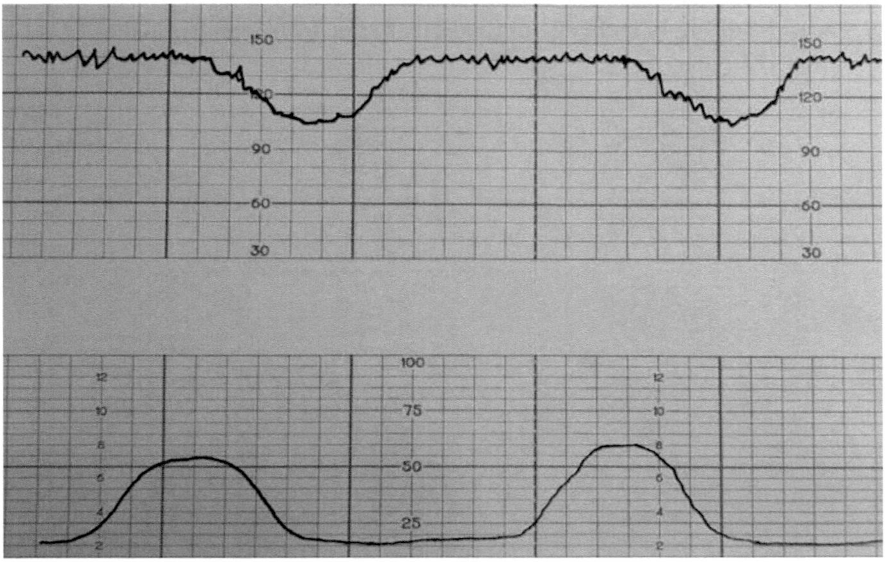

A. Early decelerations
B. Variable decelerations
C. Late decelerations
D. Sinusoidal

4. **A G1P0 parturient presents for spontaneous labor. Her pregnancy is complicated with oligohydramnios identified during a recent fetal ultrasound with an amniotic fluid index of 3 cm and a single deepest pocket of 1.5 cm. On cervical exam, she was 6 cm dilated with an intact amniotic sac. External fetal heart rate monitoring demonstrates good variability and early decelerations. The obstetric intern decided to perform an amniotomy, resulting in a change in the FHR pattern, as depicted below. What is the FHR pattern?**

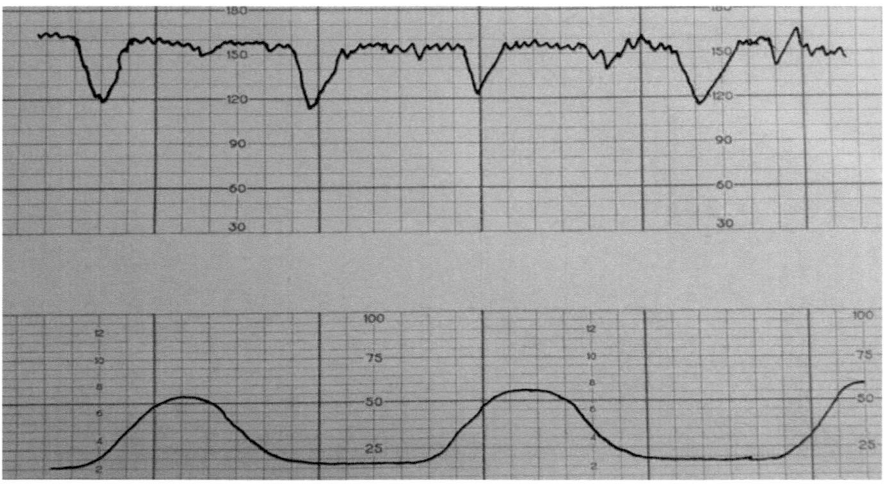

   A. Early decelerations
   B. Variable decelerations
   C. Late decelerations
   D. Sinusoidal
5. **A G1P0 parturient at term presents to the labor and delivery unit in spontaneous labor. She had no significant medical history, and her pregnancy was uncomplicated. On ultrasound, the fetus was vertex and occiput anterior. She is refusing continuous electronic fetal monitoring but accepts intermittent auscultation. Is it acceptable to use intermittent auscultation in this parturient?**
   A. Yes, intermittent auscultation can be used
   B. No, intermittent auscultation should be avoided
6. **What is true about the use of continuous electronic fetal heart rate monitoring?**
   A. The use of continuous electronic FHR monitoring in a noncomplicated pregnancy has been shown to improve both maternal and fetal outcomes
   B. The use of continuous electronic FHR monitoring is superior to intermittent auscultation in the detection of fetal distress in all pregnancies
   C. The use of continuous electronic FHR monitoring has been shown to increase both cesarean deliveries and operative vaginal deliveries

D. The use of continuous electronic FHR monitoring has been shown to improve fetal acidosis and neonatal APGAR scores

7. **A 40-year-old G2P1 parturient at term presented with severe abdominal pain and vaginal bleeding. Her current pregnancy is complicated by pre-eclampsia and active cocaine use. She had a classical cesarean delivery for her first pregnancy. A fetal heart rate tracing is demonstrated below. What category is this FHR tracing, and does it require an intervention?**

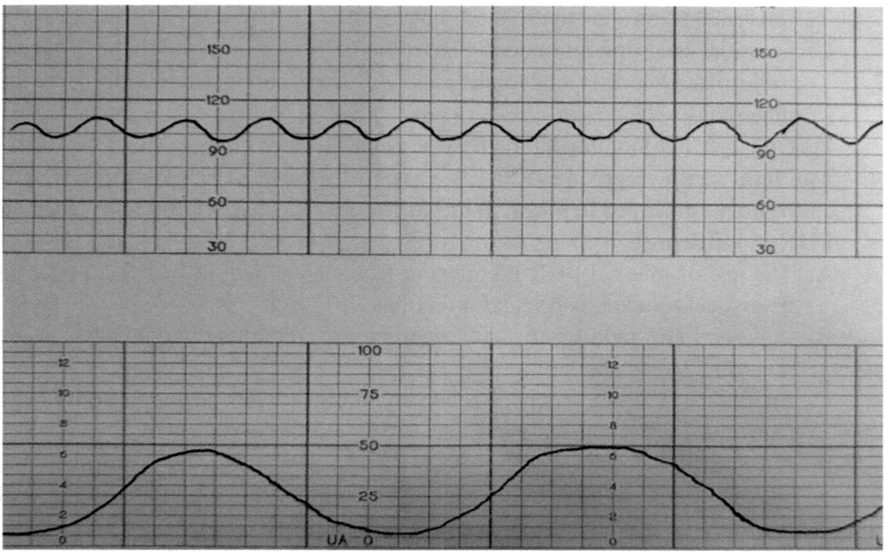

A. This is a category I tracing and requires no immediate intervention
B. This is a category I tracing and requires an emergent delivery
C. This is a category II tracing and requires no immediate intervention
D. This is a category II tracing and requires an emergent delivery
E. This is a category III tracing and requires no immediate intervention
F. This is a category III tracing and requires an emergent delivery

8. **A 22-year-old parturient at 33-week gestation presented to the main operating room for an appendectomy due to acute appendicitis. She had no past medical history, and her current pregnancy had been uncomplicated prior to this admission. What is the ACOG recommendation for nonobstetric surgery during pregnancy at this gestational age?**

A. Fetal monitoring is not necessary due to the gestational age and is not recommended
B. Electronic fetal heart rate and contraction monitoring should be performed before and after the procedure. If applicable, intraoperative continuous FHR monitoring should be utilized
C. This surgery should be postponed until after delivery
D. The obstetrician should be notified but does not have to be in or near the hospital at the time of the surgery

9. **A parturient present in spontaneous labor with rupture of membrane. External FHR monitoring has been difficult due to the patient's habitus and her inability to stay still. On exam, her cervix was noted to be 5 cm dilated with fetal head engagement in the pelvis. What other modalities can be considered to monitor the FHR?**
   A. Consider applying more pressure to the external FHR devices to compensate for maternal movement and habitus
   B. Consider inserting an internal electronic FHR monitor with both spiral and reference electrodes to the fetal scalp
   C. Consider inserting an internal electronic FHR monitor with the spiral electrode placed in the fetal scalp and the reference electrode placed on the maternal thigh
   D. Consider not monitoring the FHR during the labor course
10. **The fetal scalp electrode (FSE) is a type of internal FHR monitor that is commonly employed in labor. What are some risks associated with internal FHR monitoring?**
   A. The use of internal FHR monitoring has been shown to increase maternal fevers, cesarean delivery, and infections
   B. Internal FHR monitoring can be employed for all fetuses regardless of maternal and fetal conditions
   C. Internal FHR monitoring is a relatively benign condition and has only been shown to cause fetal scalp trauma
   D. Internal FHR monitoring has been associated with serious complications such as subgaleal hematoma, cephalohematoma, and subdural and cerebral hemorrhage
11. **A parturient at 24-week gestation presents for a routine obstetric evaluation. She is concerned about her pregnancy, as her friend recently had a stillbirth. Which viable gestational age has the highest stillbirth rate?**
   A. 32–33 weeks of gestation
   B. 27–28 weeks of gestation
   C. 39–40 weeks of gestation
   D. 42–43 weeks of gestation
12. **What are the components of the fetal biophysical profile (BPP)?**
   A. Fetal breathing, gross body movements, fetal tone, amniotic fluid volume, and nonstress test
   B. Fetal nuchal translucency, gross body movements, fetal tone, amniotic fluid volume, and nonstress test
   C. Fetal breathing, gross body movements, fetal tone, amniotic fluid volume, and baseline FHR
   D. Fetal breathing, gross body movements, fetal tone, fetal nuchal translucency, and baseline FHR
   E. Fetal breathing, gross body movements, fetal umbilical Doppler, amniotic fluid volume, and nonstress test

13. **A 33-year-old G5P4 parturient at 39 weeks presents for the onset of labor. She indicates that her "water broke" 3 h prior to presentation. She is now admitted to the labor unit for expectant management. The FHR tracing has a baseline FHR of 140 bpm and recurrent early decelerations with moderate variability. No variable or late decelerations are present. What category is the FHR tracing?**
    A. This is a category I tracing
    B. This is a category II tracing
    C. This is a category III tracing
    D. There is not enough information provided
14. **A parturient has a complicated labor course. She is noted to have a temperature of 38.4 °C, maternal heart rate of 130 bpm, foul-smelling amniotic fluid, and new onset of fetal tachycardia with an FHR of 190 bpm. The parturient is started on broad spectrum antibiotics. The neonate was delivered and required neonatal resuscitation with direct admission to the neonatal intensive care unit. An umbilical arterial cord blood gas was obtained and resulted in a pH of 6.96, pCO_2 of 50 mmHg, and a base excess (BE) of −16.3 mmol/L. What information can be deduced from the umbilical arterial cord blood gas?**
    A. There is not enough information to make a clinical decision from the umbilical arterial cord blood gas.
    B. Umbilical arterial cord blood gas is concerning. It represents severe metabolic acidosis and is associated with increased fetal morbidity and mortality.
    C. The umbilical artery provides information on maternal acid-base status.
    D. The umbilical vein provides information on the fetal acid-base status.
15. **When does most fetal neurological injury occur?**
    A. First trimester
    B. Second trimester
    C. Third trimester
    D. Prior to onset of labor
16. **A parturient present for her routine antepartum visit. External fetal monitoring is applied on the maternal abdomen. What is true regarding minimal FHR variation?**
    A. Fetal gestational age does not affect FHR variation
    B. The use of magnesium does not decrease FHR variation
    C. Minimal FHR variation does not occur with fetal sleep
    D. Maternal opioid use can cause minimal FHR variation
17. **A parturient at 30 weeks of gestation is admitted for premature rupture of membranes. She is given a course of antenatal steroids for fetal lung maturity. What effects can antenatal steroids cause on the FHR that providers should be aware of?**
    A. Antenatal steroids have no known effect on the FHR and fetal movement
    B. Antenatal steroids may cause a transient effect on FHR, including a decrease in FHR variation, a decrease in FHR accelerations, and a decrease in fetal movements
    C. Antenatal steroids may cause a transient effect on the FHR, including an increase in FHR variation, an increase in FHR accelerations, and an increase in fetal movements

18. **What is true regarding the use of fetal pulse oximetry?**
    A. Normal fetal pulse oximetry is between 30% and 70%, and it has been shown to decrease the number of cesarean deliveries
    B. A fetal pulse oximetry <30% is concerning and requires immediate attention
    C. The use of fetal pulse oximetry is a novel technique that has decreased the number of cesarean deliveries
    D. A normal fetal pulse oximetry is >70%, and the implementation of fetal pulse oximetry has not affected cesarean delivery rates

Answers and Explanations

1. **B**. Dr. Virginia Apgar was an anesthesiologist who developed the Apgar score in 1953. The Apgar score was the first reproducible scoring system that provides a rapid and reliable objective assessment of the neonate at the time of delivery. Furthermore, it allows providers to assess neonatal response to resuscitation. The Apgar score is measured by five components, and each component is scored between 0 and 2 points, with a cumulative score between 0 and 10 points. An Apgar score of ≥7 is considered reassuring. The Apgar evaluation focuses on neonatal breathing effort, heart rate, muscle tone, skin color, and stimulation reflex. Fortunately, Dr. Apgar's name can be used as a mnemonic to recall the five elements.

Apgar	0 point	1 point	2 points
Appearance (skin color)	Infant is diffusely pale or blue	Centrally pink, but the extremities are blue	Entirely pink
Pulse (heart rate)	No heartbeat present	Heart rate <100 bpm	Heart rate >100 bpm
Grimace (stimulation reflex)	No response to stimulation	Grimacing to stimulation	Crying, coughing, or sneezing to stimulation
Activity (muscle tone)	No tone/floppy	Some tone and flexion	Actively moving all extremities
Respiration (breathing effort)	No respiratory effort	Slow and irregular, weak or gasping respiratory effort	Vigorous cry

It is important to understand and calculate the Apgar score, as it will guide neonatal resuscitation efforts. The Apgar score at the 1-min mark is 3: 0 points for no muscle tone, 1 point for a pulse of 96 bpm, 0 points for grimace, 1 point for peripheral cyanosis, and 1 point for weak cry. The Apgar score at the 5-min mark is 6: 1 point for grimacing to stimulation, 2 points for a pulse of 125 bpm, 1 point for peripheral cyanosis, 1 point for minimal movement, and 1 point for irregular breathing. The Apgar score at the 10-min mark is 9: 2 points for stimulation, 2 points for an HR of 139 bpm, 1 point for peripheral cyanosis, 2 points for movement, and 2 points for vigorous crying.

2. **A**. Early decelerations are identified by the symmetrical decrease in the FHR in relation to the uterine contraction. The onset of FHR deceleration to the nadir will occur in ≥30 s, with the onset occurring with uterine contraction and the nadir occurring at the peak of uterine contraction. The change in the FHR represents a nonhypoxic autonomic response caused by uterine compression onto

the fetal head. This will lead to an increase in fetal intracranial pressure and activation of the Cushing reflex, resulting in a transient decrease in the FHR. Early decelerations are not associated with fetal hypoxia and acidosis and do not require further interventions [1].

3. **C**. Late decelerations can be identified by the delayed nature of the FHR in response to the onset of uterine contraction. FHR deceleration will occur after the start of a uterine contraction, and the FHR will reach a nadir of ≥30 s after the peak of uterine contraction. Late decelerations are a concern finding that occurs when there is uteroplacental insufficiency. The etiology for late decelerations includes fetal anemia, hypoxia, uterine tachysystole, and placental abruption. The underlying pathophysiology of late deceleration begins with uterine contraction, reducing uterine-placental perfusion and oxygen delivery to the fetus. The decrease in fetal oxygenation will cause a chemoreceptor-mediated autonomic reflex to decrease fetal PO_2, resulting in a delayed transient decrease in the FHR [2].
4. **B**. Variable decelerations are abrupt decreases in the FHR that are not associated with uterine contraction. The FHR should decrease by 15 bpm from baseline and last more than 15 s and less than 2 min. Variable decelerations can be caused by the transient compression of the umbilical cord from fetal movement or uterine contraction. The mechanical compression of the umbilical cord can indirectly cause a transient increase in the fetal arterial blood pressure that will activate the baroreceptor reflex to rapidly decrease the FHR. Another more concerning cause of variable decelerations is transient episodes of fetal hypoxia. The decrease in fetal PO_2 will activate chemoreceptors and cause a rapid decrease in the FHR. Occasional variable decelerations are usually not associated with worsening perinatal outcomes. However, if variable decelerations occur in ≥50% of uterine contractions, they are categorized as recurrent and may indicate fetal distress [3].
5. **A**. Intermittent auscultation can be utilized in healthy parturients with low-risk pregnancies. The technique is performed with a fetal stethoscope. The practitioner listens and records the FHR and the uterine contraction every 15–30 min depending on the institutional protocol. The use of intermittent auscultation has also been shown to decrease the risk of emergency cesarean deliveries in labor patients compared to other types of FHR monitoring [4].
6. **C**. Continuous electronic FHR monitoring is the most common obstetric procedure performed and used in 85% of laboring parturients in the United States. However, the use of continuous electronic FHR monitoring has not been shown to be superior to intermittent auscultation in reducing cerebral palsy, acidosis, and death in both low- and high-risk pregnancies. Instead, it has increased instrumental vaginal deliveries (RR of 1.16; 95% CI: 1.01–1.32) and operative cesarean deliveries (RR of 1.66; 95% CI: 1.30–2.13). The American College of Obstetricians and Gynecologists (ACOG) recommends that high-risk pregnancies such as preeclampsia, intrauterine growth restriction, and prior cesarean delivery be monitored with continuous electronic fetal heart rate monitoring [4, 5].

7. **F**. This FHR pattern is concerning and is a category III tracing that requires immediate attention and intervention, such as an emergent delivery. Notably, the parturient has risk factors for placental abruption or uterine rupture that can present with category III FHR tracings. The National Institute of Child Health and Human Development (NICHD) developed a three-tier classification system to standardize the definition, terminology, and interpretation of FHR patterns. A category I tracing is a reassuring FHR pattern and includes all of the following: a baseline FHR of 110–160 bpm with moderate FHR variability, presence or absence of fetal accelerations, presence or absence of early decelerations, and no variable or late deceleration. A category III is an FHR tracing that is concerning and includes one of the following: absent baseline FHR variability, recurrent late decelerations, recurrent variable decelerations, fetal bradycardia (FHR <110 bpm), or a sinusoidal pattern. The presence of a category III tracing requires immediate attention and intervention. A category II includes all FHR tracing not categorized in category I or category III [6].
8. **B**. During nonobstetric surgeries in pregnancy, the ACOG mentions that a parturient should never be denied or delayed medically necessary surgeries regardless of trimester. If the infant is considered viable, at a minimum, simultaneous electronic FHR and contraction should be performed before and after the procedure to assess fetal well-being and uterine contraction. Intraoperative continuous electronic fetal monitoring should be performed if the fetus is viable and if the planned surgery can be safely interrupted for an emergent cesarean delivery. The potential for viable preterm delivery can occur, and the administration of corticosteroids for fetal lung protection can be beneficial. The surgery should be performed at an institution where neonatal, pediatric, and obstetrical anesthesia services are immediately available in case of an emergent delivery [7].
9. **C**. The use of internal electronic fetal monitoring is preferred when there is difficulty monitoring FHR with external monitoring techniques. This can occur due to maternal habitus, early gestation, maternal and fetal movements, polyhydramnios, or multiple gestations. The use of internal electronic FHR monitoring requires several parameters to be satisfied: the cervix must be $\geq$3 cm, the fetal position is a vertex with engagement to the pelvis, and the amniotic membrane must be ruptured. The device contains a bipolar spiral electrode placed in the fetal scalp transcervically and a second reference electrode placed on the maternal thigh. This will allow for the measurement of the FHR with minimal maternal heart rate interference. This provides an alternative, accurate, and reliable method for fetal FHR monitoring.
10. **D**. The use of internal FHR monitoring, especially an FSE, has been associated with both minor scalp trauma and serious complications such as subgaleal hematoma, cephalohematoma, and subdural and cerebral hemorrhages. Internal

FHR monitoring has not been shown to increase maternal fever, infections, and cesarean delivery rates. However, there are controversies regarding the use of internal FHR monitoring compared to external FHR monitoring. The consensus is that internal FHR monitoring has not been shown to improve neonatal outcomes. Certain situations in which internal FHR monitoring should be avoided include a risk of vertical transmission (active genital herpes infection, hepatitis B, C, D, E, and HIV), suspected fetal blood dyscrasia, if artificial rupture of membrane is inappropriate, or if there is uncertainty about the presenting fetal parts [8].

11. **D**. Stillbirth is defined as a fetal demise after 20 weeks of gestation and affects 1 in 175 births. Each year, approximately 21,000 babies are stillborn in the United States. Fetal demise can be identified into three different categories: early (20–27 weeks of gestation), late (28–36 weeks of gestation), or term (37 weeks of gestation or more). Due to advances in medical technology, there has been a reduction in the incidence of late and term stillbirth. However, the rate of early stillbirth has remained relatively unchanged for the past 30 years. Stillbirth can affect any pregnancy. However, certain groups are more susceptible to stillbirth, for example, African Americans, advanced maternal age, lower socioeconomic status, multiple gestation, and history of stillbirth. Based on a 2006 study, the stillbirth rate was noted to be high at 20–22 weeks of gestation and after 41 weeks of gestation. At 20–23 weeks of gestation, the rate was noted to be 0.51–0.60 and then declined at 27–33 weeks of gestation to 0.19–0.20 and remained relatively low until 37 weeks of gestation. However, there was a dramatic increase at 43 weeks of gestation to a rate of 0.78 [9, 10].

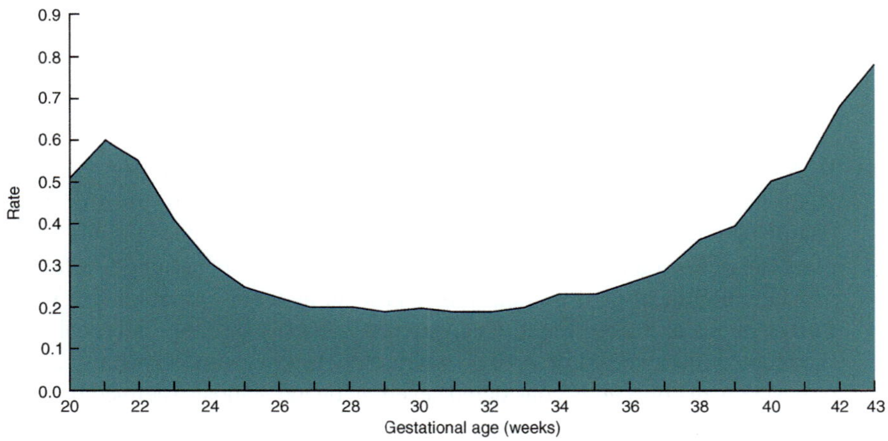

NOTE: The prospective fetal mortality rate is the number of fetal deaths at a given gestational age per 1.000 live births and fetal deaths at that gestational age or greater. SOURCE: CDC/NCHS, National Vital Statistics System.

12. **A**. The fetal biophysical profile (BPP) is a noninvasive test that begins as early as 24 weeks of gestation. It consists of measuring four parameters: fetal movement, fetal tone, fetal breathing, and amniotic fluid volume. The BPP can also be performed with a nonstress test (NST). Each parameter can be measured from 0 to 2 points with a total score of 10 points. A score of ≥8 is indicative of fetal well-being with good fetal oxygenation and normal acid-base status. A score ≤4 is concerning and is a sign of fetal compromise.

Biophysical profile test	Normal (2 points)	Abnormal (0 points)
Fetal breathing movements	≥1 episode of rhythmic fetal breathing lasting for 30 s within 30 min	No episode of fetal breathing movements lasting at least 30 s during a 30-min period
Fetal tone	≥1 episode of active extension of fetal extremities with return to flexion, or opening, or closing hand within 30 min	Slow extension with no return, or slow return to flexion of fetal extremities, or no fetal movement
Amniotic fluid volume	A single deepest vertical pocket of amniotic fluid >2 cm	A single deepest vertical pocket of amniotic fluid of <2 cm
Fetal body movement	≥3 discrete body or limb movements within 30 min	<3 body or limb movements within 30 min
Nonstress test (NST)	≥2 fetal heart rate accelerations that peak at least 15 bpm above the baseline and last at least 15 s from baseline during 20-min period	<2 accelerations of FHR after 40 min of observation

13. **A**. The FHR tracing is reassuring. The baseline FHR is currently 140 bpm, which corresponds to a normal baseline FHR. Moderate FHR variability represents the ability of the fetal autonomic nervous system to compensate for changes in the uterine environment. The presence of early deceleration is a normal physiological response to uterine contraction that is not associated with fetal hypoxemia and acidemia. The onset of uterine contraction will correlate with the initiation of the deceleration of the FHR, and the nadir of the FHR will be gradual and correspond with the peak of uterine contraction.
14. **B**. A normal umbilical artery has a pH of 7.27, pCO_2 of 50 mmHg, HCO_3 of 22 mmHg, and BE of −2.7 (mEq/L). Umbilical artery cord gas provides information on fetal well-being. Umbilical venous cord gas provides information on placental perfusion and exchange. In this case, there are concerning risk factors in which umbilical cord gas analysis is crucial, as the information will guide further neonatal management. Understanding and interpreting umbilical arterial blood gas is a vital skill. A basic interpretation starts with the pH, is it acidic or basic? A pH of 6.96 is considered severe neonatal acidosis (defined by a pH of <7.0). Next determine the etiology of the abnormal pH as metabolic, respiratory, or both. A BE of −16.3 is concerning for severe metabolic acidosis. The fetus can rapidly clear CO_2 through the placental circulation. If CO_2 is not cleared rapidly, carbonic acid (H_2CO_3) will accumulate, leading to respiratory acidemia. Interpretation of the umbilical artery blood gas demonstrates that there is no increase in pCO_2, so this is unlikely to be respiratory acidosis. The

most important information obtained from an umbilical artery blood gas is the pH and BE. A pH <7.0 and a BE >12 mmol/L correlate with fetal morbidity and mortality [11].

15. **D**. It is estimated that 70% of fetal neurologic injury occurs prior to the onset of labor. These events may include congenital abnormalities, environmental exposures, intrauterine infections (e.g., toxoplasmosis, CMV, rubella), placental dysfunction, and ischemic brain injury. Four percent of these fetal neurological injuries occur during labor, which can be attributed to uterine rupture, umbilical cord prolapse, amniotic fluid embolism, and placental abruption [12].
16. **D**. There are many factors that can decrease the variability in the FHR, including pharmacologic agents, normal fetal physiology, and pathological conditions. Pharmacological agents include opioids, barbiturates, anesthetics, and magnesium sulfate. Normal fetal physiology includes fetal sleep cycle, cyclic variation, and preterm fetus <28 weeks of gestation. Pathological conditions include preexisting fetal neurologic injury, hypoxia, and acidemia.
17. **B**. The administration of antenatal steroids has been shown to improve fetal lung maturity for at-risk preterm fetuses. However, the administration of antenatal steroids is not without risk and can cause a transient change in the FHR and fetal behavior. These changes include a decrease in the FHR variation, a decrease in the FHR acceleration, a decrease in the baseline FHR, and a decrease in the fetal movements. This effect can mimic fetal compromise, and providers should be aware of this transient phenomenon to avoid preemptive iatrogenic delivery of the fetus. These changes should resolve after day 4 of administration of antenatal steroids [13].
18. **B**. A normal fetal pulse oximetry saturation ranges between 30% and 70%. If the pulse oximetry decreases below 30%, immediate attention and intervention with maternal repositioning should be attempted. If pulse oximetry saturation remains <30% for at least 10 min in conjunction with non-reassuring FHR tracing, this can imply worsening fetal acidosis and requires urgent/emergent delivery. Unfortunately, the use of fetal oxygen saturation is reserved for certain situations and has not been shown to decrease cesarean delivery rates [14].

References

1. Choe J, Shanks AL, Mahdy H. Early decelerations [updated 2022 Aug 29]. In: StatPearls. Treasure Island, FL: StatPearls Publishing; 2022.
2. Pillarisetty LS, Bragg BN. Late decelerations [updated 2022 May 8]. In: StatPearls. Treasure Island, FL: StatPearls Publishing; 2022.
3. Sung S, Abramovitz A. Variable decelerations [updated 2022 Sep 18]. In: StatPearls. Treasure Island, FL: StatPearls Publishing; 2022.
4. Carter A, Nunes N. In low-risk pregnant women in labor, does continuous fetal heart monitoring lead to improved maternal and perinatal outcomes compared to intermittent fetal heart rate auscultation? Evid Based Pract. 2019;22(12):11–2. https://doi.org/10.1097/EBP.0000000000000445.
5. Al Wattar BH, et al. Effectiveness of intrapartum fetal surveillance to improve maternal and neonatal outcomes: a systematic review and network meta-analysis. CMAJ. 2021;193:E468.

6. National Guideline Alliance (UK). Addendum to intrapartum care: care for healthy women and babies. London: National Institute for Health and Care Excellence (NICE); 2017. Clinical Guideline, No. 190.1. Appendix J, Fetal heart rate classifications.
7. Nonobstetric surgery during pregnancy. Obstet Gynecol. 2019;133(4):e285–6. https://www.acog.org/clinical/clinical-guidance/committee-opinion/articles/2019/04/nonobstetric-surgery-during-pregnancy.
8. Harper LM, et al. The risks and benefits of internal monitors in laboring patients. Am J Obstet Gynecol. 2013;209(1):38.e1–6. https://doi.org/10.1016/j.ajog.2013.04.001.
9. MacDorman MF, Gregory ECW. Fetal and perinatal mortality: United States, 2013. Natl Vital Stat Rep. 2015;64:1–24.
10. Metz TD, et al. Management of stillbirth. Am J Obstet Gynecol. 2020;222:B2.
11. Ayres-de-Campos D, et al. Figo consensus guidelines on intrapartum fetal monitoring. Int J Gynecol Obstet. 2015;131:13. https://obgyn.onlinelibrary.wiley.com/doi/full/10.1016/j.ijgo.2015.06.020.
12. Jain S, Acharya N. Fetal wellbeing monitoring: a review article. Cureus. 2022;14(9):e29039. https://doi.org/10.7759/cureus.29039.
13. Ahmed AA, et al. Effect of dexamethasone on antepartum cardiotocography. Austin J Obstet Gynecol. 2021; https://doi.org/10.26420/austiniobstetgynecol.2021.1160.
14. East CE, et al. Fetal pulse oximetry for fetal assessment in labor. Cochrane Database Syst Rev. 2014;2014(10):CD004075. https://doi.org/10.1002/14651858.CD004075.pub4.

Point-of-Care Ultrasound in Obstetrics

Trenton G. Lum and Michael Douglas

Questions

1. **Which of the following structures is most visualized using point-of-care ultrasound during obstetric care?**
   A. Fetal heart rate monitoring
   B. Maternal bladder assessment
   C. Placental position determination
   D. Cervical dilation measurement
2. **Which mode on the ultrasound is used for fetal heart rate monitoring?**
   A. M-mode
   B. Pulse wave Doppler
   C. Color Doppler
   D. Continuous wave Doppler
3. **A 35-year-old pregnant woman presented to the labor and delivery unit with shortness of breath and fatigue. Her blood pressure was elevated, and she had pitting edema in her lower extremities. On examination, her heart sounds were distant, and there was an S3 gallop. A point-of-care ultrasound was performed, revealing a decreased left ventricular ejection fraction and dilation of the left ventricle. Which of the following additional findings is most likely to be observed in this patient with pregnancy-induced cardiomyopathy (PIC)?**
   A. Increased placental thickness
   B. Left ventricular hypertrophy
   C. Polyhydramnios
   D. Thinning of the myocardium

T. G. Lum · M. Douglas (✉)
Department of Anesthesiology and Perioperative Medicine, Riverside University Health System, Moreno Valley, CA, USA
e-mail: T.Lum@ruhealth.org; Michael.Douglas@RUHealth.org

A. C. Sinha, I. F. Pasca (eds.), *Peripartum Care of the Pregnant Patient*,
https://doi.org/10.1007/978-3-031-62756-9_13

4. **A 30-year-old pregnant woman presented to the emergency department following a motor vehicle accident. She is currently at 20-week gestation and is complaining of abdominal pain. As part of the trauma evaluation, a focused assessment with sonography for trauma (FAST) exam is performed. Which of the following findings is most likely to be assessed using the FAST exam in this pregnant patient?**
   A. Placental abruption
   B. Cervical dilation
   C. Fetal heart rate monitoring
   D. Uterine rupture
5. **A 28-year-old pregnant woman presented to the emergency department with a sudden onset of shortness of breath and pleuritic chest pain. She is currently at 34 weeks gestation. A point-of-care ultrasound is performed to assess for a suspected pulmonary embolism. Which of the following findings is most likely to indicate right heart strain in this patient?**
   A. Enlarged left atrium
   B. Hypertrophied left ventricle
   C. Dilated inferior vena cava (IVC)
   D. Thickened interventricular septum
6. **Which of the following ultrasound probes would be most suitable for cardiac evaluation during point-of-care ultrasound in an obstetric patient?**
   A. Transvaginal probe
   B. Linear probe
   C. Curvilinear probe
   D. Phased array probe
7. **A 36-year-old female G3P3003 with a history of gHTN and a history of two cesarean sections complained of shortness of breath in the recovery unit following her third C-section, which was complicated by postpartum hemorrhage requiring massive transfusion. Upon evaluation, the patient's SpO_2 was 88%, and she was tachypneic. Lung sounds were difficult to auscultate due to ambient noise from the crying baby. Which of the following are most likely to be seen on ultrasound?**
   A. Hypertrophic cardiomyopathy
   B. Retroperitoneal hematoma
   C. Pulmonary regurgitation
   D. B-lines
8. **A 22-year-old female with gHTN at 24-week gestation presents for an appendectomy for acute appendicitis. Earlier that day, the patient had presented to the ED with fever and tachycardia where she was give antibiotics, acetaminophen, and 3.5L crystalloid. However, preoperatively, the patient experienced dyspnea. Point-of-care ultrasound (POCUS) reveals B-lines throughout bilateral lung fields while the heart appears normal. How should the patient be medically optimized for the surgery?**
   A. Postpone appendectomy until after the patient delivers
   B. Give lasix
   C. Obtain a stress ECHO
   D. Give lisinopril

9. **A 36-year-old pregnant woman at 39-week gestation was admitted to the labor and delivery unit. During labor, she suddenly becomes acutely dyspneic and hypotensive. The fetal heart rate tracing shows sudden decelerations. A bedside ultrasound is performed to assess the maternal cardiac status. What findings on cardiac ultrasound are consistent with an amniotic fluid embolism (AFE)?**
   A. Visualization of a ventricular septal defect
   B. Identification of a pericardial effusion
   C. Detection of aortic dissection
   D. Visualization of right ventricular dilation and McConnell's sign
10. **A 32-year-old female presented to the emergency department with severe lower abdominal pain and vaginal bleeding. She reports a positive pregnancy test and is concerned about a possible ectopic pregnancy. Her vitals showed the following: HR, 124; BP, 89/56; RR, 21; and SpO_2, 97%. Suspecting an ectopic pregnancy, you perform a focused assessment with sonography for trauma (FAST) exam to evaluate the possibility. During the exam, which of the following ultrasound findings would be consistent with an ectopic pregnancy?**
    A. Visualization of an intrauterine gestational sac with a yolk sac
    B. Presence of an adnexal mass and free fluid in the pelvis
    C. Visualization of a thickened endometrial lining with an empty uterus
    D. Identification of multiple gestational sacs with separate fetal poles within the uterus

Answers and Explanations

1. **A**. Point-of-care ultrasound is commonly used during obstetric care to assess the well-being of the fetus. Fetal heart rate monitoring is a crucial aspect of obstetric care, and ultrasound can provide real-time visualization of the fetal heart, allowing the clinician to monitor the fetal heartrate and assess fetal well-being [1].

   While maternal bladder assessment, placental position determination, and cervical dilation measurement are important aspects of obstetric care, they are typically not the primary focus of point-of-care ultrasound during obstetric care.
2. **A**. M-mode provides a real-time representation of fetal heart motion. By freezing the M-mode wave, one can then measure the distance between peaks to determine the fetal heart rate. Doppler modes are not recommended to assess fetal heart rate, as they are associated with elevations in temperature and damage to biological tissues in vivo [2]. Compared to the M-mode, Doppler modes have 10–20 times more transmitted acoustic power. Although poorly studied, Doppler may have adverse effects on the fetus. A useful mnemonic is "Mommy-Mode" (M-mode).

3. **D**. In pregnancy-induced cardiomyopathy (PIC), the myocardium can undergo structural changes, including thinning of the heart muscle walls. This thinning occurs due to the dilation and impaired function of the left ventricle, leading to decreased contractility. The clinical vignette provided describes a patient with signs and symptoms consistent with PIC, including elevated blood pressure, edema, distant heart sounds, and an S3 gallop. The point-of-care ultrasound findings of a decreased left ventricular ejection fraction and left ventricular dilation further support the diagnosis [3]. Thinning of the myocardium is a characteristic finding in PIC and contributes to the impaired cardiac function observed in this condition.

   While increased placental thickness, left ventricular hypertrophy, and polyhydramnios are relevant in certain obstetric conditions, they are not typically associated with pregnancy-induced cardiomyopathy.
4. **A**. During a focused assessment with sonography for trauma (FAST) exam in a pregnant patient following a motor vehicle accident, one of the key structures assessed is the uterus and placenta. Placental abruption refers to the separation of the placenta from the uterine wall before delivery. It can occur as a result of trauma, leading to abdominal pain and potential fetal distress. The FAST exam can be utilized to identify the presence of free fluid in the abdominal or pelvic cavities, which can indicate bleeding from a placental abruption [4]. Detection of free fluid on ultrasound in the setting of trauma would prompt further evaluation and appropriate management.

   While cervical dilation, fetal heart rate monitoring, and uterine rupture are important considerations in obstetric emergencies, they are not specific findings assessed using the FAST exam. The FAST exam primarily focuses on identifying free fluid, which can help detect potential internal bleeding and guide further management in trauma situations.
5. **C**. In the setting of a pulmonary embolism (PE), right heart strain can be observed on point-of-care ultrasound [5]. Dilation of the inferior vena cava (IVC) is a characteristic finding associated with the right heart strain. A pulmonary embolism can cause obstruction in the pulmonary vasculature, leading to increased resistance to blood flow and subsequent right ventricular strain. This strain can result in elevated right atrial pressures, which are transmitted to the IVC, causing its dilation.

   While an enlarged left atrium, hypertrophied left ventricle, and thickened interventricular septum may be associated with other cardiac conditions, they are not specific findings indicating right heart strain in the setting of a pulmonary embolism. The dilation of the inferior vena cava is a more direct reflection of the right heart's response to the increased pressure and strain caused by the obstruction of pulmonary blood flow.
6. **D**. When performing cardiac evaluation during point-of-care ultrasound in an obstetric patient, a phased array probe is most suitable. The phased array probe is a sector probe with a small footprint and a wide field of view [6]. It is specifically designed for cardiac imaging, allowing for optimal visualization of the heart structures, including the chambers, valves, and myocardium.

Transvaginal probes are used for transvaginal ultrasound examinations and are not typically used for cardiac evaluation. Linear probes are commonly used for superficial imaging, such as musculoskeletal or vascular assessments, but they may not provide adequate depth and field of view for comprehensive cardiac evaluation. Curvilinear probes are commonly used for abdominal and obstetric imaging, but their lower frequency range may not provide the optimal resolution for detailed cardiac assessment.

In summary, the phased array probe is the most appropriate choice for cardiac evaluation during point-of-care ultrasound in an obstetric patient due to its specific design for cardiac imaging and its ability to provide a wide field of view.

7. **D**. B-lines are an ultrasound lung finding associated with pulmonary edema from volume overload, which is the most likely sequelae of MTP associated with acute orthopnea [7]. Hypertrophic cardiomyopathy, retroperitoneal hematoma, and pulmonary regurgitation are all less likely to be associated with postoperative acute orthopnea, especially following MTP.
8. **B**. Diffuse bilateral B-lines are associated with pulmonary edema from volume overload [7]. Although patients with acute appendicitis are more likely to present to the hospital as hypovolemic, overly aggressive fluid resuscitation, especially in the setting of gHTN, may precipitate volume overload. As such, diuresis would be indicated. Appendectomy is the preferred treatment option for pregnant patients presenting with appendicitis, as operative delay is associated with an increased risk of preterm labor, preterm delivery, and abortion [8]. Obtaining a stress ECHO may be performed safely in pregnant patients; however, it would not be a part of the initial medical management for a pregnant patient with B-lines and an otherwise unremarkable ECHO. ACE inhibitors, including lisinopril, are contraindicated in the second and third trimesters of pregnancy due to their association with oligohydramnios [9].
9. **D**. Amniotic fluid embolism (AFE) is a rare but life-threatening condition that can occur during childbirth. It occurs when amniotic fluid, fetal cells, or other debris enter the maternal circulation and trigger a systemic inflammatory response. This can lead to cardiovascular collapse and respiratory distress.

   In AFE, the right ventricle is typically affected due to a sudden increase in pulmonary artery pressure. As a result, right ventricular dilation can be observed on cardiac ultrasound [10]. McConnell's sign is a characteristic finding in AFE, which refers to a regional wall motion abnormality of the right ventricle, specifically the mid-portion of the free wall, while sparing the apex.

   While the other options (**A**, **B**, **C**) are cardiac conditions, they are not specific findings associated with AFE.
10. **B**. The presence of an adnexal mass and free fluid in the pelvis suggests an ectopic pregnancy [11]. An intrauterine gestational sac with a yolk sac indicates an intrauterine pregnancy. In an ectopic pregnancy, the gestational sac will be located outside the uterus. A thickened endometrial lining with an empty uterus may be seen in cases of early intrauterine pregnancy, but it does not indicate an ectopic pregnancy. The identification of multiple gestational sacs with separate fetal poles within the uterus indicates multiple gestations within the uterus and is not consistent with an ectopic pregnancy. In an ectopic pregnancy, the gestational sac will be located outside the uterus.

References

1. Hamelmann P, Vullings R, Kolen AF, et al. Doppler ultrasound technology for fetal heart rate monitoring: a review. IEEE Trans Ultrason Ferroelectr Freq Control. 2020;67(2):226–38. https://doi.org/10.1109/TUFFC.2019.2943626.
2. Quarato CMI, Lacedonia D, Salvemini M, et al. A review on biological effects of ultrasounds: key messages for clinicians. Diagnostics (Basel). 2023;13(5):855. Published 2023 Feb 23. https://doi.org/10.3390/diagnostics13050855.
3. Ricci F, De Innocentiis C, Verrengia E, et al. The role of multimodality cardiovascular imaging in peripartum cardiomyopathy. Front Cardiovasc Med. 2020;7:4. Published 2020 Feb 18. https://doi.org/10.3389/fcvm.2020.00004.
4. Fadl SA, Linnau KF, Dighe MK. Placental abruption and hemorrhage-review of imaging appearance. Emerg Radiol. 2019;26(1):87–97. https://doi.org/10.1007/s10140-018-1638-3.
5. Simcox LE, Ormesher L, Tower C, Greer IA. Pulmonary thrombo-embolism in pregnancy: diagnosis and management. Breathe (Sheff). 2015;11(4):282–9. https://doi.org/10.1183/20734735.008815.
6. Abu-Zidan FM, Hefny AF, Corr P. Clinical ultrasound physics. J Emerg Trauma Shock. 2011;4(4):501–3. https://doi.org/10.4103/0974-2700.86646.
7. Al Deeb M, Barbic S, Featherstone R, Dankoff J, Barbic D. Point-of-care ultrasonography for the diagnosis of acute cardiogenic pulmonary edema in patients presenting with acute dyspnea: a systematic review and meta-analysis. Acad Emerg Med. 2014;21(8):843–52. https://doi.org/10.1111/acem.12435.
8. Korndorffer JR Jr, Fellinger E, Reed W. SAGES guideline for laparoscopic appendectomy. Surg Endosc. 2010;24(4):757–61. https://doi.org/10.1007/s00464-009-0632-y.
9. Bullo M, Tschumi S, Bucher BS, Bianchetti MG, Simonetti GD. Pregnancy outcome following exposure to angiotensin-converting enzyme inhibitors or angiotensin receptor antagonists: a systematic review. Hypertension. 2012;60(2):444–50. https://doi.org/10.1161/HYPERTENSIONAHA.112.196352.
10. Wiseman D, Simard C, Yang SS, Koolian M, Abenhaim HA, Lipes J. Echocardiography findings in amniotic fluid embolism: a systematic review of the literature. Can J Anaesth. 2023;70(1):151–60. https://doi.org/10.1007/s12630-022-02343-9.
11. Jurkovic D, Mavrelos D. Catch me if you scan: ultrasound diagnosis of ectopic pregnancy. Ultrasound Obstet Gynecol. 2007;30(1):1–7. https://doi.org/10.1002/uog.4077.

Spinal Anesthesia

Katherine Ghobrial, Scott Nguyen, and Leonard J. Soloniuk

Questions

1. **Which is the following is NOT a physiological change to neuraxial anatomy in the parturient?**
   A. Distended thecal sac
   B. Accentuation of lumbar lordosis
   C. Softer ligamentum flavum
   D. Dilated epidural blood vessels
2. **What cephalad sensory levels are required for cesarean section when performing spinal anesthetic?**
   A. T4–T6
   B. T7–T10
   C. L1–L3
   D. S2–S4
3. **Which of the following is a guideline for neuraxial anesthesia for pregnant patients according to the American Society of Anesthesiologists (ASA)?**
   A. Required presence of qualified anesthesia and obstetric providers
   B. Immediate availability of resuscitation medication and equipment
   C. Employment and documentation of maternal vital signs and fetal heart rate monitoring
   D. Mandatory preprocedural intravenous access
   E. All of the above

K. Ghobrial · S. Nguyen
Riverside University Health System, Moreno Valley, CA, USA
e-mail: K.Ghobrial@ruhealth.org; VS.Nguyen@ruhealth.org

L. J. Soloniuk (✉)
Riverside University Health System, Moreno Valley, CA, USA

Loma Linda University, Loma Linda, CA, USA
e-mail: l.soloniuk@ruhealth.org

A. C. Sinha, I. F. Pasca (eds.), *Peripartum Care of the Pregnant Patient*,
https://doi.org/10.1007/978-3-031-62756-9_14

4. **Which spinal needle is associated with the HIGHEST incidence of post-dural puncture headache?**
   A. Whitacre
   B. Sprotte
   C. Quincke
   D. Gertie Marx
5. **Which of the following factors is most important for determining the spread and duration of subarachnoid anesthesia?**
   A. Density of local anesthetic
   B. Patient height
   C. Weight
   D. Body mass index (BMI)
6. **Which of the following most important determinant of the INITIAL spread of isobaric local anesthetic in spinal anesthesia?**
   A. Cardiac pulsations
   B. Gross patient movements (e.g., turning from lateral to supine)
   C. Bulk displacement
   D. Body mass index (BMI)
7. **A patient undergoing cesarean section receives spinal anesthesia with hyperbaric bupivacaine, morphine, and fentanyl. The procedure was uneventful, but the patient then complained of pruritus. Which medication would be MOST beneficial in treating this patient's symptoms?**
   A. Diphenhydramine
   B. Nalbuphine
   C. Metoclopramide
   D. Naloxone
8. **A pregnant patient receives a combined spinal epidural for labor analgesia using ropivacaine in the spinal solution. Although the patient reports improvement of pain, she shortly complains of chest tightness and dyspnea. The patient also complains of decreased grip strength and is only able to whisper. You are concerned about a total spinal block, and you assemble resuscitative equipment. In addition to supportive treatment, which position should you place the patient in?**
   A. Reverse Trendelenburg
   B. Trendelenburg
   C. Right lateral recumbent
   D. Flex the patient's head at the neck
9. **A postpartum patient wishes to undergo tubal ligation for sterilization, and you decide to perform a spinal anesthetic. Which local anesthetic is the best choice for this case?**
   A. Hyperbaric bupivacaine
   B. Isobaric bupivacaine
   C. Hypobaric bupivacaine
   D. Eubaric bupivacaine

10. **What are the layers that you will pass through for a spinal anesthetic using the PARAMEDIAN approach?**
    A. Skin → Subcutaneous tissue → Supraspinous ligament → Interspinous ligament → Ligamentum flavum → Dura mater
    B. Skin → Subcutaneous tissue → Supraspinous ligament → Interspinous ligament → Posterior ligament → Ligamentum flavum → Dura mater
    C. Skin → Subcutaneous tissue → Supraspinous ligament → Interspinous ligament → Anterior ligament → Ligamentum flavum → Dura mater
    D. Skin → Subcutaneous tissue → Ligamentum flavum → Dura mater
11. **A 38-year-old G1P0 patient presents for a trial of labor. On questioning, the patient reported that she had a history of rheumatic fever and was now on a prosthetic mitral valve on warfarin. Assuming a therapeutic INR, how long must the patient wait between her last dose and placement of neuraxial anesthesia?**
    A. 3 days
    B. 5–7 days
    C. 10 days
    D. No waiting time necessary
12. **A 28-year-old G3P2 patient presented for an elective cesarean section. After an uneventful spinal anesthetic and procedure, the patient reported pain in the low back and buttocks. The patient denies any other symptoms, such as saddle anesthesia, sensory/motor deficits, and no changes in symptoms with posture. What is the next BEST step of management?**
    A. Consult neurosurgery for evaluation for possible emergent laminectomy
    B. Administer nonsteroidal anti-inflammatory drugs (NSAIDs)
    C. Administer opioids
    D. Epidural blood patch
13. **A patient undergoes spinal anesthesia for cesarean section with hyperbaric bupivacaine. Shortly after lying down, she developed weakness in her upper extremity strength, lost consciousness, and was hypotensive. You suspect a total spinal. What is <u>NOT</u> the best course of action in treating this patient?**
    A. Administer vasopressors
    B. Fluid boluses
    C. Trendelenburg positioning
    D. Left uterine displacement
14. **For a patient with local anesthetic systemic toxicity (LAST), which of the following vasopressors would NOT be appropriate?**
    A. Vasopressin
    B. Phenylephrine
    C. Norepinephrine
    D. Epinephrine
15. **If a patient with LAST develops ventricular dysrhythmias, which of the following medications would be beneficial to treating this patient?**
    A. Esmolol
    B. Diltiazem

C. Amiodarone
D. Digoxin

16. **A patient with LAST is not responsive to lipid emulsion therapy and supportive treatment. What is the next best step?**
    A. Cardiopulmonary bypass
    B. Add additional pressors
    C. Fluid and/or colloid boluses
    D. Repeat lipid bolus
17. **A patient presented for tubal ligation and underwent spinal anesthesia. The spinal placement was unexpectedly difficult, and a Quincke needle was used to access the spinal space. Twelve hours after the procedure, the patient reported headache primarily at the frontal sinus, which was worse with standing and better with lying flat. What is the next best step?**
    A. Epidural blood patch
    B. Epinephrine 10 mcg
    C. Bed rest and hydration
    D. Reassurance
18. **A 28-year-old G2P2 patient presented to the emergency department for severe headache, fever, neck stiffness, and altered mental status. Of note, the patient received a spinal anesthetic 2 weeks prior to cesarean section. On workup, the patient was suspected to have meningitis. Which of the following is the MOST likely cause of the meningitis?**
    A. Inadequate preparation with chlorhexidine/iodine
    B. Medication and/or equipment contamination
    C. Maskless clinician during procedure
    D. Skin flora
19. **You are performing a spinal anesthetic for a cesarean section. You obtain cerebrospinal fluid through your spinal needle, but the patient reports a sudden paresthesia radiating down her right leg. What is the next BEST step?**
    A. Inject medication and proceed with the procedure
    B. Stop and assess the presence of CSF in the needle hub
    C. Inject half of the planned dose into the spinal space
    D. Conversion to general anesthesia as continuing with the procedure increases the risk of nerve damage
20. **A 32-year-old G2P1 patient presented for a repeat cesarean section. The patient reports that the only complication from her prior anesthetic is that she recalls is pruritis, which was treated with IV medications. Which dosage of fentanyl is enough to provide adequate analgesia while reducing the risk for intrathecal opioid-induced pruritus?**
    A. 5–10 mcg
    B. 11–15 mcg
    C. 16–20 mcg
    D. 21–25 mcg

Answers and Explanations

1. **A**. Uterine enlargement and vena caval compression cause engorgement of the epidural veins, which would DECREASE the spinal canal space for the thecal sac. Furthermore, the vertebral foraminal veins and epidural veins are also enlarged, which compresses the thecal sac and displaces the CSF into the thoracolumbar region. The CSF specific gravity in pregnant patients is also decreased. As such, pregnant women generally have lower spinal anesthesia requirements than the general population. Three changes cause increased lordosis: (1) the pelvis rotates on the long axis of the spine, (2) there is less space between lumbar spinous processes, and (3) the apex of the lumbar lordosis is shifted inferiorly during pregnancy. Hormonal changes in pregnancy affect ligamentous structures such as the ligamentum flavum, making it softer [1].
2. **A**. T4 to T6 sensory levels must be achieved for cesarean sections due to additional pain pathways involved in the procedure. Usually, a horizontal incision is used, which requires coverage of T11–12, but the stretching and visceral pain involved in the procedure involves four or more levels/dermatomes higher [1].
3. **E**. The American Society of Anesthesiologists (ASA) established guidelines for providing neuraxial anesthesia for obstetric patients. Important points of the guidelines include (1) required the presence of qualified anesthesia and obstetric providers, (2) immediate availability of resuscitation medication and equipment, (3) employment and documentation of maternal vital signs and fetal heart rate monitoring, and (4) mandatory preprocedural intravenous access. One of the serious complications of neuraxial anesthesia is total spinal anesthesia, which results in spinal blockade above T3 that may be associated with life-threatening apnea, hypotension, bradycardia, and paralysis without always decreasing maternal cognition and awareness. Treatment for total spinal generally involves supportive care, including securing the airway with intubation and medications for hemodynamic support. As such, it is recommended to have medications and equipment available such as induction medications (e.g., propofol, succinylcholine), resuscitation medications (e.g., epinephrine, atropine, sodium bicarbonate), airway equipment (e.g., laryngoscope with blades, endotracheal tubes, bag, and mask). Maternal monitoring includes an automatic blood pressure cuff (measured every 1–2 min after test dose and therapeutic doses, otherwise every 15–30 min), and continuous pulse oximeter. Per the ASA task force on obstetric anesthesia, fetal heart patterns should be monitored before and after neuraxial anesthesia. Continuous monitoring may not be possible during neuraxial placement and may not be necessary [1].
4. **C**. The Quincke needle tip has a cutting bevel and is associated with a higher incidence of postdural puncture headaches. The most commonly used spinal needles today are the noncutting "pencil tip" needles, such as the Whitacre, Sprotte, and Gertie Marx needles. A widely accepted standard is to use needles gauge or smaller [1].

5. **A**. The density and dose are the most important factors in determining the spread and length of action of subarachnoid anesthesia. Patient height, weight, BMI, and vertebral column length had no clinically significant effect on the spread of local anesthetic [2].
6. **C**. Bulk displacement determines the initial spread of isobaric local anesthetics. The final spread of the block is influenced next by the gross patient movements and cardiac pulsations [2].
7. **B**. Pruritus is a common side effect of neuraxial opioids. It is more common with intrathecal administration as compared to the epidural route. The mechanism of pruritus is currently unknown; however, it is unlikely to be caused by histamine release. Nalbuphine is an opioid antagonist (2.5–5 mg IV or 10 mg subcutaneous) used to treat pruritus secondary to intrathecal opioids. Nalbuphine is preferred over naloxone because it is less likely to reverse the analgesic effects of the administered opioids. As discussed above, the mechanism of neuraxial opioid pruritus is unlikely to be due to histamine release, but diphenhydramine (an antihistaminergic) could still be used for light sedation [1].
8. **D**. Flexing the patient's head will help prevent further spread of the anesthetic to the cervical region. Although it may be tempting to place the patient in the reverse Trendelenburg position to reduce the height of the block, it will cause blood to pool in the legs and worsen the hypotension. Furthermore, the reverse Trendelenburg position will decrease cerebral blood flow. Placing the patient in the Trendelenburg position would cause worsening of the total spinal, especially with a hyperbaric solution. The right lateral position would worsen aortocaval compression, causing reduced venous return and exacerbation of hypotension [2].
9. **A**. Baricity is defined as the ratio between two densities, and in the context of neuraxial anesthesia, it is used to compare the densities of local anesthetic and CSF. Hyperbaric solutions of local anesthetics are those that are denser than CSF and will "sink" to gravity. In a supine patient, this will cause the local anesthetic to settle in the sacrum and thoracic regions. Hyperbaric bupivacaine results in more predictable spread of anesthesia than other baricities. To make hyperbaric solutions, the local anesthetic is generally mixed with dextrose [2].
10. **D**. The paramedian approach for neuraxial techniques is usually used for patients with difficult placement. Unlike the median approach (choice **A**), the paramedian approach does not pass through the interspinous ligament but instead goes from subcutaneous tissue straight to the ligamentum flavum and ultimately the dura mater. The needle does not pass through the posterior or anterior ligament in any neuraxial technique [2].
11. **B**. A potential complication of neuraxial anesthesia in the setting of anticoagulants is a spinal hematoma. For patients on warfarin, the current recommendation is to hold the medication for 5 days and to have a normal INR. Patients on oral Xa inhibitors such as rivaroxaban and apixaban are to wait 3 days or to have normal anti-Xa levels prior to neuraxial procedures. Clopidogrel requires 5–7 days before neuraxial procedures and ticlopidine requires 10 days. NSAIDs do not need a waiting period [3].

12. **B**. Common symptoms of transient neurologic syndrome (TNS) include pain in the legs and/or buttocks a few hours after anesthesia. First-line treatment is NSAIDs, followed by opioids in refractory cases (**B**). Major risk factors for TNS include intrathecal lidocaine, lithotomy position, and ambulatory anesthesia. If the patient also complained of other neurologic symptoms, such as motor weakness, bowel/bladder dysfunction, or saddle anesthesia, it may be signs of more serious complications, such as cauda equina syndrome or hematoma. In such a case, urgent neurosurgery consultation and intervention would be needed (**A**). An epidural blood patch (**D**) is usually used to treat postdural puncture headache that is refractory to conservative management, such as fluids and NSAIDs. Postdural headaches are also associated with symptoms that change with posture (i.e., worse with standing, better when supine) [3].
13. **C**. The patient developed a total spinal block following a spinal anesthetic with hyperbaric bupivacaine. Considering hyperbaric solutions "'sink" to gravity, placing the patient in the Trendelenburg position is not a reasonable course of action because it would cause worsening of the total spinal condition as the local anesthetic drifts cephalad. Classic symptoms of total spinals include rapid sensory-motor blockade, dyspnea, inability to phonate, loss of consciousness (from lack of brain perfusion), and decreased upper extremity muscle tone (e.g., decreased grip strength). Generally, the first-line treatments are supportive. For hypotension, immediate pressors and fluid boluses are warranted. Left uterine displacement is also important to improve circulation. In many cases, it is important to secure the airway with endotracheal intubation [4].
14. **A**. Vasopressin should be avoided in local anesthetic systemic toxicity. Epinephrine, if needed, should be used in low amounts [4].
15. **C**. Ventricular dysrhythmia secondary to LAST should be treated with amiodarone, especially if bupivacaine was the offending agent to elicit the episode. Calcium channel blockers (e.g., diltiazem) and beta-blockers (e.g., esmolol) should be avoided and they can worsen the cardiac symptoms of LAST [4].
16. **A**. If a patient with suspected LAST does not improve with supportive treatment and/or ACLS, then the next best step would be cardiopulmonary bypass [4].
17. **C**. The patient exhibited symptoms of postdural puncture headache (PPD), which occurred when cerebrospinal fluid leaks through the dura. The choice of equipment influences the rate of PPD. For example, needles 16 gauge and larger have an approximately 70% chance of PPD, whereas smaller needles (e.g., 25 or 26 gauge) have an incidence of less than 1%. The risk for PPD also increases with cutting tip needles such as Quincke needles versus pencil point needles such as the Whitacre or Sprotte needles. The initial treatment for PPD is generally conservative (choice **C**), consisting of bed rest, hydration (IV and/or oral), and simple analgesics such as ibuprofen. Caffeine (500 mg IV or 400 mg orally) could also be used. If the patient continues to have symptoms of PPD for 24 h and fails conservative treatment (choice **A**), an epidural blood patch may be performed. The procedure involves withdrawing 20 cc of the patient's own blood using aseptic technique and injecting it in the epidural space [4].

18. **B**. Although infection from neuraxial procedures is relatively rare, it is a feared complication that clinicians need to be aware of. Meningitis secondary to spinal anesthetics is most frequently caused by contamination of medications and/or equipment from the provider's nasopharyngeal flora. As such, proper PPE is very important when performing neuraxial procedures. Epidural abscesses are commonly caused by contamination of the skin flora. Therefore, proper skin preparation is also important [4].
19. **B**. Transient paresthesiae is common (13.5% occurrence) and usually due to brief spinal nerve root contact during needle insertion. While some authors recommend needle withdrawal and redirection after paresthesias, others recommend first assessing for good CSF flow before dosing [5].
20. **A**. 5–10 mcg of fentanyl is enough to provide analgesic effects while reducing the risk of pruritus. Unlike the histamine release caused by systemic opioids, the mechanism of intrathecal opioid pruritus is thought to be caused by activation of mu opioid signals in superficial/deep dorsal horn neurons and the medulla oblongata. Due to this mechanism, antihistamines such as diphenhydramine are unlikely to be effective. Instead, agents such as nalbuphine (due to its mu receptor agonism-antagonism) or naloxone (mu receptor antagonism) may be used [6].

References

1. Chestnut DH, et al. Ch. 12: Spinal, epidural, and caudal anesthesia: anatomy, physiology and technique. In: Chestnut's obstetric anesthesia: principles and practice. 6th ed. Elsevier; 2019.
2. Barash PG, et al. Ch. 35: Neuraxial anesthesia: anatomy. In: Clinical anesthesia. 8th ed. Wolters Kluwer; 2017.
3. Gropper M, et al. Patient blood management: coagulation. In: Miller's anesthesia. 9th ed. Elsevier; 2019. p. 1598–9. E-book.
4. Barash PG, et al. Ch. 41: Obstetric anesthesia: anesthetic complications. In: Clinical anesthesia. 8th ed. Wolters Kluwer; 2017.
5. Pong RP, Gmelch BS, Bernards CM. Does a paresthesia during spinal needle insertion indicate intrathecal needle placement? Reg Anesth Pain Med. 2009;34(1):29–32. https://doi.org/10.2097/AAP.0b013e3181933eed.
6. Ganesh A, Maxwell LG. Pathophysiology and management of opioid-induced pruritus. Drugs. 2007;67(16):2323–33. https://doi.org/10.2165/00003495-200767160-00003.

Epidural Anesthesia

Sindhuja R. Nimma, Nigel Gillespie, and Asaf Gans

Questions

1. **An urgent cesarean section is scheduled for failure to progress. She has many signs of a difficult airway. There are no concerns about fetal well-being. She had an L3–4 epidural that was placed without difficulty, and the patient was comfortable during her labor course. Upon arrival at the operating room, her epidural was bolused multiple times with local anesthetic, but she did not develop a surgical level. Fetal heart tones were normal. The decision is made to perform a spinal anesthetic to help avoid a general anesthetic. Which of the following is the patient at risk of developing?**
   A. High spinal
   B. Postdural puncture headache
   C. Bezold-Jarisch reflex
   D. All the above
2. **What is the correct order of the structures passed on the way to the lumbar epidural space via the midline approach?**
   A. **Ligamentum flavum**
   B. **Interspinous ligament**
   C. **Supraspinous ligament**
   D. **Skin**
   E. **Subcutaneous fat**
   F. **Arachnoid mater**
   G. **Paraspinous muscle**

S. R. Nimma (✉) · N. Gillespie · A. Gans
Department of Anesthesia and Perioperative Medicine, Mayo Clinic, Jacksonville, FL, USA
e-mail: Nimma.Sindhuja@mayo.edu; gillespie.nigel@mayo.edu

A. C. Sinha, I. F. Pasca (eds.), *Peripartum Care of the Pregnant Patient*,
https://doi.org/10.1007/978-3-031-62756-9_15

A. D, E, C, B, A, F
B. D, E, C, B, A
C. D, E, G, C, B, A
D. D, E, B, C, A

3. **What is a potential disadvantage of combined spinal-epidural (CSE)?**
   A. Ineffective analgesia
   B. Unproven efficacy of the epidural catheter
   C. Decreased success rate of epidural placement
   D. Prolongation of stage 1 of labor
4. **Which of the following patients should have a platelet count checked prior to epidural placement?**
   A. A morbidly obese G1P0 who has been inpatient for a radius and ulna fracture and receiving heparin 5000 U TID for 4 days with her last dose 6 h prior
   B. Type 1 diabetic G2P1 taking ASA 81 mg daily
   C. A G3P2 with BP 160/90 with headache
   D. A G1P0 with platelet count throughout pregnancy between 120 and 130
5. **The patient is a 32-year-old G1P0 parturient female who weighs 95 kg and is otherwise healthy, except for a history of lower extremity deep venous thromboembolism (DVT). She is currently on 40 mg of subcutaneous enoxaparin once a day for DVT prophylaxis. She is scheduled for induction of labor next week and would like an epidural prior to starting oxytocin. Prior to epidural placement, when should she discontinue enoxaparin**?
   A. 40 mg enoxaparin is a prophylactic dose and needs to be discontinued for 12 h prior to epidural placement
   B. 40 mg enoxaparin is a therapeutic dose, so the last dose can be 24 h prior to epidural placement
   C. 40 mg enoxaparin is a therapeutic dose and should be continued as she is at a high risk for DVT
   D. The patient can continue enoxaparin, but she needs an INR and platelet count prior to epidural placement
6. **The patient was a 24-year-old G1P0 parturient female with a BMI of 19 who was discharged from the hospital 2 days after an uncomplicated vaginal delivery under epidural anesthesia. Today, she returns to the emergency room (ER) complaining of a positional headache that is worse in the upright position and better when reclined. What is the most likely diagnosis and treatment?**
   A. Exacerbation of chronic headache, no treatment is indicated
   B. Epidural hematoma requires urgent neurosurgery consultation for possible intervention
   C. Postdural puncture headache, start with conservative management such as hydration, acetaminophen, and caffeine
   D. Postdural puncture headache (PDPH), she needs urgent MRI of the brain and spine and neurosurgery consultation

7. **Pick the order of sensitivity of nerve fibers to local anesthetic in the epidural space from highest sensitivity to lowest sensitivity.**
   A. Sensory C-fibers > sensory A-delta fibers > preganglionic sympathetic fibers > sensory A-beta fibers > motor A-alpha fibers
   B. Preganglionic sympathetic fibers > sensory C-fibers > sensory A-delta fibers > sensory A-beta fibers > motor A-alpha fibers
   C. Motor A-alpha fibers > sensory A-delta fibers > sensory A-beta fibers > preganglionic sympathetic fibers > sensory C-fibers
   D. Sensory C-fibers > sensory A-delta fibers > sensory A-beta fibers > preganglionic sympathetic fibers > motor A-alpha fibers
8. **What are the respiratory effects seen with a high epidural block?**
   A. Vital capacity is increased and expiratory reserve volume is decreased due to loss of intercostal and abdominal muscles
   B. Loss of function of the diaphragm and accessory respiratory muscles
   C. Vital capacity is reduced due to a reduction in expiratory reserve volume related to abdominal muscle paralysis
   D. A high epidural block never affects respiratory effort
9. **A 27-year-old female parturient received an epidural catheter for labor analgesia. After the epidural infusion was started, she was comfortable for several hours and then started to complain of a patchy block on the left side, extensive sensory block with minimal motor block, and hypotension despite adequate resuscitation. What is the likely diagnosis?**
   A. Epidural hematoma
   B. Accidental spinal
   C. Subdural block
   D. Air in the epidural space
10. **Which of the following statements is true about epidural catheter placement in the obese parturient?**
    A. Ultrasound-guided placement is the standard of care in patients with BMI>40
    B. Dural puncture using a spinal needle through the Tuohy needle prior to epidural catheter insertion increases the efficacy of labor analgesia
    C. Obese patients have a higher rate of epidural catheter failure than patients without obesity
    D. CT scan of the lumbar spine should be performed prior to any neuraxial attempt in these patients
11. **The dermatomal spread of an epidural is most likely associated with what?**
    A. Volume
    B. Local anesthetic baricity
    C. Speed of injection
    D. Needle direction
12. **A 26-year-old female presented with induction of labor at 40 weeks and 2 days. Her pregnancy has been uncomplicated. She had a history of intermittent asthma and relapsing remitting multiple sclerosis (MS). Her initial**

presentation of MS was at age 21 with monocular vision loss. Her most recent flare was 1 year ago and was characterized by paresthesias in her lower extremities. Which of the following statements is true if counseling her about labor analgesia options?

A. Neuraxial anesthesia is contraindicated
B. Combined spinal-epidural anesthesia is the preferred method of labor analgesia
C. Magnetic resonance imaging of her spine prior to the neuraxial procedure is necessary
D. Local anesthetic in the epidural or intrathecal space could potentially precipitate symptoms

13. **You are observing a colleague perform a lumbar epidural on a healthy patient scheduled for induction of labor at the L4/L5 interspace. After careful advancement of the Tuohy needle and loss of resistance to saline, there is rapid and continuous return of clear fluid when the syringe is disconnected from the needle. Your colleague immediately removes the Tuohy needle. The patient is in a seated position, tolerating the procedure well, and the fetal monitors continue to have a reassuring tracing. This was your colleagues' first attempt, and the trajectory to the epidural space was straightforward. What is the next best step?**

   A. Abort the procedure
   B. Perform a single-injection spinal block at the L4/L5 interspace
   C. Lay the patient flat for 2 h before reattempting
   D. Attempt epidural placement at the L2/L3 interspace

14. **You are evaluating a 29-year-old nonbinary patient who is postpartum day 1 after cesarean delivery under epidural anesthesia. They complained of a severe headache that started at the time of their epidural placement. Their first epidural placement was characterized by patchy sensory blockade, minimal motor blockade, and pronounced hypotension. Their second epidural functioned appropriately. There were no other complications noted. The patient does not notice any change in the quality of headache with changes in position. They had no history of chronic headaches. Which of the following would suggest their symptoms are related to neuraxial procedure?**

   A. Epidural insertion using loss of resistance to air technique
   B. Enlarged third ventricle without any other findings on computed tomography (CT) venogram
   C. Papilledema on magnetic resonance cerebral venography (MRV) without any other findings
   D. Epidural insertion using loss of resistance to saline

15. **A postpartum patient complained of difficulty ambulating 2 days after spontaneous vaginal delivery with epidural analgesia. Her epidural placement required four attempts, and there were no complications or paresthesias noted during placement. Her labor was complicated by prolonged first and second stages of labor requiring use of a vacuum assistive device and**

reduction of a shoulder dystocia. Her BMI is 43. Her vitals are HR-87 BP-124/82 RR-10 SpO_2 97% on room air. She reported mild perineal soreness and uterine cramping that were well controlled with NSAIDs. On exam, she had some numbness in the anteromedial thigh and weakness in leg extension on the left. Her right lower extremity had no sensory or motor deficits. Which of the following most likely contributed to these findings?

A. Prolonged first stage of labor
B. Prolonged second stage of labor
C. Use of vacuum assistive device
D. Multiple epidural attempts

Answers and Explanations

1. **D**. The situation described occurs when a previously placed epidural is insufficient for surgical anesthesia. The benefits of regional anesthesia over general anesthesia are well-documented and include avoidance of airway manipulation, experience of childbirth, decreased blood loss, reduced maternal mortality, improved postoperative pain control, and the ability to use fewer intraoperative drugs [1]. Risks of utilizing regional anesthesia include hypotension, postdural puncture headache, local anesthetic systemic toxicity, need to convert epidural anesthesia to general anesthesia, and intraoperative discomfort [2]. The risk of postdural puncture headache after a single-shot uncomplicated spinal is 3–9% [3], and headache after an unintended dural puncture with an epidural Touhy needle between 81% and 88% [4]. As with all spinal anesthetics, there is a risk of hypotension with bradycardia, which is known as the Bezold-Jarisch reflex. This is a parasympathetically mediated reflex where the stretch receptors in the left ventricle respond to a decrease in preload, resulting in bradycardia and decreased contractility, which has been postulated to be a protective reflex to allow for increased left ventricular filling [5]. The Bezold-Jarisch reflex occurs due to the sympathectomy associated with cardiac acceleratory fibers that occur at T1–T4 [6]. It has been reported that a high or total spinal can occur when a spinal is performed on a patient with a preexisting epidural. One explanation can be that the injection of the fluid epidurally increases the pressure in the epidural space and thus the cerebral spinal fluid; therefore, spinal medication may be displaced cranially leading to a high block [7].
2. **B**. The correct order for the midline approach to the lumbar epidural space is skin → subcutaneous tissue → supraspinous ligament → interspinous ligament → ligamentum flavum [8]. The arachnoid mater is deep into the epidural space and passing through the arachnoid mater signifies passing into the intrathecal space. Via the midline approach, the epidural needle does not pass through the paraspinous muscle. The option showing the order skin → subcutaneous fat → paraspinous muscle → ligamentum flavum shows the route of the epidural needle via the paramedian approach [8].

3. **B**. Combined spinal-epidural is a neuraxial technique that incorporates the benefits of both a spinal and an epidural. It has a quick onset because of the spinal portion of the procedure and extended analgesia because of the ability to leave an epidural catheter in place. Combined spinal-epidurals produce very effective analgesia and have been shown to have improved sacral spread when compared to epidural anesthesia alone [9]. One potential explanation for this is the movement of local anesthetic from the epidural space into the cerebral spinal fluid via the dural puncture site [10]. It has been proposed that the combined spinal-epidural technique has a higher rate of success because the confirmation of return of cerebral spinal fluid through the spinal needle helps ensure that the Touhy needle is in the correct (epidural) space. The return of CSF helps ensure that the loss of resistance felt was a true loss of resistance and not a false loss [11]. While the success rate of placement of the epidural portion of the procedure was higher compared to the epidural technique alone, the functionality of the epidural has not been tested, as the initial analgesia is from the intrathecal medication. The only true way to prove that the epidural catheter is functioning appropriately is to reevaluate the patient after the spinal medication has worn off. Neuraxial anesthesia does not prolong the duration of stage 1 of labor but does prolong stage 2 of labor by approximately 15 min [12, 13].
4. **C**. This question alludes to the broader topic of coagulation status and neuraxial catheter placement and the risk of epidural hematoma. (**A**) Has two components that must be discussed. Prophylactic heparin dosing should be held between 4 and 6 h prior to neuraxial catheter placement. The other aspect of this answer that should be discussed is whether she is at risk for developing heparin-induced thrombocytopenia (HIT). The risk factors for HIT include heparin administration for >5 days, hemodialysis, autoimmune disease, gout, and heart failure [14]. The patient in (**A**) has only been receiving heparin for 4 days and therefore has a lower risk of developing HIT. Therefore, the patient in (**A**) does not need to have a platelet count checked prior to neuraxial catheter placement. According to the American Society of Regional Anesthesia, there are no restrictions on placement of a neuraxial catheter on an individual who is currently taking aspirin. In the absence of other risk factors, such as the patient in (**D**), a platelet count of 80–90 is considered safe for placing a lumbar epidural [15]. However, the risks and benefits of the procedure in the context of the potential for an epidural hematoma should be discussed with the patient [16]. In this patient with a stable mild thrombocytopenia of 120–130, a platelet count does not need to occur. (**C**) Has vital signs and symptoms that are concerning for preeclampsia with severe features. Features that take a patient from preeclampsia to preeclampsia with severe features include systolic blood pressure >160 or diastolic blood pressure >110, hepatic dysfunction or right upper quadrant pain, new onset headache or visual disturbance, platelet count <100, or pulmonary edema [17]. It is imperative to rule out a dropping platelet count (which can occur with preeclampsia) prior to placement of an epidural catheter due to the risk of epidural hematoma and resultant neurologic injury [18].

5. **A**. The prophylactic dose of enoxaparin (low-molecular-weight heparin/lovenox) is <0.5 mg/kg dosed every 24 h (QD). Therapeutic enoxaparin is either dosed every 12 h (BID) or each injection dose is >0.5 mg/kg. According to ASRA guidelines on anticoagulation and neuraxial blocks, a prophylactic dose of enoxaparin should be discontinued for 12 h prior to placement of an epidural catheter or spinal block placement or epidural catheter removal. Once the epidural is removed, you must wait 12 h to reinitiate therapy. If a patient is on a therapeutic dose of enoxaparin, it should be discontinued 24 h (**B**) prior to placement of a neuraxial block (spinal, epidural, paravertebral, etc.). If enoxaparin has been used for >4 days, the risk of heparin-induced thrombocytopenia (HIT) is higher, so the patient will need a platelet count prior to epidural catheter insertion. It is important to note that pregnancy itself leads to a hypercoagulable state, and often patients at high risk of thromboembolic events (such as a previous history of DVT) may be started on unfractionated heparin or low-molecular-weight heparin (enoxaparin), so knowing when to stop these medications prior to a neuraxial intervention is important. Coagulopathy is a relative contraindication to epidural placement in all patients (**C**). Anticoagulants can increase the risk of epidural hematoma, with the highest risk at the time of insertion and removal and should be held according to the ASRA guidelines. Choice (**D**) is incorrect because she should not continue her anticoagulant due to the risk of bleeding and hematoma with epidural catheter placement [19–21].
6. **C**. The scenario describes a postdural puncture headache and treatment starts with conservative management such as hydration, acetaminophen, and caffeine. Headaches after accidental dural puncture are a common complication after an epidural. PDPH has the highest occurrence in young, thin females. Women who deliver by cesarean delivery have a lower incidence of headache after dural puncture than those who deliver vaginally. The ultimate treatment for PDPH is an epidural blood patch (EBP); however, symptoms are initially managed with IV fluids, caffeine, lying in a supine position, and a multimodal pain regimen. If unresolving or if the headaches severely debilitate the ability of the mother to care for her infant, an EBP can be offered. An EBP involved injection of up to 20 mL of autologous blood into the epidural space either at the same spine level as the initial dural puncture or a few levels below. Autologous blood is withdrawn in a sterile fashion and injected into the epidural space until the patient feels fullness and pressure in her back or the headache is resolved. Typically, the recommended volume of blood in the EBP is 20 mL. Other causes of postpartum headache include stress, preeclampsia, caffeine withdrawal, pain, chronic migraine, and breastfeeding. It is important to differentiate between PDPH and other causes because treatment is vastly different. An EBP is the last resort for treatment because it can lead to rare but devastating complications. Without treatment, PDPH typically resolved in 2 weeks. The smaller the needle gauge, the lower the chance for a PDPH after accidental dural puncture [22–24].

7. **B**. Preganglionic sympathetic fibers > sensory C-fibers > sensory A-delta fibers > sensory A-beta fibers > motor A-alpha fibers. Local anesthetic in the epidural space disrupts nerve transmission, and sites of neural blockage include the spinal cord, spinal nerve roots, and epidural spaces. The sensitivity of nerve fibers to local anesthesia is affected by size and myelination. The most sensitive fibers, and therefore the first to be affected by local anesthetics, are preganglionic sympathetic fibers. Sensory C-fibers have moderate sensitivity and affect temperature and sensation followed by the sensory A-fibers. Next sensitive are the A-delta fibers, responsible for pinprick sensation, and A-beta fibers, responsible for touch sensation. The most resistant and therefore least sensitive to local anesthetics are the large, heavily myelinated motor A-alpha fibers. When performing an epidural procedure, there is also a differential block based on this sensitivity [25]. The highest level will be a sympathetic block (anesthesia to cold sensation). Anesthesia to pinprick sensation will be two dermatome levels lower, and anesthesia to touch sensation will be 1–2 dermatomes lower than pinprick. Therefore, if you have anesthesia to cold sensation at T4, anesthesia to pinprick will be at T6. It is important to note how you test an epidural, especially prior to an urgent or emergent delivery [25–27].
8. **C**. Vital capacity is reduced due to a reduction in expiratory reserve volume related to abdominal muscle paralysis. Respiratory changes due to a higher-than-expected epidural spread of local anesthetic are usually of little consequence. Due to abdominal muscle paralysis, you can expect a decrease in expiratory reserve volume leading to a decreased vital capacity. Generally, blockage of the intercostal and abdominal muscles does not adversely affect respiratory effort; however, in patients with baseline respiratory disease, this could be problematic. A high spinal, however, can lead to respiratory arrest due to hypoperfusion of the respiratory center in the brainstem. The diaphragm is innervated by C3/C4/C5, so unless the local spreads to the cervical levels, the diaphragm is unaffected. Rather, the feeling of shortness of breath is experienced due to blockade of the abdominal and other accessory respiratory muscles [28–31].
9. **C**. Accidental subdural injection during epidural catheter placement can occur and can lead to several adverse effects. The subdural space is located between the dural and arachnoid spaces. Typically, either the epidural needle traumatically punctures the subdural space, or the needle tip is in the epidural space, but the epidural catheter is either threaded into or migrates to the subdural space. The incidence of a subdural block is less than 1%. Symptoms of a subdural block are initially difficult to recognize due to delayed and gradual onset of symptoms [32, 33]. Typically, patients present with an extensive sensory block and can sometimes have patchy deficits and minimal motor blockade. The motor blockage is minimal due to the subdural space being larger posteriorly, minimizing anterior spread to block the motor fibers. Greater hypotension is also seen than expected with an epidural block [32–34]. It is important to note that if the local anesthetic in the subdural space tracks cephalad, it can cause slow-onset dyspnea and even loss of consciousness.

10. **C**. Real-time ultrasound-guided neuraxial techniques are not the standard of care. Some practitioners use ultrasound to find and mark interspinous spaces before proceeding with the landmark technique to help facilitate the initial needle trajectory [35]. The dural puncture technique has shown mixed results in the literature. Procedurally, it confirms Tuohy placement in the epidural space at the time of puncture. Data are conflicting about whether this approach improves the quality or decreases the rate of block failure in patients [36, 37]. Obese patients have a higher rate of catheter failure than nonobese patients associated with more challenging placement, increased distance to the epidural space, and more subcutaneous tissue allowing for increased catheter movement after placement [38]. Obesity alone is not an indication for obtaining spine imaging in the parturient. Exposing a fetus to ionizing radiation from a CT scan without emergent indications is not appropriate [38].
11. **A**. There are numerous factors to consider when attempting to achieve an adequate dermatomal level for either surgical anesthesia or postoperative analgesia. The most important factors in determining dermatomal spread are the volume of local anesthetic administered and the location of epidural placement. It has been shown that 1–2 mL of local anesthetic in the epidural space at the lumbar area can expand dermatomal coverage by approximately 1 dermatomal level [39]. The goal of initial epidural placement, in addition to successful placement, is placing the epidural close to the anticipated incision or location of analgesia needed. In this way, a lower volume and amount of drug is needed to achieve successful analgesia. It has been shown that as patients age, less local anesthetic is needed to achieve the same level of blockade, likely secondary to the size and compliance of the epidural space [39, 40]. Height also plays a role in the height of the expected epidural spread, with shorter individuals requiring less volume. Last, patient positioning also plays an integral part in the epidural spread of local anesthetics [39, 40]. This effect is less substantial than that seen in spinal anesthetics, but there will be a higher density of blockade in the dependent site (i.e., left lateral decubitus will have higher density on the left side, and a sitting patient will have a higher density block in the lower lumbar/sacral levels. The speed of injection seems to have a very small effect on the distribution of sensory blockade, but the main contribution is the volume of local anesthetic [41]. Spinal administration of local anesthetic results in spread based on the baricity of the anesthetic solution, patient positioning, drug dosage, site of injection, age, needle direction, and pregnancy status [42].
12. **D**. Multiple sclerosis (MS) is an autoimmune disease that affects the central nervous system, causing demyelination and plaque-like or sclerotic lesions. Patients have varying degrees of neurologic deficits based on lesion location and severity. The disease course and prognosis vary from person to person [43]. Neuraxial anesthesia is not contraindicated in these patients. Prospective and retrospective studies have not demonstrated an increased incidence of MS flares or changes in disease progression in parturients after receiving epidural anesthesia [44, 45]. Early case report literature described worsening symptoms after spinal anesthesia, but more recent small-sized retrospective studies have

demonstrated no worsening of symptoms or disease progression. Some expert opinions suggest that because local anesthetics are already neurotoxic, it is best to avoid spinal anesthesia and pursue epidural deposition of the medication, which decreases the concentration present in spinal cord white matter [46]. Imaging is not required prior to neuraxial procedures in these patients.

13. **D**. Unintentional dural puncture (UDP) is a known complication of epidural insertion, and it is not necessary to abort the procedure after UDP following a single attempt. There are multiple management strategies present in the literature after UDP that include intrathecal catheter placement, insertion of the epidural catheter after slow withdrawal of the Tuohy needle until cerebrospinal fluid stops flowing, and removal of the needle and replacement of the epidural catheter [47, 48]. There are no studies comparing subsequent epidural catheter placement above, below, or at the same level where UDP occurred for any outcome. There are studies that suggest continuous epidural infusion for 24 h after UDP decreases the rate of dural puncture headache, and one study intentionally replaced the epidural one vertebral interspace above the level of UDP [49, 50]. A single-injection spinal block is not appropriate analgesia for this scenario as the patient is not in labor or near the second stage of labor. Laying the patient flat before replacing the epidural does not offer any patient benefit.
14. **A**. Headache related to neuraxial procedures is generally related to dural puncture, pneumocephalus, or very rarely meningitis and dural venous thrombosis [51, 52]. Epidural insertion using loss of resistance to air can introduce air into the CNS and cranial vault if the needle is subdural or subarachnoid at the time of placement, causing pneumocephalus. Pneumocephalus typically has an acute onset of headache very shortly after or even during the procedure. Other symptoms can include decreased level of consciousness, focal neurologic deficit, seizures, and respiratory arrest with severity dependent on the amount and location of air and change in intracranial pressure [53, 54]. The patient's first epidural is descriptive of subdural catheter placement. An enlarged third ventricle and papilledema are nonspecific findings in hydrocephalus. Both imaging modalities are appropriate for the detection of dural venous thrombosis. Loss of resistance to saline technique is protective against pneumocephalus.
15. **B**. The first stage of labor has a latent phase (cervical dilation from 0 to 5 cm) and an active phase (6 to 10 cm dilation). Obese patients have a risk of prolonged first stage of labor, but this does not carry risk of postpartum neurapraxia [37]. The second stage of labor consists of full dilation to delivery of the neonate. Obesity does not increase the risk of a prolonged second stage of labor but does increase the risk of fetal macrosomia, which can contribute to shoulder dystocia and complicate delivery [37, 38]. Prolonged time in hip flexion during neonatal delivery or extreme hip flexion maneuvers to facilitate reduction of shoulder dystocia can cause compression of the femoral nerve by the inguinal ligament, leading to neurapraxia. The use of external assistive devices to facilitate delivery of the neonatal head does not increase the risk of neurapraxia, but intravaginal devices such as forceps can potentially compress or injure the lumbar plexus [55]. Multiple epidural attempts can increase the risk of hematoma

formation in patients at risk of bleeding. Bilateral neurologic deficits with saddle anesthesia and incontinence would be findings more consistent with this pathology. Epidural hematoma requires emergent imaging and surgical intervention [55]. This patient appears to have left femoral nerve neurapraxia from inguinal ligament compression due to prolonged or extreme hip flexion during the second stage of labor. These injuries are self-limited, with improvement and resolution seen in most patients on the order of weeks to months after presentation. Other peripheral nerves at risk are the lateral femoral cutaneous nerve and common peroneal nerves. It is rare but possible for bilateral peripheral nerve neurapraxias to be present in a patient.

References

1. Spielman FJ, Corke BC. Advantages and disadvantages of regional anesthesia for cesarean section. A review. J Reprod Med. 1985;30(11):832–40.
2. Rollins M, Lucero J. Overview of anesthetic considerations for cesarean delivery. Br Med Bull. 2012;101(1):105–25. https://doi.org/10.1093/bmb/ldr050.
3. DelPizzo K, Cheng J, Dong N, Edmonds CR, Kahn RL, Fields KG, Curren J, Rotundo V, Zayas VM. Post-dural puncture headache is uncommon in young ambulatory surgery patients. HSS J. 2017;13(2):146–51. https://doi.org/10.1007/s11420-017-9541-0. Epub 2017 Mar 16.
4. Sprigge JS, Harper SJ. Accidental dural puncture and post dural puncture headache in obstetric anaesthesia: presentation and management: a 23-year survey in a district general hospital. Anaesthesia. 2008;63(1):36–43. https://doi.org/10.1111/j.1365-2044.2007.05285.x.
5. Warltier DC, Campagna JA, Carter C. Clinical relevance of the Bezold–Jarisch reflex. Anesthesiology. 2003;98:1250–60. https://doi.org/10.1097/00000542-200305000-00030.
6. Huang WA, Boyle NG, Vaseghi M. Cardiac innervation and the autonomic nervous system in sudden cardiac death. Card Electrophysiol Clin. 2017;9(4):665–79. https://doi.org/10.1016/j.ccep.2017.08.002.
7. Gupta A. Spinal anesthesia after failed epidural anesthesia. Anesth Analg. 1996;82(1):214.
8. Teng W-N, Tsou M-Y, Chang W-K, Ting C-K. Eyes on the needle: identification and confirmation of the epidural space. Asian J Anesthesiol. 2017;55(2):30–4.
9. Wong C, Scavone B, Peaceman A, et al. The risk of cesarean delivery with neuraxial analgesia given early versus late in labor. N Engl J Med. 2005;352:655–65.
10. Suzuki N, Koganemaru M, Onizuka S, et al. Dural puncture with a 26G spinal needle affects spread of epidural anesthesia. Anesth Analg. 1996;82:1040–4.
11. Norris MC. Are combined spinal-epidural catheters reliable? Intl J Obstet Anesth. 2000;9:3–6.
12. Zhang J, Yancey MK, Klebanoff MA, Schwarz J, Schweitzer D. Does epidural analgesia prolong labor and increase risk of cesarean delivery? A natural experiment. Am J Obstet Gynecol. 2001;185(1):128–34. https://doi.org/10.1067/mob.2001.113874.
13. Grant EN, Tao W, Craig M, McIntire D, Leveno K. Neuraxial analgesia effects on labour progression: facts, fallacies, uncertainties and the future. BJOG. 2015;122(3):288–93. https://doi.org/10.1111/1471-0528.12966. Epub 2014 Aug 4.
14. Kato S, Takahashi K, Ayabe K, Samad R, Fukaya E, Friedmann P, Varma M, Bergmann SR. Heparin-induced thrombocytopenia: analysis of risk factors in medical inpatients. Br J Haematol. 2011;154(3):373–7. https://doi.org/10.1111/j.13652141.2011.08746.x. Epub 2011 May 26.
15. Regional anesthesia in the patient receiving antithrombotic or thrombolytic therapy. Reg Anesth Pain Med. 2018;43(5):566.

16. Van Veen JJ, Nokes TJ, Makris M. The risk of spinal haematoma following neuraxial anaesthesia or lumbar puncture in thrombocytopenic individuals. Br J Haematol. 2010;148(1):15–25. https://doi.org/10.1111/j.1365-2141.2009.07899.x. Epub 2009 Sep 22.
17. Leeman L, Dresang LT, Fontaine P. Hypertensive disorders of pregnancy. Am Fam Physician. 2016;93(2):121–7.
18. Ankichetty SP, Chin KJ, Chan VW, Sahajanandan R, Tan H, Grewal A, Perlas A. Regional anesthesia in patients with pregnancy induced hypertension. J Anaesthesiol Clin Pharmacol. 2013;29(4):435–44. https://doi.org/10.4103/0970-9185.119108.
19. Horlocker TT, Wedel DJ, Rowlingson JC, et al. Regional anesthesia in the patient receiving antithrombotic or thrombolytic therapy: American Society of Regional Anesthesia and Pain Medicine evidence-based guidelines (third edition). Reg Anesth Pain Med. 2010;35:64–101.
20. Vandermeulen EP, Van Aken H, Vermylen J. Anticoagulants and spinal-epidural anesthesia. Anesth Analg. 1994;79:1165–77.
21. Jacobson B, Rambiritch V, Paek D, Sayre T, Naidoo P, Shan J, Leisegang R. Safety and efficacy of enoxaparin in pregnancy: a systematic review and meta-analysis. Adv Ther. 2020;37(1):27–40. https://doi.org/10.1007/s12325-019-01124-z. Epub 2019 Oct 31.
22. Apfel CC, Saxena A, Cakmakkaya OS, et al. Prevention of postdural puncture headache after accidental dural puncture: a quantitative systematic review. Br J Anaesth. 2010;105:255–63.
23. Oedit R, van Kooten F, Bakker SL, et al. Efficacy of the epidural blood patch for the treatment of post lumbar puncture headache BLOPP: a randomised, observer-blind, controlled clinical trial. BMC Neurol. 2005;5:12.
24. Gaiser RR. Postdural puncture headache: an evidence-based approach. Anesthesiol Clin. 2017;35(1):157–67. https://doi.org/10.1016/j.anclin.2016.09.013.
25. de Jong RH. Differential nerve block by local anesthetics. Anesthesiology. 1980;53(6):443–4. https://doi.org/10.1097/00000542-198012000-00003.
26. Yanagidate F, Strichartz GR. Local anesthetics. Handb Exp Pharmacol. 2007;177:95–127. https://doi.org/10.1007/978-3-540-33823-9_4.
27. Berde C, Strichartz G. Chapter 30: Local anesthetics. In: Miller's anesthesia. 7th ed. Churchill Livingstone; 2009. p. 913–41.
28. O'Toole SM, Kramer J. Unilateral diaphragmatic paralysis [updated 2023 Jan 26]. In: StatPearls. Treasure Island, FL: StatPearls Publishing; 2023. Available from: https://www.ncbi.nlm.nih.gov/books/NBK557388/.
29. Bonica JJ. Maternal respiratory changes during pregnancy and parturition. Clin Anesth. 1974;10(2):1–19.
30. Sundberg A, Wattwil M, Arvill A. Respiratory effects of high thoracic epidural anaesthesia. Acta Anaesthesiol Scand. 1986;30(3):215–7. https://doi.org/10.1111/j.1399-6576.1986.tb02399.x.
31. Yun E, Topulos GP, Body SC, Datta S, Bader AM. Pulmonary function changes during epidural anesthesia for cesarean delivery. Anesth Analg. 1996;82(4):750–3. https://doi.org/10.1097/00000539-199604000-00013.
32. Collier CB. Accidental subdural injection during attempted lumbar epidural block may present as a failed or inadequate block: radiographic evidence. Reg Anesth Pain Med. 2004;29(1):45–51.
33. Alshoubi A, Newhide D. Inadvertent subdural catheter placement: a rare complication in obstetric anesthesia. Cureus. 2022;14(7):e27252. https://doi.org/10.7759/cureus.27252.
34. Agarwal D, Mohta M, Tyagi A, Sethi AK. Subdural block and the anaesthetist. Anaesth Intensive Care. 2010;38(1):20–6. https://doi.org/10.1177/0310057X1003800105.
35. Zhou Y, Chen W, Zhou S, et al. Comparison of different approaches to combined spinal epidural anesthesia (CSEA) under the guidance of ultrasound in cesarean delivery of obese patients: a randomized controlled trial. Eur J Med Res. 2021;26:106. https://doi.org/10.1186/s40001-021-00577-9.
36. Tan HS, Reed SE, Mehdiratta JE, Diomede OI, Landreth R, Gatta LA, Weikel D, Habib AS. Quality of labor analgesia with dural puncture epidural versus standard epidural technique in obese parturients: a double-blind randomized controlled study. Anesthesiology. 2022;136(5):678–87. https://doi.org/10.1097/ALN.0000000000004137.

37. Yurashevich M, Taylor CR, Dominguez JE, Habib AS. Anesthesia and analgesia for the obese parturient. Adv Anesth. 2022;40(1):185–200. https://doi.org/10.1016/j.aan.2022.07.004.
38. Hansen W, Moshiri M, Paladin A, Lamba R, Katz DS, Bhargava P. Evolving practice patterns in imaging pregnant patients with acute abdominal and pelvic conditions. Curr Probl Diagn Radiol. 2017;46(1):10–6. https://doi.org/10.1067/j.cpradiol.2016.06.002. Epub 2016 Jun 22.
39. Brown DL. Spinal, epidural, and caudal anesthesia. In: Miller RD, editor. Miller's anesthesia. 6th ed. Philadelphia: Elsevier Churchill Livingstone; 2005.
40. Burn JM, Guyer PB, Langdon L. The spread of solutions injected into the epidural space. A study using epidurograms in patients with the lumbosciatic syndrome. Br J Anaesth. 1973;45(4):338–45. https://doi.org/10.1093/bja/45.4.338.
41. Visser WA, Lee RA, Gielen MJ. Factors affecting the distribution of neural blockade by local anesthetics in epidural anesthesia and a comparison of lumbar versus thoracic epidural anesthesia. Anesth Analg. 2008;107(2):708–21. https://doi.org/10.1213/ane.0b013e31817e7065.
42. Sakura S. [Factors influencing the level of spinal anesthesia: (II). Patient characteristics and technique of injection]. Masui. 2000;49(2):150–8. Japanese.
43. Dighriri IM, Aldalbahi AA, Albeladi F, Tahiri AA, Kinani EM, Almohsen RA, Alamoudi NH, Alanazi AA, Alkhamshi SJ, Althomali NA, Alrubaiei SN, Altowairqi FK. An overview of the history, pathophysiology, and pharmacological interventions of multiple sclerosis. Cureus. 2023;15(1):e33242. https://doi.org/10.7759/cureus.33242.
44. Confavreux C, Hutchinson M, Hours MM, Cortinovis-Tourniaire P, Moreau T. Rate of pregnancy-related relapse in multiple sclerosis. Pregnancy in Multiple Sclerosis Group. N Engl J Med. 1998;339:285–91.
45. Harazim H, Štourač P, Janků P, Zelinková H, Frank K, Dufek M, Štourač P. Obstetric anesthesia/analgesia does not affect disease course in multiple sclerosis: 10-year retrospective cohort study. Brain Behav. 2018;8(9):e01082. https://doi.org/10.1002/brb3.1082. Epub 2018 Jul 25.
46. Kopp SL, Jacob AK, Hebl JR. Regional anesthesia in patients with preexisting neurologic disease. Reg Anesth Pain Med. 2015;40:467–78.
47. Antunes MV, Moreira A, Sampaio C, Faria A. Punção Acidental da Dura e Cefaleia Pós-punção da Dura na População Obstétrica: Oito Anos de Experiência [Accidental dural puncture and post-dural puncture headache in the obstetric population: eight years of experience]. Acta Med Port. 2016;29(4):268–74. https://doi.org/10.20344/amp.6815. Portuguese. Epub 2016 Apr 29.
48. Van de Velde M, Schepers R, Berends N, Vandermeersch E, De Buck F. Ten years of experience with accidental dural puncture and post-dural puncture headache in a tertiary obstetric anaesthesia department. Int J Obstet Anesth. 2008;17(4):329–35. https://doi.org/10.1016/j.ijoa.2007.04.009. Epub 2008 Aug 8.
49. Cesur M, Alici HA, Erdem AF, Silbir F, Celik M. Decreased incidence of headache after unintentional dural puncture in patients with cesarean delivery administered with postoperative epidural analgesia. J Anesth. 2009;23(1):31–5. https://doi.org/10.1007/s00540-008-0690-7. Epub 2009 Feb 22.
50. Somaya E, Ghada G. Sequential higher epidural catheter re-insertion after accidental dural puncture ameliorates the frequency and severity of post-dural puncture headache. Egypt J Anaesth. 2010;26(4):261–5. ISSN: 1110-1849. https://doi.org/10.1016/j.egja.2010.04.001.
51. Zhou Y, Geng Z, Song L, Wang D. Epidural hydroxyethyl starch ameliorating postdural puncture headache after accidental dural puncture. Chin Med J. 2023;136:88. https://doi.org/10.1097/CM9.0000000000001967. Epub ahead of print.
52. Halliday L, Nelson SM, Kearns RJ. Epidural analgesia in labor: a narrative review. Int J Gynaecol Obstet. 2022;159(2):356–64. https://doi.org/10.1002/ijgo.14175. Epub 2022 Mar 21
53. Pires AF, Mendes TM, Reis AA, Pacheco AF, Fagundes V, Mesquita M. Symptomatic pneumocephalus as a complication of lumbar epidural anaesthesia. Eur J Case Rep Intern Med. 2020;7(2):001425. https://doi.org/10.12890/2020_001425.
54. Jayakumaran JS, Thomas U, Schuster M. Diagnosis airhead: a case of pneumocephalus in labor. Am J Obstet Gynecol. 2019;221(4):361. https://doi.org/10.1016/j.ajog.2019.02.057. Epub 2019 Mar 5.
55. Boyce H, Plaat F. Post-natal neurological problems. Contin Educ Anaesth Crit Care Pain. 2013;13(2):63–6. https://doi.org/10.1093/bjaceaccp/mks057.

Combined Spinal Epidural and Dural Puncture Epidural

Avoumia Marcus and Leonard J. Soloniuk

Questions

1. **Compared to the use of CEA for labor analgesia, a DPE epidural using a 25-gauge needle is associated with which of the following?**
   A. An increase in the fentanyl dose needed for satisfactory analgesia
   B. Preservation of sacral nerve root function
   C. More rapid onset of analgesia
   D. An increase in epidural catheter replacement rates
2. **Compared to CEA, the use of the CSE technique is more likely to be associated with:**
   A. Maternal hypotension
   B. Cesarean delivery
   C. Adverse maternal outcomes
   D. Adverse fetal outcomes
3. **Which epidural technique is associated with the highest risk for fetal bradycardia?**
   A. CEA
   B. DPE
   C. CSE
   D. The risks are equivalent between the techniques.

A. Marcus
A.T. Still University School of Osteopathic Medicine, Mesa, AZ, USA

L. J. Soloniuk (✉)
Riverside University Health System, Moreno Valley, CA, USA

Loma Linda University, Loma Linda, CA, USA
e-mail: l.soloniuk@ruhealth.org

A. C. Sinha, I. F. Pasca (eds.), *Peripartum Care of the Pregnant Patient*,
https://doi.org/10.1007/978-3-031-62756-9_16

4. **For the initiation of labor analgesia, a DPE technique requires what percent of the local anesthetic that is needed for a CEA technique?**
   A. 30%
   B. 65%
   C. 100%
   D. 125%
5. **When performing a CSE, which spinal levels should be targeted for epidural catheter placement?**
   A. Caudad to T10
   B. Caudad to T12
   C. Caudad to L1
   D. Caudad to L2
6. **Which of the following statements are true regarding the technique used for DPE placement?**
   A. A pencil-point spinal needle is less uncomfortable than a cutting-point spinal needle.
   B. There is less discomfort using saline for loss-of-resistance identification of the epidural space than using air.
   C. Use of a 25-gauge spinal needle rather than a 27-gauge spinal needle results in a higher block.
   D. Use of a pencil-point spinal needle smaller than 25-gauge will reduce the incidence of post-dural puncture headache compared to a 25-gauge pencil point needle.
7. **Compared to CEA, when using PIEB (programmed intermittent bolus) drug delivery in patients with DPE, the bolus volume needed for satisfactory analgesia is shown to require:**
   A. Less bolus volume is needed with DPE
   B. Equal bolus volume with DPE
   C. Greater bolus volume is needed with DPE
8. **With epidural conversion for cesarean delivery after established labor analgesia, which of the following is most correct about using an epidural placed with a DPE technique compared to a CEA?** (Epidural conversion is when an existing epidural is dosed to produce a surgical level of anesthesia.)
   A. Faster onset of adequate anesthesia
   B. Increased risk of a high spinal
   C. Increased risk of hypotension
   D. Less reliable quality of anesthesia
9. **Which technique offers the most rapid onset of labor analgesia?**
   A. CSE
   B. DPE
   C. CEA
   D. The techniques do not have statistically different times of onset.
10. **True or False: The use of the DPE technique yields a better quality of analgesia in obese parturient patients compared to the use of CEA.**

11. **A CSE can be performed at different spinal levels for the spinal puncture and the epidural catheter placement (double-space technique) or can be done with a needle-through-needle technique at a single spinal level. Compared to the needle-through-needle technique, the double-space technique is superior in which way?**
    A. Faster onset of block
    B. Further rostral extension of anesthesia
    C. Less risk of hypotension
    D. None of the above
12. **Which of the following is an absolute contraindication for use of a CSE?**
    A. Patent foramen ovale
    B. Elevated intracranial pressure
    C. Aortic stenosis
    D. Chorioamnionitis
13. **When using the combined spinal-epidural (CSE) technique with hyperbaric bupivacaine for cesarean delivery, compared to placement in the sitting position, placement in the lateral position is associated with which of the following:**
    A. Less hypotension
    B. Less paresthesiae
    C. Faster onset of sensory block to T6
    D. Increased need for epidural supplementation
    E. Improved neonatal outcomes

Answers and Explanations

1. **C.** The use of DPE is associated with a lower requirement for epidural medication, improved anesthetic coverage of the sacral roots, and faster onset of analgesia [1]. The DPE technique is also associated with a reduced rate of epidural catheter replacement [2].
2. **A.** Maternal hypotension is more common with the use of the CSE technique than CEA or DPE. The use of a CSE technique is not associated with a higher frequency of cesarean delivery. Adverse maternal and fetal outcomes with the use of CSE techniques are comparable to the use of CEA [3].
3. **C.** The CSE technique has a 14.6% risk of prolonged decelerations or fetal bradycardia, much higher than the risk associated with CEA and DPE techniques [4].
4. **B.** To attain satisfactory pain control, a DPE requires 65% of the dose needed for a CEA [5].
5. **D.** For the dural puncture during a CSE, the spinal needle should be placed below the L2 interspace to avoid trauma to the spinal cord [3]. Targeting spinal levels rostral to L2 carries the risk of damage to the spinal cord.

6. **B.** The use of a pencil-point spinal needle produces more patient reactions than the use of a cutting-point spinal needle [6]. If identification of the epidural space is done with loss-of-resistance using air, 80% of patients will have a negative reaction during dural puncture, such as moving, grimacing, or reporting paresthesiae. There are fewer negative reactions with a loss-of-resistance using saline [7]. Using a 25-gauge spinal needle rather than a 27-gauge needle results in slightly faster onset of analgesia but no increase in block height [8]. Unlike cutting-point needles, using a smaller gauge pencil-point needle does not reduce the risk of post-dural puncture headache [9].
7. **B.** The bolus volume needed with PIEB pumps is equivalent between the CEA technique and the DPE technique [10].
8. **A.** For epidural conversion, the use of a DPE technique during catheter placement is associated with a faster onset of surgical anesthesia. There is no significant difference in the risk of a high spinal or hypotension. The use of a DPE technique is associated with a more reliable quality of anesthesia after epidural conversion [11].
9. **A.** CSE offers the most rapid onset of analgesia compared to DPE and CEA [12].
10. **False.** DPE has not been shown to offer a higher analgesic quality during labor for obese parturients when compared to the CEA [13].
11. **D.** For time of onset and incidence of side effects, there is no significant difference between the needle-through-needle technique and the double-level technique [14].
12. **B.** The dural puncture used as part of the DPE and CSE techniques makes increased intracranial pressure an absolute contraindication to these techniques [15]. Aortic stenosis is a relative contraindication, leaving it up to the physician's discretion to perform a dural puncture or not. Chorioamnionitis is not an absolute contraindication to any type of epidural.
13. **C.** Compared to the sitting position, placement of a CSE in the lateral position is associated with more hypotension and paresthesiae. There is faster onset of sensory block to T4 with placement in the lateral position and the position is associated with less need for epidural supplementation. There is no difference in neonatal outcomes between sitting and lateral positions [16, 17].

References

1. Song Y, Du W, Zhou S, Zhou Y, Yu Y, Xu Z, Liu Z. Effect of dural puncture epidural technique combined with programmed intermittent epidural bolus on labor analgesia onset and maintenance: a randomized controlled trial. Anesth Analg. 2021;132(4):971–8. https://doi.org/10.1213/ANE.0000000000004768.
2. Berger AA, Jordan J, Li Y, Kowalczyk JJ, Hess PE. Epidural catheter replacement rates with dural puncture epidural labor analgesia compared with epidural analgesia without dural puncture: a retrospective cohort study. Int J Obstet Anesth. 2022;52:103590. https://doi.org/10.1016/j.ijoa.2022.103590. Epub 2022 Aug 2.
3. Roofthooft E, Rawal N, Van de Velde M. Status of the combined spinal-epidural technique in obstetrics and surgery. Best Pract Res Clin Anaesthesiol. 2023;37(2):189–98. ISSN: 1521-6896. https://doi.org/10.1016/j.bpa.2023.04.004.

4. Okahara S, Inoue R, Katakura Y, Nagao H, Yamamoto S, Nojiri S, Takeda J, Itakura A, Sumikura H. Comparison of the incidence of fetal prolonged deceleration after induction of labor analgesia between dural puncture epidural and combined spinal epidural technique: a pilot study. BMC Pregnancy Childbirth. 2023;23(1):182. https://doi.org/10.1186/s12884-023-05473-0.
5. Maeda A, Villela-Franyutti D, Lumbreras-Marquez MI, Murthy A, Fields KG, Justice S, Tsen LC. Labor Analgesia Initiation With Dural Puncture Epidural Versus Conventional Epidural Techniques: A Randomized Biased-Coin Sequential Allocation Trial to Determine the Effective Dose for 90% of Patients of Bupivacaine. Anesth Analg. 2024;138(6):1205–14. https://doi.org/10.1213/ANE.0000000000006691. Epub 2023 Oct 12. PMID: 37824436.
6. van den Berg AA, Ghatge S, Armendariz G, Cornelius D, Wang S. Responses to dural puncture during institution of combined spinal-epidural analgesia: a comparison of 27 gauge pencil-point and 27 gauge cutting-edge needles. Anaesth Intensive Care. 2011;39(2):247–51. https://doi.org/10.1177/0310057X1103900215.
7. van den Berg AA, Ghatge S, Wang S. Loss of resistance to saline reduces responses accompanying spinal needle insertion during institution of 'needle-through-needle' combined spinal-epidural analgesia. Anaesth Intensive Care. 2010;38(6):1013–7. https://doi.org/10.1177/0310057X1003800608.
8. Contreras F, Morales J, Bravo D, Layera S, Jara Á, Riaño C, Pizarro R, De La Fuente N, Aliste J, Finlayson RJ, Tran DQ. Dural puncture epidural analgesia for labor: a randomized comparison between 25-gauge and 27-gauge pencil point spinal needles. Reg Anesth Pain Med. 2019;44:rapm-2019-100608. https://doi.org/10.1136/rapm-2019-100608. Epub ahead of print.
9. Zorrilla-Vaca A, Healy R, Zorrilla-Vaca C. Finer gauge of cutting but not pencil-point needles correlate with lower incidence of post-dural puncture headache: a meta-regression analysis. J Anesth. 2016;30(5):855–63. https://doi.org/10.1007/s00540-016-2221-2. Epub 2016 Jul 28.
10. Xiao F, Yao HQ, Qian J, Deng JL, Xu ZF, Liu L, Chen XZ. Determination of the optimal volume of programmed intermittent epidural bolus when combined with the Dural puncture epidural technique for labor analgesia: a random-allocation graded dose-response study. Anesth Analg. 2023;137:1233. https://doi.org/10.1213/ANE.0000000000006451. Epub ahead of print.
11. Sharawi N, Williams M, Athar W, Martinello C, Stoner K, Taylor C, Guo N, Sultan P, Mhyre JM. Effect of dural-puncture epidural vs standard epidural for epidural extension on onset time of surgical anesthesia in elective cesarean delivery: a randomized clinical trial. JAMA Netw Open. 2023;6(8):e2326710. https://doi.org/10.1001/jamanetworkopen.2023.26710.
12. Chau A, Bibbo C, Huang CC, Elterman KG, Cappiello EC, Robinson JN, Tsen LC. Dural puncture epidural technique improves labor analgesia quality with fewer side effects compared with epidural and combined spinal epidural techniques: a randomized clinical trial. Anesth Analg. 2017;124(2):560–9. https://doi.org/10.1213/ANE.0000000000001798.
13. Tan HS, Reed SE, Mehdiratta JE, et al. Quality of labor analgesia with dural puncture epidural versus standard epidural technique in obese parturients: a double-blind randomized controlled study. Anesthesiology. 2022;136(5):678–87. https://doi.org/10.1097/ALN.0000000000004137.
14. Chun EH, Cho S, Woo JH, Kim YJ. A randomized double-blind comparison of the double-space technique versus the single-space technique in combined spinal-epidural anesthesia for cesarean section. BMC Anesthesiol. 2020;20(1):29. https://doi.org/10.1186/s12871-020-0948-7.
15. Waters JFR. Neurologic complications of obstetric anesthesia. Continuum (Minneap Minn). 2022;28(1):162–79. https://doi.org/10.1212/CON.0000000000001073.
16. Patel M, Samsoon G, Swami A, Morgan B. Posture and the spread of hyperbaric bupivacaine in parturients using the combined spinal epidural technique. Can J Anaesth. 1993;40(10):943–6. https://doi.org/10.1007/BF03010097.
17. Tan ED, Günaydın B. Comparison of maternal and neonatal effects of combined spinal epidural anaesthesia in either the sitting or lateral position during elective cesarean section. Turk J Anaesthesiol Reanim. 2014;42(1):23–32. https://doi.org/10.5152/TJAR.2013.55. Epub 2013 Aug 29.

Pudendal, Lumbar Paravertebral Sympathetic, and Paracervical Nerve Blocks

Alan Iwahashi and Minh Chau Joe Tran

Questions

1. **The pudendal nerve originates from the anterior divisions of which spinal nerve roots?**
   A. T12–L1
   B. L1–L2
   C. L2–L4
   D. S2–S4
2. **While performing a transvaginal pudendal nerve block, the obstetrician will feel for which procedural landmark?**
   A. Sacrospinous ligament
   B. Ischial tuberosity
   C. Lateral edge of the cervix
   D. Ischial spine
3. **A pudendal nerve block provides appropriate analgesia when placed during which stage of labor?**
   A. First stage
   B. Second stage
   C. Third stage
   D. Limited use in episiotomy repairs
4. **Which of the following would be the safest choice of anesthetic for a pudendal block?**
   A. 0.5% bupivacaine
   B. 2% lidocaine
   C. 3% 2-chloroprocaine

A. Iwahashi
Loma Linda University Medical Center, Loma Linda, CA, USA

M. C. J. Tran (✉)
VA Loma Linda Health Care, Loma Linda, CA, USA

A. C. Sinha, I. F. Pasca (eds.), *Peripartum Care of the Pregnant Patient*,
https://doi.org/10.1007/978-3-031-62756-9_17

D. 1% lidocaine

5. **Bilateral pudendal nerve blocks are administered to a 70 kg patient using 10 mL of 2% 2-chloroprocaine without epinephrine on each side shortly before vaginal delivery. The patient experiences adequate pain control within 10 minutes. If repeated doses are needed, what is the maximum total amount of 2-chloroprocaine that can safely be used?**
   A. 8 mg/kg
   B. 11 mg/kg
   C. 14 mg/kg
   D. 20 mg/kg
6. **Of the structures listed, which does not border the lumbar paravertebral space?**
   A. Vertebral bodies
   B. Intervertebral discs
   C. Psoas major muscle
   D. Costotransverse ligament
7. **Which level is the procedural target to produce the intended labor analgesia in a lumbar paravertebral block?**
   A. L1
   B. L2
   C. L3
   D. L4
   E. L5
8. **Which of the following local anesthetics is generally not used for lumbar (or thoracic) paravertebral blocks?**
   A. 0.5% bupivacaine
   B. 0.5% ropivacaine
   C. 0.5% levobupivacaine
   D. 2% 2-chloropropane
9. **Several hours after a successful lumbar paravertebral block, a patient reported worsening left-sided back pain with vague, abnormal sensations on the anterior thigh. Vital signs are essentially unchanged from before the block; however, HR is mildly increased. Which test should be ordered?**
   A. CT of the abdomen and pelvis without contrast
   B. CT of the abdomen and pelvis with contrast
   C. MRI of the lumbar spine without contrast
   D. Transvaginal ultrasound
10. **A young mother (height 158 cm) received bilateral lumbar paravertebral blocks at L2 with 10 mL of 0.5% bupivacaine on each side. After a negative aspiration test for blood, the second block is placed, and the patient lies down to rest. Soon after, supine hypotension (74/28 mmHg) ensued with relative bradycardia (72 BPM) and drowsiness. The patient experienced no seizures, tremors, or abnormal sensations of taste. Inadvertent injection into which space is most likely?**
    A. Intravascular

B. Epidural
C. Intrathecal
D. Intraneural

11. **Which of the following blocks is associated with the highest risk of fetal bradycardia?**
A. Paracervical
B. Paravertebral
C. Pudendal
D. Lumbar epidural

12. **Which nerve(s) are the target of a paracervical block?**
A. S2–S4 ventral rami
B. Lumbar spinal nerve roots
C. Superficial somatic nerve endings
D. Paracervical ganglion

13. **Which position around the cervix, by palpation, serves as the target for a paracervical block?**
A. Superior fornix
B. Inferior fornix
C. Lateral fornix
D. Sacrospinous ligament

14. **Twenty minutes after a bilateral paracervical block with a total of 20 mL of 3% 2-chloroprocaine, marked fetal bradycardia ensued. After assuming the left lateral decubitus position with supplemental oxygenation, what is the most appropriate next step in patient management?**
A. Immediately perform cesarean delivery
B. Discontinue oxytocin and alert OR team for possible emergent cesarean delivery
C. Administer an extra dose of oxytocin
D. Administer atropine

15. **Which of the following is NOT a mechanism of fetal bradycardia?**
A. Reflex bradycardia
B. Direct fetal central nervous and myocardial depression
C. Increased uterine activity
D. Increased uterine or umbilical arterial vasospasm and reduced uteroplacental perfusion
E. Neonatal seizures due to hyponatremia

16. **Due to the proximity of the paracervical block to the fetal head (risk of fetal bradycardia), anesthesia practitioners will often use less potent local anesthetics, such as lidocaine or 2-chloroprocaine. What chemical property most heavily influences local anesthetic potency?**
A. pKa
B. Hydrophobicity
C. Protein binding
D. Molecular weight

17. **A 25-year-old mother complained of new mild persistent back and leg pain 3 hours after a difficult left-sided lumbar paravertebral block. Left-sided straight leg raise is positive. The left patellar reflex is diminished with a normal Achilles reflex. Which procedural complication is suspected?**
    A. Iliopsoas hematoma
    B. Cauda equina syndrome due to epidural hematoma
    C. Uncontrolled labor pain due to failed block
    D. Sacral neuropathy
18. **A 33-year-old female had a history of lumbar fusion surgery after being involved in a car accident 12 years ago. Neuraxial access has been attempted multiple times without success. She also had gestational diabetes and pre-eclampsia with a normal platelet count. Which of the adjunctive blocks would be best suited for this mother for the first stage of labor?**
    A. Lumbar paravertebral block
    B. Paracervical block
    C. Pudendal block
    D. Perineal infiltration
19. **Alternative regional obstetric blocks (i.e., paracervical and pudendal) are close in proximity to the fetal head and are in areas surrounded by rich vascular beds. Which local anesthetic carries the highest risk for neonatal cardiovascular toxicity?**
    A. 2-Chloroprocaine
    B. Lidocaine
    C. Ropivacaine
    D. Bupivacaine
20. **A 33-year-old parturient had a history of motor vehicle collision 8 years prior, resulting in the need for lumbar fusion. The patient is being bridged with an unfractionated heparin drip for pregnancy-related DVT. As she enters the first stage of labor, epidural analgesia is initially attempted but ultimately aborted in favor of bilateral lumbar paravertebral blocks, which provide her with adequate pain control. Which of the following is the correct guideline-based management of heparin for this block?**
    A. Hold 3 hours, resume in 3 hours
    B. Hold 5 hours, resume in 3 hours
    C. Hold 3 hours, resume in 1 hour
    D. Hold 5 hours, resume in 1 hour

Answers and Explanations

1. **D.** The ventral rami of S2–S4 form the pudendal nerve and the pelvic splanchnic nerves. The pudendal nerve exits the pelvis via the greater sciatic foramen (i.e., below the piriformis, medial to the pudendal artery, and lateral to the ischial spine) and then enters the perineum via the lesser sciatic foramen and Alcock's canal. The pudendal nerve splits into the inferior rectal, perineal, and

dorsal nerves. In females, sensory coverage includes the labia minora, posterior labia majora, and lower fifth of the vaginal canal. Motor functions include control of the external anal sphincter, bladder continence, and tone of the pelvic and perineal muscles.

T12–L1 forms the ilioinguinal nerve, which provides motor function to the transverse abdominis and internal obliques. Sensory coverage includes the upper anteromedial thigh and labia majora in females. Ilioinguinal neuralgia may result from entrapment injury after lower abdominal surgeries (hernias, appendectomies, etc.)

The L1–L2 branches of the lumbar plexus form the genitofemoral nerve. After descending over the psoas muscle, the genitofemoral divides into femoral (sensory) and genital (motor) branches. Sensation is provided to the mons pubis and labia majora in females.

L2–L4 roots form the femoral nerve. The most lateral member of the femoral triangle, the femoral nerve, splits into anterior, and posterior divisions (approximately at the deep iliac circumflex artery takeoff). The anterior division splits into the medial cutaneous sensory nerve and the motor nerve to the sartorius. Posteriorly, lie the sensory saphenous nerve and the motor nerve to the quadriceps. The femoral nerve and its branches supply sensation to the anterior thigh, knee, and medial leg below the knee. Clinical relevance includes femoral and saphenous nerve blocks, often in orthopedic and vascular surgeries [1–3].

2. **D.** The sacrospinous ligament (**A**) is a relevant structure and will be pierced by the needle's path during a pudendal block. However, the target procedural landmark is the ischial spine. The ischial tuberosity (**B**) is too posterior and caudal. The lateral edge of the cervix (**C**) is the landmark for a paracervical nerve block.

   In the transvaginal approach, the obstetrician palpates along the lateral wall of the vaginal canal for the ischial spine (**D**), which lies (anteroposterior) between the anus and vagina. Once a finger is securely anchored onto the ischial spine, the operator's other hand will then introduce the anesthetic needle, covered in a protective needle guide (Kobak, or Iowa trumpet). The needle will be aimed just medial and posterior to the ischial spine and then advanced out of the needle guide so that it protrudes 1–1.5 cm. Recall from question 1 that the pudendal artery is closely medial to the nerve, so syringe aspiration must precede injection to confirm that the needle is not intravascular [4, 5].
3. **B.** (**A**) The first stage is too early. During cervical dilation, most of the regions anesthetized by the pudendal block do not experience significant pain. A paracervical block is appropriate for first-stage labor discomfort. (**B**) The pudendal nerve block is intended to anesthetize the lower vaginal canal and the more external perineal tissues that stretch during delivery. It is offered when neuraxial anesthesia is contraindicated or refused, although it is overall less effective than neuraxial options. Because of the pudendal nerve's motor capacity (pelvic and perineal muscles), blockade can theoretically prolong the second stage of labor. An earlier trial concluded that pudendal nerve blocks only slightly prolonged the second stage. European obstetricians generally perform the

pudendal block earlier during the second stage, while American practitioners perform the block slightly later, for this reason. A suggested compromise is to perform the block in the second stage when the patient first begins complaining of vaginal and perineal pain so that there will be ample time for onset. By the third stage (**C**) of labor, most of the benefit from a pudendal nerve block will have been missed. (**D**) Some randomized data show that pudendal block is inferior to neuraxial anesthesia and provides inadequate relief during labor. However, for episiotomy and repair, an accurately placed pudendal block is quite effective [5, 6, 7].

4. **D.** The principle is to use a less concentrated local anesthetic while being mindful of the total volume injected due to the high vascularity of the surrounding tissues. Pudendal blocks are rapidly taken up, and some previous studies have shown detectable levels of local anesthetic in maternal venous and fetal scalp blood in just 5 minutes. To reduce the risk of maternal and fetal local anesthetic toxicity, less concentrated formulations of 2% 2-chloroprocaine (duration ~0.5–1 hour, max dose 11 mg/kg) and 1% lidocaine (duration ~0.75–1.5 hours, max dose 4.5 mg/kg, or 7 mg/kg with epinephrine) are preferred. Studies have not conclusively shown that added epinephrine improves the effect of anesthesia. Because they are also shorter acting, they are ideally administered closer to delivery [5].
5. **B**. (**A**) 8 mg/kg is less than the recommended maximum dose cutoff. (**B**) 11 mg/kg is the weight-based maximum allowable dose for 2-chloroprocaine without epinephrine, which in this patient would be 770 mg. Recall that 2% is 20 mg/mL. Thus, 20 ml (for two 10 mL injections) would equal 400 mg total, which is well within the safe range. For very obese patients, an absolute maximum dose recommendation is set at 800 mg. (**C**) 14 mg/kg is the weight-based maximum allowable dose for 2-chloroprocaine with epinephrine. For a 70 kg patient, the weight-based maximum (980 mg) would exceed the absolute limit of 800 mg. (**D**) 20 mg/kg exceeds the toxic dose cutoff for both epinephrine- and norepinephrine-containing formulations [8].
6. **D.** Answers **A, B, and C** pertain to the lumbar paravertebral space. Its borders are the vertebral bodies, intervertebral discs and foramen medially; the transverse processes and connecting ligaments posteriorly; and the psoas major muscle anterolaterally. The (**D**) costotransverse ligaments (and transverse processes) form the posterior border of the thoracic paravertebral space. Some noteworthy differences between the thoracic and lumbar paravertebral spaces are that the thoracic spinous processes are angled more inferiorly than in the lumbar region. The palpable portion of a given spinous process in the thoracic spine may be at the same vertical level as the transverse process from the next level below. The lumbar paravertebral space also communicates medially with the epidural space, while the thoracic paravertebral space communicates with both the epidural and the intercostal spaces [5, 9].
7. **B.** This is a question about sensory dermatomes. (**A**) L1 covers the upper hips and lower abdomen. (**C**) L3 covers the middle thigh, (**D**) L4 covers the lower thigh, and (**E**) L5 covers the lower lateral thigh. Answer (**B**) L2 is the suggested

target level for a lumbar paravertebral block in the setting of labor, as the cervical and lower uterine afferent sensory fibers travel through the lumbar sympathetic chain via L2-L3. The iliac crest corresponds to the L3–L4 interspace, and with palpation, the L2 spinous process can be located. The center of the spinous process defined the midline, and the needle entry point was 2.5 cm lateral to the midline. The lesser angulation of the lumbar spinous processes may mean that to be closest to the corresponding nerve root, the needle should be "walked" underneath the transverse process rather than above, as in the thoracic region. A common practice is to advance the needle a predetermined distance (1.5–2.0 cm) past the transverse process (usually 4–6 cm deep), and after negative aspiration for CSF or blood, inject 5–10 mL of local anesthetic per side at the desired spinal level [9, 10].

8. **D**. Answers **A–C** are more potent and longer acting, which is desired for lumbar paravertebral blocks. Unlike paracervical and pudendal blocks, the lumbar paravertebral block is further away from the fetus, reducing the risk of fetal exposure and bradycardia. Anesthesia (absent sensation) may develop in less than 30 minutes and last up to ~5 hours. Analgesia may last much longer (up to ~12–18 hours) and, when combined with a multimodal pain regimen, may reduce postdelivery opiate use. A prior study safely used injection totals as large as 20 mL of 0.5% bupivacaine (with 1:200,000 epinephrine) [5, 9].
9. **C**. The focal nature of symptoms should prompt consideration of a more structural procedural consequence. Nonstructural complications of a lumbar paravertebral block include intrathecal injection and sympathectomy, intravascular injection, and LAST. These would be less likely in the absence of more prominent hemodynamic changes and neurological symptoms. A key procedural step in the lumbar paravertebral block is to avoid the medial direction of the needle (i.e., toward the vessels and CSF). Given focal symptoms, retroperitoneal or psoas hematoma and lumbar plexopathy and spinal epidural hematoma and cauda equina syndrome were considered. Although this could also be a case of psoas hematoma with plexopathy, as suggested by the laterality (left), one cannot rule out a spinal epidural hematoma without an MRI (**C**). Spinal decompression has been shown to yield better neurological outcomes if performed in <12 hours. (**A**) A noncontrast CT would rapidly show a retroperitoneal hematoma, but this diagnosis is not as time-sensitive as a spinal epidural hematoma because it does not require decompressive surgery. (**B**) The benefit of venous contrast would mainly be to look for a psoas abscess, which is not consistent with the onset time. (**D**) Considering fetal well-being is important at all times, but an ultrasound would not reveal the diagnosis here [5, 9, 11].
10. **C.** This case describes accidental intrathecal injection and ascending spinal-induced hypotension. Among the risk factors for spinal hypotension are spinal puncture at or above the L2–L3 interspace and blockade at or above T5. In this case, the young mother received an L2 intrathecal injection of bupivacaine, which ascended to affect the levels involving the thoracic sympathetic chain. The major factors that affect block height include dermatomal level of injection, CSF volume, age, pregnancy, baricity and dose, patient positioning, and

epidural injection postspinal. Unlike LAST, where there is an antidote (intralipid), treatment of a high spinal is purely supportive: IV fluids, LUD to maximize preload, vasopressors, airway management, and intubation if necessary. (**A**) Intravascular injection is less likely with repeated negative aspiration tests, although a learning point is that the official method of testing for intravascular injection during (planned) epidural anesthesia is the epidural test dose (usually 15 μg epinephrine/3 ml lidocaine, which produces changes in vitals that serve as a marker). (**B**) Epidural placement may be suspected if the patient has mild hypotension with a bilateral, symmetric anesthetic pattern. The mother, despite potentially receiving an effective analgesic, should be monitored for specific complications of epidural anesthesia (i.e., LAST and epidural hematoma). (**D**) Intraneural injection to a lumbar nerve root would be painful but not create the hemodynamic instability seen in a high spinal [5, 12, 13].

11. **A**. Of the alternative regional blocks in this chapter, paracervical block has been associated with the highest risk of fetal bradycardia due to its proximity to the fetal head and the uterus. Fetal bradycardia from paracervical blocks has been hypothesized to result from drug-induced vasospasm. It typically develops within 2–10 minutes of injection and self-resolves within 5–10 minutes (some have lasted as long as 30 minutes); thus, some providers recommend observing 10 minutes before safely anesthetizing the contralateral side. Not surprisingly, the severity and duration of bradycardia correlate with the degree of neonatal acidosis and depression. The duration of fetal bradycardia is very relevant clinically, as operative delivery is recommended if bradycardia persists >10 minutes. Rates of fetal bradycardia with paracervical block vary widely in the literature (between 0–2%, 24%, and up to 70%), yet causality has not yet been established between this block and reduced Apgar scores or rates of emergency cesarean section. Nevertheless, paracervical blocks are generally reserved for healthy term parturients without uteroplacental insufficiency or fetal compromise who are not markedly dilated (8 cm or more) due to the close proximity to the fetal head. (**B**) The main risk posed to the fetus is if systemic hypotension ensues from sympathectomy leading to decreased uterine perfusion. Paravertebral blocks are considered to have a lower risk for fetal bradycardia. (**C**) Fetal harm from a pudendal nerve block primarily results from direct fetal trauma from the needle and direct anesthetic injection causing fetal LAST. The risk of fetal bradycardia in uncomplicated pudendal blocks is generally low. (**D**) A lumbar epidural, similar to the paravertebral block, poses fetal risk primarily if systemic hypotension arises due to sympathectomy [5, 8].
12. **D.** (**A**) S2–S4 ventral rami are the target of the pudendal nerve block, distal to the confluence of roots, and proximal to the pudendal nerve's dividing point into terminal branches. (**B**) Lumbar spinal nerve roots are the target for the lumbar paravertebral and lumbar epidural blocks. (**C**) Superficial somatic nerve endings are anesthetized via perineal infiltration, often concurrently performed with the pudendal nerve block due to the latter's higher failure rate. (**D**) Paracervical ganglion is correct (a.k.a. Frankenhauser's ganglion). It is a synapse point immediately posterolateral to the cervicouterine junction, comprised of visceral afferent

fibers from the cervix, lower uterine segment, and upper vagina that join the lumbar sympathetic chain at L2–L3, ascend, and then enter the spinal cord at T10-L1. Because these fibers are purely sensory visceral, there is no somatic coverage (i.e., sensation to the vagina, vulva, and perineum that is covered with the pudendal block) or motor blockade that will slow the progress of labor. Because of the paracervical block's limitations in coverage, it is specifically for analgesia during the first stage of labor (i.e., cervical dilation) [5].

13. **C.** The lateral fornix at the 4 o'clock and 8 o'clock positions are the sites of local anesthetic injection. 5–10 mL of dilute (e.g., 2% 2-chloroprocaine) injected 2–3 mm deep (with the needle protected by needle guide to reduce risk of fetal injury) will bathe the paracervical ganglion. The injection is most effective when placed just lateral to the uterosacral ligaments, where it is able to anesthetize the uterovaginal plexus. Due to the close proximity of the injection site to the cervix, as previously mentioned, paracervical block is not recommended with significant cervical dilation (8 cm or more) due to protrusion of the fetal head. (**A**, **B**) The superior and inferior fornices would miss the collection of intended nerves described in (**C**) and would result in inadequate analgesia. (**D**) The sacrospinous ligament lies just medial and posterior to its connection with the ischial spine and is the target site for pudendal nerve block [5, 8].
14. **B**. By discontinuing oxytocin, uterotonic uterine contractions will decrease, which will also decrease uterine oxygen consumption. Ensuring normal blood pressure and maximizing oxygen delivery attempts to compensate for the mechanism of local anesthetic-induced fetal bradycardia, which is placental vasospasm and reduced fetal perfusion. It would be prudent to notify the OR team simultaneously, should the bradycardia remain refractory. Cesarean delivery is recommended for refractory bradycardia persisting >10 minutes (**A**). **C** would worsen placental oxygen demand. **D** would be the treatment for symptomatic maternal bradycardia. If maternal hemodynamic instability (with neurological symptoms and seizures) is thought to be the trigger for fetal bradycardia, consider LAST, stabilize ABCs, and initiate empiric treatment with a 1.5 mL/kg bolus of intralipid [5, 13].
15. **E.** Answers **A–D** are all proposed mechanisms of fetal bradycardia, with **D** being predominant in serious or refractory cases. **A** is usually seen with manipulation of the uterus, fetal head, or uterine vessels during a procedure. Because of the rapidity of a local anesthetic's ability to cross the placenta, large volume injection close to the fetus may result in direct myocardial suppression via sodium channel blockade (**B**). Various studies have analyzed fetal versus maternal timed serum concentrations of local anesthetic to assess mechanisms of toxicity. Local anesthetic injected near the uterine vasculature may cause regional vasospasm and reduced uteroplacental perfusion (**D**). Because the common mechanism of fetal bradycardia is a reduction in placental perfusion, it is recommended to perform a paracervical block with left lateral uterine displacement and without the addition of epinephrine to maximize regional blood flow. When fetal bradycardia is encountered, discontinuing uterotonics (**C**) reduces uterine oxygen consumption. Unintended injection or diffusion of local

anesthetic may cause fetal cardiotoxicity from sodium channel blockade, not an absolute deficit in sodium (**E**). While seizures may occur, the main mechanism of fetal bradycardia is thought to be compromised perfusion [5].

16. **B.** Hydrophobicity is nearly synonymous with lipophilicity. Lipophilicity is partly affected by pKa, but multiple properties also contribute in vivo (anesthetic charge, hydrophobicity, i.e., membrane diffusion, and degree of local vasodilation/constriction). For example, in Miller Table 29.2, procaine (an ester) has a very high pKa (8.9, a weak acid) and a hydrophobicity of 100 (low), whereas tetracaine has a very high hydrophobicity (5822) with a slightly lower pKa (8.4). Notice that the higher potency locals (tetracaine, bupivacaine, etidocaine) tend to be amides. Lidocaine and mepivacaine are also amides and are in the intermediate potency group (a group shared by esters and amides). Hydrophobicity is the primary determinant of intrinsic potency, as the sodium blocking ability is produced by the anesthetic binding to a hydrophobic site on the sodium channel. pKa partially influences potency (via its effect on hydrophobicity), but it is more associated with the speed of onset (**A**). From organic chemistry, pKa is the −log(Ka), the acid dissociation constant in which the numerator represents the dissociation from an acid. A greater numerator means that the acid is stronger because it donates more H+ (the definition of an acid). In a table of local anesthetics and their pKa values, all pKa values are >7.45 (physiologic pH). The pKa is the pH value at which a chemical species will accept or donate a proton. If the pKa of a substance is greater than ambient pH, the substance will tend to accept an H+ (i.e., becoming protonated). The positive charge conferred by its protonation will make the molecule less able to pass through the cell membrane, which favors the passage of one uncharged molecule. Because all local anesthetic pKa values are greater than 7.4, pKa values closer to physiologic will be lower and less likely to accept H+ ions and become protonated by the environment. Lower pKa anesthetics will be more likely to exist in a nonprotonated form (i.e., as a conjugate base) and be able to pass more easily through the cell membrane. Some books designate the conjugate base as an anion (e.g., A−) and the conjugate base as HA, whereas local anesthetic conjugate bases are thought of as neutral ("A") with their conjugate protonated acid existing as HA+. Protein binding affects the degree (availability) of free drug (**C**). This affects the speed of onset, but onset is primarily determined by pKa, and again, hydrophobicity primarily defines potency. Smaller-molecular-weight particles more easily diffuse through a membrane and have a smaller influence on onset time (**D**). As a final note, it has been observed that the volume of injected anesthetic is also important to local anesthetic spread (especially in neuraxial blocks) and not just the total mass in (gram, mg, mcg). For example, 30 mL of 1% lidocaine will likely distribute further than 10 mL of 3% lidocaine, even though the same amount (300 mg) of drug was delivered [14–16].
17. **A.** This case is of lumbar plexopathy due to a retroperitoneal hematoma, which can present with psoas and quadriceps weakness (hip flexion knee extension, respectively) and anteromedial thigh numbness. The femoral nerve (L2–L4)

runs along the anterior edge of the iliopsoas muscle; thus, a positive straight leg raise may indicate a sizable proximal hematoma, as it is usually generated by the lower lumbar nerve roots (i.e., L5). Hematomas can be diagnosed with non-contrast CT, but MRI is preferred to visualize individual nerve roots. The prognosis of hematoma-related plexopathies is generally good, and most retroperitoneal hematomas can be managed noninvasively. Even with early unilateral symptoms, this should always be on the differential for new neurological complaints after a paravertebral block, as unintended epidural injection can be encountered with the medial direction of the needle (**B**). Straight leg raise indicates lumbosacral nerve root irritation and is not sufficiently sensitive or specific to differentiate epidural hematoma versus a more distal lesion. This patient likely will undergo testing for both diagnoses (epidural hemorrhage and for a retroperitoneal hematoma if MRI is negative). Notably, isolated iliopsoas hematoma has been reported as a complication of epidural catheter placement. Labor pain should not present with focal neurological findings, as described (**C**). Recall that the target of the lumbar paravertebral block is at L2 (**D**). Sacral involvement (suggested by a diminished ankle jerk reflex) would not be expected here [17, 18].

18. **A**. Bilateral lumbar paravertebral blocks are an option for first-stage labor pain when epidural analgesia is not possible. The distance from the fetus makes it safer to use longer acting, more potent anesthetics such as ropivacaine and bupivacaine, as the risk of fetal bradycardia is much lower than the paracervical block. The block interrupts the sympathetic roots of L2–L3 to innervate the lower uterine segment and the cervix while avoiding somatic and motor blockade. A key point is that it does not cover second-stage labor pain, and a pudendal nerve block will be necessary. Although the paracervical would cover first-stage pain, it is contraindicated when at risk for uteroplacental insufficiency (here with gestational diabetes and preeclampsia) (**B**). The pudendal nerve block does not cover cervical and lower uterine sensation (making the paracervical and lumbar paravertebral the alternates for first stage pain) (**C**). **D** does not offer coverage for the first-stage labor pain. However, it may be used for episiotomy repair [5].
19. **D.** All local anesthetics carry respectable risk for cardiac and neurologic toxicity to the mother and to the fetus. However, bupivacaine is especially risky. Bupivacaine has a lower minimum dose to produce irreversible cardiotoxicity and is more likely to induce refractory ventricular arrhythmias than lidocaine. Patients are more sensitive to local anesthetics when pregnant, and bupivacaine is among the more potent local anesthetics; for this reason, bupivacaine 0.75% is no longer used for obstetric anesthesia. Newborn infants also have immature liver enzymes and are more prone to the accumulation of amides (lidocaine, bupivacaine, and ropivacaine). Chloroprocaine, even in preterm neonatal use, is rapidly cleared, making it desirable from a safety perspective for paracervical and pudendal blocks. However, its short duration of action may present a clinical challenge to provide lasting relief for parturients and may require repeated dosing [14].

20. **D.** ASRA recommends holding treatment dose IV heparin for 4–6 hours (SC 8–12 hours) before a neuraxial block and resuming 1 hour after puncture, catheter manipulation, or catheter removal. SC prophylactic heparin should be held 4–6 hours and resumed 1 hour postprocedure. Lovenox (LMWH) should be held before puncture (12 hours for prophylaxis, 24 hours for treatment dose) and resumed 4 hours after placement. The guidelines also list hold/resume times for NOACs (and anti-platelet agents); however, most mothers will be bridged with UFH/LMWH in the peripartum period. If the parturient was covered with argatroban due to a history of HIT, the hold time was 4 hours, and the time to resumption was 2 hours [19].

References

1. Elsakka KM, Das J, Allam AE. Ilioinguinal neuralgia. [Updated 2022 Oct 10]. In: StatPearls [Internet]. Treasure Island (FL): StatPearls Publishing; 2022 Jan-. https://www.ncbi.nlm.nih.gov/books/NBK538256
2. Gupton M, Varacallo M. Anatomy, abdomen and pelvis, genitofemoral nerve. [Updated 2022 Oct 24]. In: StatPearls [Internet]. Treasure Island (FL): StatPearls Publishing; 2022 Jan-. https://www.ncbi.nlm.nih.gov/books/NBK430733
3. Sykes Z, Pak A. Femoral nerve block. [Updated 2022 Jul 25]. In: StatPearls [Internet]. Treasure Island (FL): StatPearls Publishing; 2022 Jan-. https://www.ncbi.nlm.nih.gov/books/NBK546704
4. Seif J. Pudendal nerve block. In: Farag E, Mounir-Soliman L, Brown D, editors. Brown's atlas of regional anesthesia, vol. 46. 6th ed. Elsevier; 2021. p. 291–2.
5. Chestnut D. Alternative regional analgesic techniques for labor and vaginal delivery. In: Chestnut's obstetric anesthesia, vol. 24. 6th ed. Elsevier; 2020. p. 540–52.
6. Pace MC, Aurilio C, Bulletti C, Iannotti M, Passavanti MB, Palagiano A. Subarachnoid analgesia in advanced labor: a comparison of subarachnoid analgesia and pudendal block in advanced labor: analgesic quality and obstetric outcome. Ann N Y Acad Sci. 2004;1034:356–63. https://doi.org/10.1196/annals.1335.037.
7. Zador G, Lindmark G, Nilsson BA. Pudendal block in normal vaginal deliveries. Clinical efficacy, lidocaine concentrations in maternal and fetal blood, fetal and maternal acid–base values and influence on uterine activity. Acta Obstet Gynecol Scand Suppl. 1974;(34):51–64.
8. Obstetrical analgesia and anesthesia. In: Cunningham F, Leveno KJ, Dashe JS, Hoffman BL, Spong CY, Casey BM (eds). Williams obstetrics, 26e. McGraw Hill; 2022. Accessed 15 Feb 2023. https://accessmedicine.mhmedical.com/content.aspx?bookid=2977&sectionid=249763743
9. Karmakar M, Greengrass R, Latmore M, and Levin M. Thoracic and lumbar paravertebral block—landmarks and nerve stimulator technique. NYSORA (New York School of Regional Anesthesia). 2023. Accessed 15 Feb 2023.
10. Cleland JGP. Paravertebral anaesthesia in obstetrics experimental and clinical basis. Surv Anesthesiol. 1981;25(5):341.
11. Lawton MT, Porter RW, Heiserman JE, Jacobowitz R, Sonntag VKH, Dickman CA. Surgical management of spinal epidural hematoma: relationship between surgical timing and neurological outcome. J Neurosurg. 1995;83(1):1–7. https://thejns.org/view/journals/j-neurosurg/83/1/article-p1.xml. Accessed 16 Feb 2023
12. Brull R, MacFarlane JR, Chan V. Spinal, epidural, and caudal anesthesia. In: Miller's anesthesia, vol. 45. 9th ed. Elsevier; 2020. p. 1413–49.

13. Borshoff D, Lighthall G. Total spinal. In: The anesthetic crisis manual. Leeuwin Press; 2017. Section 16A-B.
14. Lirk P, Berde CM. Local anesthetics. In: Miller's anesthesia, vol. 29. 9th ed. Elsevier; 2020. p. 865–90.
15. Kahn Academy Organic Chemistry. Organic acid–base chemistry, unit 2, lesson 3. Kahn Academy; 2023. Accessed 15 Feb 2023.
16. Taylor A, McLeod G. Basic pharmacology of local anesthetics. BJA Educ. 2020;20(2):34–41. https://doi.org/10.1016/j.bjae.2019.10.002. Epub 2019 Dec 4. Erratum in: BJA Educ. 2020 Apr;20(4):140.
17. Camino Willhuber GO, Piuzzi NS. Straight leg raise test. [Updated 2022 Jun 22]. In: StatPearls [Internet]. Treasure Island (FL): StatPearls Publishing; 2022 Jan-. https://www.ncbi.nlm.nih.gov/books/NBK539717/
18. Crosby ET, Reid DR, DiPrimio G, Grahovac S. Lumbosacral plexopathy from iliopsoas hematoma after combined general-epidural anesthesia for abdominal aneurysmectomy. Can J Anaesth. 1998;45(1):46–51. https://doi.org/10.1007/BF03011992.
19. Horlocker TT, Vandermeuelen E, Kopp SL, et al. Regional anesthesia in the patient receiving antithrombotic or thrombolytic therapy: american society of regional anesthesia and pain medicine evidence-based guidelines (Fourth Edition). Regional Anesth Pain Med. 2018;43:263–309.

In Vitro Fertilization

Rashmi Thapa and Bashu Dev Parajuli

Questions

1. **All are the goals of anesthesia during oocyte retrieval procedure, except**
   A. Immobilization
   B. Sedation
   C. Analgesia
   D. Paralysis
2. **Which type of anesthesia is most often used for oocyte retrieval?**
   A. General anesthesia
   B. Sedation
   C. Regional Anesthesia
   D. Paracervical block
3. **Why is conscious sedation preferred over general anesthesia (GA) for oocyte retrieval procedure?**
   A. Conscious sedation provides eco-friendly when compared with GA
   B. Conscious sedation is always safe for patients over GA in full stomach
   C. Conscious sedation never requires airway instrumentation, unlike GA
   D. Conscious sedation provides the same degree of comfort to patients and anesthesiologists
4. **When should regional anesthesia be used for oocyte retrieval?**
   A. Patient chooses to be awake
   B. Contraindication to sedation
   C. Patient has an allergy to common anesthetic agent
   D. All the above
5. **Typical duration of oocyte retrieval is**
   A. 15–30 min

R. Thapa · B. D. Parajuli (✉)
Department of Anaesthesiology, Tribhuvan University Teaching Hospital, Maharajgunj Medical Campus, Institute of Medicine, Maharajgunj, Kathmandu, Nepal

A. C. Sinha, I. F. Pasca (eds.), *Peripartum Care of the Pregnant Patient*,
https://doi.org/10.1007/978-3-031-62756-9_18

   B. 30–60 min
   C. 60–90 min
   D. >90 min
6. **What is the primary aim of paracervical block in oocyte retrieval?**
   A. To ensure immobility during the procedure
   B. To provide unconsciousness during the procedure
   C. To alleviate pain and discomfort associated with the procedure
   D. To reduce the consumption of the anesthetic agent
7. **The most painful stimulus during the oocyte retrieval is**
   A. Insertion of transvaginal USG probe
   B. Needle piercing through the cervix/lateral vaginal wall
   C. Aspiration of ovum
   D. Positioning
8. **All the following drugs accumulate in follicular fluid, <u>except</u>:**
   A. Fentanyl
   B. Remifentanil
   C. Propofol
   D. Midazolam
9. **Which factor may influence the choice of anesthesia for oocyte retrieval?**
   A. Patient's age
   B. Patients weight
   C. Number of retrieved oocytes
   D. Surgeons' preference
10. **Which patient population requires special consideration during anesthesia for oocyte retrieval?**
    A. Young and healthy women
    B. Women with a history of multiple pregnancy
    C. Patient with known allergy to anesthesia drug,
    D. Women with a low ovarian reserve
11. **All the following are the drugs that are most used as procedural sedation during oocyte retrieval, <u>except</u>:**
    A. Fentanyl
    B. Propofol
    C. Isoflurane
    D. Midazolam
12. **What is the primary concern while selecting anesthetic agent for oocyte retrieval?**
    A. Its effect on embryo cleavage and pregnancy rates
    B. Its penetration into follicular fluid
    C. Its potential for room contamination
    D. Its effect on the success of in vitro fertilization
13. **Which type of anesthetic agent is considered safe and effective for induction and maintenance of general anesthesia?**
    A. Propofol
    B. Thiopental

C. Ketamine
D. Isoflurane

14. **Which opioid is preferred in clinical settings for oocyte retrieval in terms of its duration of action and success rate of pregnancy?**
    A. Fentanyl
    B. Sufentanil
    C. Morphine
    D. Remifentanil
15. **What is the primary mechanism of action of opioids for oocyte retrieval?**
    A. Blocking GABA receptors
    B. Acting as agonist at opioid μ receptor
    C. Modifying chloride ionophores
    D. Facilitate the action of acetylcholine
16. **Why is propofol considered a suitable anesthetic drug for outpatient surgery?**
    A. It has potent analgesic effects
    B. It offers the benefit of antiemetic properties along with faster onset and short duration of action
    C. It does not penetrate follicular fluid
    D. It has a long duration of action, ensuring patient comfort after surgery
17. **Which anesthetic agents are known to have a potential negative impact on the success rate of in vitro fertilization?**
    A. Propofol
    B. Fentanyl
    C. Inhalational agents
    D. Ketamine
18. **Which drug is contained in follicular fluid proportionally to the total dose injected in the patient?**
    A. Midazolam
    B. Fentanyl
    C. Sodium thiopentone
    D. Propofol
19. **What is the primary concern related to nitrous oxide use as an anesthetic agent for oocyte retrieval?**
    A. Its potential for operation room contamination
    B. Its more beneficial effects than regional anesthesia
    C. Its solubility with oocyte fluid and exposure to oocyte decreases thymidine
    D. Its potential to cause hangover effects following surgery
20. **Which anesthetic agent is selectively modified to cause hyperpolarization of cell membrane and functional inhibition of postsynaptic neurons in the central nervous system?**
    A. Fentanyl
    B. Ketamine
    C. Propofol
    D. Midazolam

Answers and Explanations

1. **D**. Paralysis is not required for the oocyte retrieval. Sedation and analgesia are sufficient for immobility, anxiolysis, and analgesia. Paralysis is usually reserved for procedures where oocyte retrieval is planned laparoscopically. Transvaginal oocyte retrieval can be conducted under conscious sedation. The duration of the procedure is usually 15–30 min. The combination of short-acting sedatives, analgesics will help to achieve the goals. Besides, this is a day-care procedure and patients are mostly discharged to home [1].
2. **B.** In the UK, monitored sedation is used by 46% of centers, general in 28%, regional with sedation in 12%, and some other combination in 14%. Monitored sedation is preferred over other forms of anesthesia. General anesthesia (GA) is not superior to conscious sedation, and inhaled anesthetic agents have been detected in follicular fluid causing many clinicians to avoid its use in oocyte retrieval even though levels did not reach toxic levels. There is insufficient evidence that the mode of anesthesia impacts pregnancy rates [1–3].
3. **D.** Conscious sedation provides the same degree of comfort to patients and anesthesiologists when compared with GA. Conscious sedation can achieve the goals of anesthesia which include analgesia, patient comfort, and immobility. Shorter-acting agents like propofol, midazolam, and fentanyl maintain vitals, including oxygenation and ventilation without necessitating intubation. Inhalational agents can decrease cleavage rates and increase abortion [4–6].
4. **D.** Regional anesthesia is not the typical choice of anesthesia for oocyte retrieval. However, this can be offered to patients who have a contraindication to other forms of anesthesia (sedation or general anesthesia) like full stomach, new onset pulmonary infection, known anesthetic allergy, or who want to be awake throughout the procedure [4].
5. **A.** The duration of retrieval is around 15–30 min [4].
6. **C.** The goal is to alleviate pain and discomfort associated with the procedure. Paracervical block helps as an adjunct for the procedure to alleviate pain [1]. However, in many cases, particularly when oocyte retrieval is anticipated to be complicated, a single paracervical block may not be sufficient and often cannot be the sole anesthetic technique. It can be used in conjunction with conscious sedation to reduce the need of anesthetic medications [4].
7. **B.** Needle piercing through the cervix and lateral vaginal wall. Vaginal innervation is supplied by the pudendal nerve and the sacral nerve roots. It is the most painful structure [3]. Pain is usually felt while piercing the needle through the vagina toward the oocyte, which can cause jerky leg movement leading to the displacement of the needle which can increase the risk of piercing the vascular structures [4]. Other options are mainly associated with the discomfort rather than the pain.
8. **B.** Anesthetic agents (propofol, thiopental, midazolam, fentanyl, and alfentanil) can accumulate in the follicular fluid. This can be used only as an indirect index of potential toxicity but cannot prove any real toxic effect on the outcome.

However, intravenous infusion of remifentanil does not interfere in the quality and number of oocytes retrieved and makes the pick-up of oocytes easier [7].

9. **C.** Number of retrieved oocytes. The choice of anesthetic agent during oocyte retrieval mainly depends on its pharmacokinetic properties, whether the substance enters the follicular fluid, and its toxic effects on fertilization, cleavage, and pregnancy rates [1].
10. **D.** Women with low ovarian reserve require special consideration during anesthesia for oocyte retrieval.
11. **C.** Most of the studies have demonstrated the deleterious effect of halogenated fluorocarbons on IVF outcomes resulting in decreased cleavage rates and increased abortions [4].
12. **B.** The primary concern when selecting anesthetic agents for oocyte retrieval is the drug's penetration into the follicular fluid. The longer duration of exposure to anesthetic drugs causes a linear increase of its concentrations in follicular fluid, which may lead to an increased risk of low fertilization rate [8].
13. **A.** Propofol is used either alone or in combination with midazolam and fentanyl for oocyte retrieval due to its highly lipophilic nature, faster onset, and short and predictable duration of action. It offers the extra benefits of antiemetic property and speedier recovery [4].
14. **D.** Due to quick onset and quick recovery, Remifentanil and alfentanil are preferred to fentanyl in clinical settings. Remifentanil caused a considerably greater pregnancy rate than fentanyl [7]. There are no negative effects of alfentanil or remifentanil on the rate of fertilization, embryo development, or clinical pregnancy rates [1].
15. **B.** Acting as agonists at opioid μ receptors, opioids exert antinociceptive effects by acting as agonists at specific opioid receptors at presynaptic and postsynaptic locations in the central nervous system (primarily in the brainstem and spinal cord) [9].
16. **B.** It offers the benefit of antiemetic properties along with faster onset, short duration of action. It is a safe and effective drug for induction and maintenance of general anesthesia. It is used either alone or in combination with midazolam and fentanyl for oocyte retrieval due to its highly lipophilic nature, faster onset, and short and predictable duration of action [4]. Follicular fluid contained steadily rising propofol levels proportional to the total dose given. Although earlier research had shown that increased exposure to propofol had negative effects on the cleavage of oocytes, a more recent study found that, despite a rise in propofol follicular concentration, there was no difference in the rates of mature to immature oocytes [8].
17. **C.** Gonen et al. discovered that N_2O had a negative impact on the success of IVF. Compared to the epidural or sedation groups, the N_2O group had significantly lower clinical pregnancy rates [10]. Methionine synthetase is inactivated by N_2O, which lowers the quantity of thymidine accessible for DNA synthesis in proliferating cells. Isoflurane and sevoflurane are two frequently used volatile agents in other cases. Most research has shown that halogenated fluorocarbons have a negative impact on the success rate of IVF, leading to decreased

cleavage rates and increased abortions. However, propofol, ketamine, and fentanyl proved to be safe for oocyte retrieval despite some level of drugs that can penetrate follicular fluid [10].

18. **D.** Numerous studies have been done on how propofol affects the rates of pregnancy, embryo cleavage, and fertilization. Follicular fluid contains steadily rising propofol levels proportional to the total dose given. Although earlier research has shown that increased exposure to propofol had negative effects on the cleavage of oocytes, a more recent study found that despite a rise in propofol follicular concentration, there was no difference in the rates of mature to immature oocytes [8]. However, prolonged anesthetic medication exposure can result in low fertilization rates.
19. **C.** N_2O has a negative impact on the success of IVF. Compared to epidural or sedation groups, the N_2O group has significantly lower clinical pregnancy rates [10]. Methionine synthetase is inactivated by N_2O, which lowers the quantity of thymidine accessible for DNA synthesis in proliferating cells. This deleterious effect manifests itself only after embryo transfer and leads to lower pregnancy and delivery rates [10].
20. **C.** Propofol selectively modifies GABA-A receptors, causing hyperpolarization of cell membranes, and functional inhibition of the postsynaptic neurons in the central nervous system [9]. It is a safe and effective drug for induction and maintenance of general anesthesia. It is used either alone or in combination with midazolam and fentanyl for oocyte retrieval due to its highly lipophilic nature, faster onset, and short and predictable duration of action [4].

References

1. Jain D, et al. Anaesthesia for in vitro fertilisation. Indian J Anaesth. 2009;53(4):408–13.
2. Matsota P, Kaminioti E, Kostopanagiotou G. Anesthesia related toxic effects on in vitro fertilization outcome: burden of proof. Biomed Res Int. 2015;2015:475,362.
3. Kwan I, et al. Pain relief for women undergoing oocyte retrieval for assisted reproduction. Cochrane Database Syst Rev. 2013;1:Cd004829.
4. Sharma A, Borle A, Trikha A. Anesthesia for in vitro fertilization. J Obstet Anaesth Crit Care. 2015;5(2):62–72.
5. Hadimioglu N, et al. Comparison of various sedation regimens for transvaginal oocyte retrieval. Fertil Steril. 2002;78(3):648–9.
6. Thanikachalam P, Govindan DK. Pain management during ultrasound guided transvaginal oocyte retrieval—a narrative review. J Hum Reprod Sci. 2023;16(1):2–15.
7. Jarahzadeh MH, et al. Remifentanil versus fentanyl for assisted reproductive technologies: effect on hemodynamic recovery from anesthesia and outcome of ART cycles. Int J Fertil Steril. 2011;5(2):86–9.
8. Ben-Shlomo I, et al. The effect of propofol anaesthesia on oocyte fertilization and early embryo quality. Hum Reprod. 2000;15(10):2197–9.
9. Shafer SLRJPFP. Stoelting's pharmacology and physiology in anesthetic practice. Wolters Kluwer; 2015.
10. Gonen O, et al. The impact of different types of anesthesia on in vitro fertilization-embryo transfer treatment outcome. J Assist Reprod Genet. 1995;12(10):678–82.

Anesthesia for Multiparity, Multiple Gestation, and Breech Presentation

Jessica Chan and Joseph Villaluz

Questions

1. **All of the following are risk factors for postpartum dural puncture headache, EXCEPT:**
   A. Female sex
   B. Multiparity
   C. Use of Quincke needle
   D. Obesity
2. **Grand multiparity is defined by live births greater than or equal to:**
   A. 3
   B. 4
   C. 5
   D. 10
3. **All of the following are independent risk factors for developing gallstones during pregnancy, EXCEPT:**
   A. Family history
   B. Diabetes mellitus
   C. Low body mass index
   D. Multiparity
4. **Literature strongly links multiparity and the following obstetric complications, EXCEPT:**
   A. Placenta previa
   B. Postpartum urinary retention

J. Chan (✉)
Kaweah Health Medical Center, Visalia, CA, USA
e-mail: jechan@kaweahhealth.org

J. Villaluz
University of California Irvine, Irvine, CA, USA
e-mail: jvillalu@kaweahhealth.org

A. C. Sinha, I. F. Pasca (eds.), *Peripartum Care of the Pregnant Patient*,
https://doi.org/10.1007/978-3-031-62756-9_19

   C. Lumbopelvic pain
   D. Gestational hypertension
5. **All of the following are prognostic factors for peripartum cardiomyopathy, EXCEPT:**
   A. Age greater than 35
   B. Multiparity
   C. Race
   D. Smoking
6. **Studies associate multiparity increasing the risk of which of the following long-term maternal complications:**
   A. Pelvic organ prolapse
   B. Breast cancer
   C. Endometrial cancer
   D. Osteoporosis
7. **What is the rate of primary cesarean deliveries among multiparous women in the United States?**
   A. 4%
   B. 11%
   C. 22%
   D. 35%
8. **Risk factors for multiple gestation include all of the following, EXCEPT:**
   A. Multiparity
   B. Delayed childbearing
   C. Use of assisted reproductive technologies
   D. Gestational diabetes
9. **Compared to a singleton pregnancy, multiple gestation leads to the following physiologic and anatomic changes, EXCEPT:**
   A. Increased cardiac output
   B. Decreased lower esophageal sphincter (LES) competence
   C. Increased creatinine
   D. Decreased functional residual capacity (FRC)
10. **What is the rate of preterm labor in pregnant women carrying twins from in vitro fertilization?**
   A. 10%
   B. 22%
   C. 35%
   D. 52%
11. **All of the following are the different types of breech presentation, EXCEPT:**
   A. Complete breech
   B. Incomplete breech
   C. Starling breech
   D. Frank breech
12. **What is the first-line approach to a full-term baby in breech presentation?**
   A. Urgent cesarean delivery
   B. Emergent vaginal delivery

C. External cephalic version
D. None of the above

13. **Which anesthetic technique has been shown to improve the success of the external cephalic version?**
A. General anesthesia
B. Neuraxial anesthesia
C. Monitored anesthesia care (MAC)
D. None of the above

14. **All of the following are risk factors associated with breech presentation, EXCEPT:**
A. Uniparity
B. Polyhydramnios
C. Multiple gestation
D. Anencephaly

15. **All of the following are complications associated with breech presentation, EXCEPT:**
A. Intrapartum fetal death
B. Umbilical cord prolapse
C. Fetal head entrapment
D. Vernix caseosa

16. **Which type of breech presentation has a higher risk for umbilical cord prolapse?**
A. Frank breech
B. Complete breech
C. Incomplete breech
D. Starling breech

17. **What gestational age is fetal head entrapment from breech presentation more likely to occur?**
A. 31-week gestation
B. 34-week gestation
C. 37-week gestation
D. 40-week gestation

Answers and Explanations

1. **D**. Female sex (**A**), multiparity (**B**), and Quincke needle use (**C**) are associated with increased risk for postpartum dural puncture headache (PDPH). Obesity (**D**) is associated with lower risk of postpartum dural puncture headache [1].
2. **C**. Grand multiparity is defined by the delivery of five or more births (**C**). Multiparity is defined as the delivery of two or more births. Grand grand multiparity (**D**) is defined as the delivery of ten or more births. Answer choices (**A**) and (**B**) are incorrect [2].
3. **C**. Risk factors for developing gallstones during pregnancy are family history (**A**), diabetes mellitus (**B**), and multiparity (**D**). Obesity, not low body mass

index (**C**), is associated with an increased risk of developing gallstones during pregnancy [3].

4. **D**. Multiparity is a risk factor for placenta previa (**A**), postpartum urinary retention (**B**), and lumbopelvic pain (**C**). However, there is limited consensus as to whether multiparity is a risk factor for gestational hypertension (**D**) [4–6].
5. **D**. Prognostic factors for peripartum cardiomyopathy include worse New York Heart Association functional class, left ventricular ejection fraction <25%, age >35 (**A**), multiparity (**B**), and race (i.e., African American) (**C**). Smoking is not a prognostic factor for peripartum cardiomyopathy [7].
6. **A**. Literature associates pelvic organ prolapse with multiparity. A prospective cohort study following over 17,000 females over the course of 17 years showed a significant increase in risk for pelvic organ prolapse. When compared to nulliparity, the second birth showed an eightfold increase in risk for pelvic organ prolapse. Some data have associated multiparity with decreasing the risk for both breast and endometrial cancer (**B**) (**C**). There is mixed data with multiparity and osteoporosis with some data showing no risk and others showing an increased risk (**D**) [8–11].
7. **B**. In a retrospective cohort study of over 38,000 primary cesarean deliveries in the United States between the years 2002 and 2008, the primary cesarean rate was 30.8% for primiparous women and 11.5% for multiparous women. Answer choices (**A**), (**C**), and (**D**) are incorrect [12].
8. **D**. Risk factors for multiple gestation include multiparity (**A**), delayed childbearing (**B**), and use of assisted reproductive technologies (**C**) [4].
9. **C**. Compared to singleton pregnancy, multiple gestation leads to increased cardiac output (**A**), decreased lower esophageal sphincter competence (**B**), and decreased functional residual capacity (**D**). Renal, hepatic, and central nervous systems of multiple gestation women mirror those of a woman with a singleton pregnancy [4].
10. **D**. Patients with multiple gestation are at a high risk for preterm labor. Preterm labor occurs in women with spontaneous twins at a rate of 22% (**B**), while preterm labor in women with twins from in vitro fertilization occurs at a rate of 52%. Answer choices (**A**) and (**C**) are incorrect [13].
11. **C**. Starling breech is not a type of breech presentation. The three different types of fetal breech presentation include complete breech, incomplete breech, and frank breech. Complete breech (**A**) occurs when the hips and knees are flexed. Incomplete breech (**B**), also known as footling, occurs when one or both hips and knees are extended. Lastly, frank presentation (**D**) occurs when the legs are flexed at the hips and extended at the knees [14].
12. **C**. External cephalic version (ECV) is the first-line approach to a full-term baby in breech presentation. The American College of Obstetricians and Gynecologists (ACOG) recommends that "all women near term with breech presentations should be offered external cephalic version, if there are no contraindications." There is no consensus in the literature about the contraindications of ECV. However, one of the most commonly cited contraindications is oligohydramnios. Successful ECV reduces perinatal complications and the risk

associated with ECV is small. ECV should be offered after 37 weeks gestation. Emergent and urgent deliveries are not indicated as they are associated with a higher risk of complications (**A**) (**B**) [4, 15].

13. **B**. The first-line approach to breech presentation is the external cephalic version (ECV). Studies have shown that neuraxial anesthesia helps improve the success of ECV through pain relief. In addition, neuraxial anesthesia helps with the inhibition of the parturient pushing during the first stage of labor and allows the option to extend the anesthesia in case of emergent cesarean delivery. In contrast, intravenous sedation (**C**) does not help with the outcome of ECV. General anesthesia (**A**) is associated with higher maternal and fetal complications and would not be the preferred anesthetic of choice [4, 16].
14. **A**. Uniparity is not a risk factor associated with breech presentation. Risk factors associated with a breech presentation include uterine distension (e.g., multiple gestation (**C**), polyhydramnios (**B**), multiparity), maternal pelvic abnormalities (e.g., pelvic tumors, uterine anomalies), and fetal abnormalities (e.g., anencephaly (**D**), hydrocephalus) [14].
15. **D**. Complications associated with breech presentation include intrapartum asphyxia, umbilical cord prolapse (**B**), spinal cord injuries, preterm delivery, fetal heart rate (FHR) abnormalities, fetal head entrapment (**C**), and even intrapartum fetal death (**A**) [4]. Vernix caseosa is not a complication of breech presentation but rather a waxy white coating that protects the skin of the fetus and can develop in the last trimester of pregnancy.
16. **C**. Even though frank breech makes up approximately half of all the breech presentations, incomplete breech, also known as footling, is associated with a higher risk for umbilical cord prolapse with risk of 15–18%. Umbilical cord prolapse occurs when the umbilical cord exits the cervical os before the fetal presenting part. In incomplete breech, the smaller fetal presenting part compared to the other types of breeches allows for the umbilical cord to enter the cervical os, and it may result in compression of the umbilical cord. After incomplete breech, complete breech (**B**) is the next highest risk at 4–6%. Frank breech (**A**) is the lowest risk at 0.5%. Starling breech (**D**) is not one of the three breech presentations [4, 17].
17. **A**. Fetal head entrapment from breech presentation is more likely to occur before 32-week gestation. The fetal head may be entrapped due to suboptimal cervical dilatation, relatively large fetal head, or undeveloped fetal skull that may not be able to mold to the maternal pelvis. Answer choices (**B**), (**C**), and (**D**) are incorrect [4].

References

1. Orbach-Zinger S, Ashwal E, Hazan L, Bracco D, Ioscovich A, Hiersch L, Khinchuck A, Aviram A, Eidelman LA. Risk factors for unintended Dural puncture in obstetric patients: a retrospective cohort study. Anesth Analg. 2016;123(4):972–6. https://doi.org/10.1213/ANE.0000000000001510.
2. Alsammani MA, Jafer AM, Khieri SA, Ali AO, Shaaeldin MA. Effect of grand multiparity on pregnancy outcomes in women under 35 years of age: a comparative study. Med Arch. 2019;73(2):92–6. https://doi.org/10.5455/medarh.2019.73.92-96.
3. Liu B, Beral V. Balkwill a; million women study collaborators. Childbearing, breastfeeding, other reproductive factors and the subsequent risk of hospitalization for gallbladder disease. Int J Epidemiol. 2009;38(1):312–8. https://doi.org/10.1093/ije/dyn174. Epub 2008 Sep 4.
4. Chestnut DH. Chestnut's obstetric anesthesia: principles and practice. Elsevier; 2020.
5. Al JF. Grandmultiparity: a potential risk factor for adverse pregnancy outcomes. J Reprod Med. 2012;57(1–2):53–7.
6. Nassar AH, Fayyumy R, Saab W, Mehio G, Usta IM. Grandmultiparas in modern obstetrics. Am J Perinatol. 2006;23(6):345–9. https://doi.org/10.1055/s-2006-947158. Epub 2006 Jul 13.
7. Kao DP, Hsich E, Lindenfeld J. Characteristics, adverse events, and racial differences among delivering mothers with peripartum cardiomyopathy. JACC Heart Fail. 2013;1(5):409–16. https://doi.org/10.1016/j.jchf.2013.04.011.
8. Mant J, Painter R, Vessey M. Epidemiology of genital prolapse: observations from the Oxford Family Planning Association Study. Br J Obstet Gynaecol. 1997;104(5):579–85. https://doi.org/10.1111/j.1471-0528.1997.tb11536.x.
9. Högnäs E, Kauppila A, Pukkala E, Tapanainen JS. Cancer risk in women with 10 or more deliveries. Obstet Gynecol. 2014;123(4):811–6. https://doi.org/10.1097/AOG.0000000000000182.
10. Peker N, Tosun ÖÇ. Is grand multiparity a risk factor for the development of postmenopausal osteoporosis? Clin Interv Aging. 2018;13:505–8. https://doi.org/10.2147/CIA.S155793.
11. Turan V. Grand-grand multiparity (more than 10 deliveries) does not convey a risk for osteoporosis. Acta Obstet Gynecol Scand. 2011;90(12):1440–2. https://doi.org/10.1111/j.1600-0412.2011.01250.x. Epub 2011 Oct 10.
12. Boyle A, Reddy UM, Landy HJ, Huang CC, Driggers RW, Laughon SK. Primary cesarean delivery in the United States. Obstet Gynecol. 2013;122(1):33–40. https://doi.org/10.1097/AOG.0b013e3182952242.
13. American College of Obstetricians and Gynecologists. Practice Bulletin No. 169: Multifetal gestations: twin, triplet, and higher-order multifetal pregnancies. Obstet Gynecol. 2016;128:e131–46.
14. Pratt SD. Anesthesia for breech presentation and multiple gestation. Clin Obstet Gynecol. 2003;46(3):711–29.
15. Shanahan MM, Gray CJ. External cephalic version. [updated 2022 Jul 4]. In: StatPearls [internet]. Treasure Island (FL): StatPearls Publishing; 2023. https://www.ncbi.nlm.nih.gov/books/NBK482475/
16. Pollack KL, Chestnut DH. Anesthesia for complicated vaginal deliveries. Anesthesiol Clin North Am. 1990;8(1):115–29. https://doi.org/10.1016/s0889-8537(21)00157-7.
17. Boushra M, Stone A, Rathbun KM. Umbilical Cord Prolapse. [Updated 2022 Jun 5]. In: StatPearls [Internet]. Treasure Island (FL): StatPearls Publishing; 2023 Jan. https://www.ncbi.nlm.nih.gov/books/NBK542241/

Suggested Reading

Chestnut DH, Wong CA, Tsen LC, et al. Chestnut's obstetric anesthesia: principles and practice. 6th ed. Elsevier; 2020. Kacmar RM, Gaiser R (eds).

Cervical Cerclage and Tubal Ligation

Lenorre Clarke

Questions

1. **Cerclage may be indicated in which of the scenarios:**
   A. History of pregnancy loss due to painless cervical dilation in the second trimester
   B. Painless cervical dilation before 24 weeks gestation
   C. Short cervical length (<25 mm) by ultrasound before 24 weeks gestation with a history of preterm birth
   D. All the above
2. **Which of the following is false regarding the reactivation of labor epidural for postpartum tubal ligation?**
   A. Reactivation should be attempted within 24 h of placement of the epidural catheter
   B. Bilateral T6–T8 block is recommended
   C. After attempting reactivation, assess the level of the block after 5–10 min
   D. If there is evidence of a unilateral sensory block, remove the catheter completely and administer an alternative neuraxial anesthesia technique
3. **What level of sensory block is recommended for postpartum tubal ligation?**
   A. T4–T6
   B. T6–T8
   C. T8–T10
   D. T10–T12
4. **Which of the following physiologic changes occur in the immediate postpartum setting?**
   A. Airway edema resolves

L. Clarke (✉)
Riverside University Health System, Moreno Valley, CA, USA

Loma Linda University, Loma Linda, CA, USA
e-mail: l.clarke@ruhealth.org

A. C. Sinha, I. F. Pasca (eds.), *Peripartum Care of the Pregnant Patient*,
https://doi.org/10.1007/978-3-031-62756-9_20

B. Functional residual capacity decreases
C. Cardiac output increases
D. Aspiration risk returns to baseline

5. **True or false. The local anesthetic requirement for neuraxial anesthesia is increased in pregnancy and remains in this way in the postpartum setting.**
6. **The benefits of tubal ligation include:**
   A. Reduced risk of ovarian cancer
   B. Permanent sterilization
   C. Reduced risk of pelvic inflammatory disease
   D. A and B
   E. A, B, and C
7. **True or false. Minilaparotomy is generally the preferred surgical approach for postpartum and interval sterilization procedures.**
8. **Mortality rates in the USA for tubal sterilization are estimated to be:**
   A. 2/1000
   B. 2/10,000
   C. 2/100,000
   D. 2/1000,000
9. **What percentage of pregnancies achieved after tubal sterilization will result in ectopic pregnancy?**
   A. 25%
   B. 33%
   C. 50%
   D. 75%
10. **What is the recommended antibiotic choice for laparoscopic tubal sterilization?**
    A. Cefazolin
    B. Doxycycline
    C. Clindamycin
    D. Not recommended
11. **Which of the following should <u>not</u> be included in counseling prior to tubal sterilization?**
    A. Risks and benefits of anesthesia
    B. The procedure is reversible
    C. Alternative forms of contraception
    D. Benefits of sterilization
12. **True or false. When compared to tubal sterilization, vasectomy is safer, more effective, and less expensive.**
13. **What risk factor is associated with the highest risk of regret after tubal sterilization?**
    A. Procedure performed post abortion
    B. Low parity
    C. Young age <30
    D. Unmarried status

14. **What level of sensory block is recommended for transvaginal cervical cerclage?**
    A. T4–T6
    B. T6–T8
    C. T8–T10
    D. T10–T12
15. **Which of the following is correct regarding postpartum tubal ligation?**
    A. The procedure is considered urgent
    B. The Medicaid consent form must be signed 72 h prior to the procedure
    C. The Medicaid consent form does not have to be available at the time of the procedure
    D. There are no known clinical biases that increase the rate of unfulfilled tubal ligation requests

Answers and Explanations

1. **D.** Cerclage may be indicated in each of the following situations: (**A**) there is a history indicated cerclage [1], (**B**) there is a physical exam indicating cerclage [2, 3], and (**C**) there is an ultrasound indicating cerclage [3].
2. **D.** If there is evidence of a unilateral sensory block, withdraw the epidural catheter 1–2 cm before administering an additional epidural bolus. (**A**), (**B**), and (**C**) are correct statements [4].
3. **B.** (**A**) is too high of a block. (**B**) will provide adequate anesthesia for postpartum tubal ligation. (**C**) and (**D**) will not provide adequate anesthesia for postpartum tubal ligation [5].
4. **C.** (**A**) Airway edema seen in pregnancy does not resolve immediately [6]. (**B**) Functional residual capacity increases immediately after delivery [7]. (**C**) Cardiac output does increase in the immediate postpartum setting [8]. (**D**) Increased aspiration risk seen in pregnant women is still seen in the immediate postpartum setting, often when tubal ligation is performed [9].
5. **False**. Local anesthetic requirement for neuraxial anesthesia is decreased in pregnancy but may return to baseline within 24 h postpartum. Patients undergoing postpartum tubal ligation may require a higher dose of local anesthetics than patients undergoing a cesarean section [7].
6. **E.** All the above are benefits of tubal ligation [10–12].
7. **False**. Minilaparotomy is typically used for postpartum procedures, whereas laparoscopy is used for interval procedures [13].
8. **C.** The mortality rate for tubal sterilization in the USA is estimated to be 2/100,000. Most deaths are secondary to complications of general anesthesia such as hypoventilation or cardiopulmonary arrest [14].
9. **B.** Pregnancy after tubal sterilization is rare, but of those, one-third of post-sterilization pregnancies are ectopic [15].
10. **D.** When entry into the bowel or vagina is not anticipated, antibiotic prophylaxis is not recommended for diagnostic or operative laparoscopy [16].

11. **B.** Patients should be informed that sterilization is permanent and not intended to be reversible [17]. (**A**), (**C**), and (**D**) should be part of the preoperative counseling.
12. **True.** Vasectomy is safer, more effective, and less expensive than tubal sterilization [18].
13. **C.** Women who have tubal sterilization before age 30 are 4 times more likely to regret sterilization. Despite this, age should not be a barrier to sterilization, barring legal age limits dictated by each state. Postabortion sterilization was not associated with increased regret. Low parity and unmarried status have been associated with regret, but not as much as young age [19].
14. **C.** The recommended sensory block for transvaginal cervical cerclage is T8–T10 (**A**). T6–T8 (**B**) level is too high of a block for cerclage. Levels at or above T4 can result in cardiopulmonary complications. T10–T12 (**D**) would not provide adequate anesthesia for a transvaginal cerclage [20].
15. **A.** Postpartum tubal ligation is considered urgent and should not delay hospital discharge [21]. Medicaid consent form (**B**) must be signed at least 30 days prior to the procedure and available (**C**) at the time of the procedure. (**D**) Clinical biases toward patients who are young, black, and/or unmarried increase the risk of unfulfilled tubal ligation requests [22, 23].

References

1. Lazar P, Gueguen S, Dreyfus J, Renaud R, Pontonnier G, Papiernik E. Multicentred controlled trial of cervical cerclage in women at moderate risk of preterm delivery. Br J Obstet Gynaecol. 1984;91:731–5.
2. Althuisius SM, Dekker GA, Hummel P, Bekedam DJ, vanGeijn HP. Results of the cervical incompetence prevention randomized cerclage trial (CIPRACT): therapeutic cerclage with bed rest versus bed rest alone. Am J Obstet Gynecol. 2001;185:1106–12.
3. Kurup M, Goldkrand JW. Cervical incompetence: elective, emergent, or urgent cerclage. Am J Obstet Gynecol. 1999;181:240–6.
4. Guzman ER, Forster JK, Vintzileos AM, Ananth CV, Walters C, Gipson K. Pregnancy outcomes in women treated with elective versus ultrasound-indicated cervical cerclage. Ultrasound Obstet Gynecol. 1998;12:323–7.
5. McKenzie C, Akdagli S, Abir G, Carvalho B. Postpartum tubal ligation: a retrospective review of anesthetic management at a single institution and a practice survey of academic institutions. J Clin Anesth. 2017;43:39–46. https://doi.org/10.1016/j.jclinane.2017.09.006. Epub 2017 Oct 3.
6. Vincent RD Jr, Reid RW. Epidural anesthesia for postpartum tubal ligation using epidural catheters placed during labor. J Clin Anesth. 1993;5(4):289–91. https://doi.org/10.1016/0952-8180(93)90120-4.
7. Vanner RG, Goodman NW. Gastro-oesophageal reflux in pregnancy at term and after delivery. Anaesthesia. 1989;44(10):808–11. https://doi.org/10.1111/j.1365-2044.1989.tb09096.x.
8. Cugell DW, Frank NR, Gaensler EA, Badger TL. Pulmonary function in pregnancy. I. Serial observations in normal women. Am Rev Tuberc. 1953;67(5):568–97. https://doi.org/10.1164/art.1953.67.5.568.

9. Robson SC, Dunlop W, Moore M, Hunter S. Combined Doppler and echocardiographic measurement of cardiac output: theory and application in pregnancy. Br J Obstet Gynaecol. 1987;94(11):1014–27. https://doi.org/10.1111/j.1471-0528.1987.tb02285.x.
10. Bucklin BA, Smith CV. Postpartum tubal ligation: safety, timing, and other implications for anesthesia. Anesth Analg. 1999;89(5):1269–74.
11. Irwin KL, Weiss NS, Lee NC, Peterson HB. Tubal sterilization, hysterectomy, and the subsequent occurrence of epithelial ovarian cancer. Am J Epidemiol. 1991;134:362–9.
12. Kost K, Singh S, Vaughan B, Trussell J, Bankole A. Estimates of contraceptive failure from the 2002 National Survey of family growth. Contraception. 2008;77:10–21.
13. Green MM, Vicario SJ, Sanfilippo JS, Lochhead SA. Acute pelvic inflammatory disease after surgical sterilization. Ann Emerg Med. 1991;20:344–7.
14. Westhoff C, Davis A. Tubal sterilization: focus on the U.S. experience. Fertil Steril. 2000;73:913–22.
15. Peterson HB, DeStefano F, Rubin GL, Greenspan JR, Lee NC, Ory HW. Deaths attributable to tubal sterilization in the United States, 1977 to 1981. Am J Obstet Gynecol. 1983;146:131–6.
16. Peterson HB, Xia Z, Hughes JM, Wilcox LS, Tylor LR, Trussell J. The risk of ectopic pregnancy after tubal sterilization. U.S. Collaborative Review of Sterilization Working Group. N Engl J Med. 1997;336:762–7.
17. Morrill MY, Schimpf MO, Abed H, Carberry C, Margulies RU, White AB, et al. Antibiotic prophylaxis for selected gynecologic surgeries. Society of Gynecologic Surgeons Systematic Review Group. Int J Gynaecol Obstet. 2013;120:10–5. (Systematic Review).
18. Shreffler KM, McQuillan J, Greil AL, Johnson DR. Surgical sterilization, regret, and race: contemporary patterns. Soc Sci Res. 2015;50:31–45.
19. Bartz D, Greenberg JA. Sterilization in the United States. Rev Obstet Gynecol. 2008;1:23–32.
20. Curtis KM, Mohllajee AP, Peterson HB. Regret following female sterilization at a young age: a systematic review. Contraception. 2006;73:205–10.
21. Aaronson J, Goodman S. Obstetric anesthesia: not just for cesareans and labor. Semin Perinatol. 2014;38(6):378–85. https://doi.org/10.1053/j.semperi.2014.07.005. Epub 2014 Aug 19.
22. Committee on Health Care for Underserved Women. Committee opinion no. 530: access to postpartum sterilization. Obstet Gynecol. 2012;120(1):212–5.
23. Seibel-Seamon J, Visintine JF, Leiby BE, Weinstein L. Factors predictive for failure to perform postpartum tubal ligations following vaginal delivery. J Reprod Med. 2009;54(3):160–4.

Non-obstetric Surgery in Pregnancy

Benjamin Kuo

Questions

1. **Which of the following is the best positioning during surgery for a pregnant patient in the 2nd or 3rd trimester?**
   A. Supine
   B. Left lateral tilt at a 15-degree angle
   C. Right lateral tilt at a 15-degree angle
   D. Reverse Trendelenburg
2. **Which of the following is the most appropriate induction plan for a 33-year-old G2P1, 16-week-old pregnant woman who is otherwise healthy with a reassuring airway exam and is going for a laparoscopic appendectomy?**
   A. Awake fiberoptic intubation with Precedex infusion
   B. Rapid sequence induction with propofol and succinylcholine
   C. Regular induction with 0.6 mg/kg rocuronium
   D. Regular induction without any paralytics
3. **A completely elective surgery in a parturient should be performed:**
   A. First trimester
   B. Second trimester
   C. Third trimester
   D. Post pregnancy
4. **Which of the following diagnoses and treatments, when diagnosed in the first trimester, should be postponed until the second trimester?**
   A. Perforated peptic ulcer

B. Kuo (✉)
Department of Anesthesiology, Riverside University Health System,
Moreno Valley, CA, USA

Department of Anesthesiology and Perioperative Medicine, University of California, Irvine,
Orange, CA, USA
e-mail: B.Kuo@ruhealth.org

A. C. Sinha, I. F. Pasca (eds.), *Peripartum Care of the Pregnant Patient*,
https://doi.org/10.1007/978-3-031-62756-9_21

   B. Necrotizing fasciitis of the lower extremity
   C. Dental abscess causing airway compromise
   D. None of the above
5. **Which of the following is NOT an appropriate setting for non-obstetric surgery to be performed on a parturient?**
   A. A large academic tertiary referral hospital
   B. Small community hospital with an obstetric, neonatal, and pediatric service readily available
   C. Stand-alone surgery center
   D. Outpatient surgery center attached to a tertiary care hospital
6. **If the fetus is viable when the parturient is undergoing a procedure under anesthesia, which of the following monitors should be utilized perioperatively?**
   A. Standard ASA monitors
   B. Electronic fetal heart monitor
   C. Contraction monitoring
   D. All of the above
7. **Which of the following medications has been shown to be clearly hazardous to the human fetus?**
   A. Propofol
   B. Fentanyl
   C. Rocuronium
   D. None of the above
8. **A catecholamine surge due to inadequate depth of anesthesia in a parturient may be harmful to the fetus because it may cause:**
   A. Fetal awareness
   B. Impaired uteroplacental perfusion
   C. Increased bleeding risk
   D. Oligohydramnios
9. **Studies have shown an increase in the incidence of the following in pregnant patients undergoing non-obstetric surgeries:**
   A. Spontaneous abortion
   B. Premature labor
   C. Preterm delivery
   D. All of the above
10. **Which of the following prophylactic measures in a pregnant patient undergoing surgery has NOT been shown to have proven benefit and thus should not be routinely administered?**
   A. Perioperative antibiotics
   B. Venous thromboembolism mechanical or chemical prophylaxis
   C. Tocolytic prophylaxis
   D. Aspiration prophylaxis
11. **Fetal heart rate monitoring first becomes practical and should be utilized perioperatively after what weeks of gestation?**
   A. 8 weeks

B. 12 weeks
C. 20 weeks
D. 28 weeks

12. **Which of the following intracranial tumors present a unique challenge in pregnant patients due to their ability to rapidly increase in size during pregnancy?**
    A. Meningioma
    B. Glioblastoma
    C. Glioma
    D. Lymphoma
13. **Maternal airway edema begins at what stage?**
    A. First trimester
    B. Second trimester
    C. Third trimester
    D. Beginning of labor
14. **What type of anesthesia is most performed for non-obstetric surgeries in pregnant patients?**
    A. Regional anesthesia
    B. Spinal anesthesia
    C. Deep sedation
    D. General anesthesia
15. **Which of the following is an indication for the EXIT (ex utero intrapartum) procedure?**
    A. Fetal cervical mass
    B. Fetal mediastinal mass
    C. Tracheal atresia
    D. All of the above

Answers and Explanations

1. **B.** Left lateral tilt in a pregnant patient decreases aortocaval compression by the gravid uterus compared with the supine position, which in turn improves venous return and helps with hemodynamic stability. Many times, a pillow or a bump is placed under the right hip to aid with this left tilt.
2. **B**. Patients with a gravid uterus are automatically considered to have a high aspiration risk and are not properly NPO. Therefore, rapid sequence induction is the recommended plan to secure the airway for surgery, regardless of whether the patient has been NPO for greater than 8 h.
3. **D.** A completely elective surgery should be postponed until after delivery of the fetus. Any surgery during pregnancy can pose a risk in terms of premature labor, preterm delivery, and other unwanted risks. Medically necessary surgery should be offered regardless of the trimester due to increased risks to the mother and fetus if delayed.

4. **D.** Peptic ulcer perforation, lower extremity necrotizing fasciitis, and Ludwig's angina are all life-threatening, emergent surgical conditions. Therefore, they should all be performed as soon as possible without any delays. Life-threatening surgeries should not be delayed due to pregnancy status because a delay will increase the risk to both the mother and the fetus.
5. **C.** Due to the risk of premature labor, fetal compromise, and preterm delivery, non-obstetric surgeries performed on pregnant patients should be in a setting where there is an obstetrician with privileges to perform a C-section and a pediatrician and neonatologist readily available.
6. **D**. In addition to standard ASA monitors, after the fetus becomes viable, it is routine practice to perform electronic fetal heart monitoring and contraction monitoring perioperatively to monitor for fetal well-being and signs of preterm labor with a possibility of emergent delivery.
7. **D.** Although ethically challenging to perform studies and research on medications and their effects on the fetus, no evidence to date has proven any anesthetic medication to be clearly hazardous to the human fetus.
8. **B**. The fetal circulation is primarily dependent on uteroplacental perfusion, as is evident for all disease processes that compromise uteroplacental perfusion. Thus, physiologic effects induced by light anesthesia can cause a catecholamine surge that will potentially lead to detrimental effects on uteroplacental perfusion and harm the fetus.
9. **D**. It is well-known that surgical interventions during pregnancy for non-obstetric procedures increase the risk of spontaneous abortion, premature labor, and preterm delivery. The underlying cause is multifactorial and includes surgical manipulation of the uterus.
10. **C.** The pregnant patient poses various unique challenges to the anesthesiologist, including risk of aspiration, venous thromboembolism, and preterm labor. Many of these risks have evidence-based strategies for mitigation, such as rapid sequence induction to secure the airway and VTE prophylaxis via mechanical or chemical measures. However, prophylactic tocolytic administration has not been shown to benefit pregnancy, nor does it have supporting evidence that it prevents or mitigates preterm labor.
11. **C.** Perioperative fetal heart rate and contraction monitoring becomes meaningful after approximately 18–22 weeks of gestation. At that point, fetal heart rate and contraction monitoring can help in fetal delivery management decisions by both the anesthesiologists and obstetricians. Hence, it is part of the routine monitoring for perioperative management of a parturient going for surgery. If the fetus is previable, the heart rate should be monitored with a doppler at minimum before and after the surgery or more frequently if individualized care can impact fetal well-being.
12. **A**. "Gestational meningioma" has been described as a phenomenon where a meningioma increases in size very rapidly in comparison to a nonpregnant patient with a similar grade meningioma. The cause of the rapid growth is likely multifactorial, although many studies have looked into the presence of estrogen and progesterone receptors present on these meningiomas.

13. **A**. Maternal airway management is well-known to challenge in anesthesiology. Manipulation of the airway is avoided as much as possible, as the risk of inability to secure an airway is much higher compared to the general population. The causes of the increased difficulty of the airway include airway edema, increased soft tissue, increased vasculature of the oropharynx, and changes in chest/abdomen physiology. These changes occur very early in pregnancy, starting in the first trimester.
14. **D.** Although neuraxial techniques are most used for C-sections, the most common anesthetic type used for non-obstetric-related surgeries is general anesthesia.
15. **D.** Fetal cervical mass, fetal mediastinal mass, and tracheal atresia are all indications for the EXIT procedure.

Further Readings

1. American College of Obstetricians and Gynecologists. Nonobstetric surgery during pregnancy. ACOG Committee Opinion No. 775. Obstet Gynecol. 2019;133:e285–6.
2. Upadya M, Saneesh PJ. Anesthesia for nonobstetric surgery during pregnancy. Indian J Anaesth. 2016;60(4):234–41. https://doi.org/10.4103/0019-5049.179445.
3. Haggerty E, Daly J. Anesthesia and nonobstetric surgery in pregnancy. BJA Educ. 2021;21(2):42–3. https://doi.org/10.1016/j.bjae.2020.11.002.
4. Hortobágyi T, Bencze J, Murnyák B, Kouhsari MC, Bognár L, Marko-Varga G. Pathophysiology of meningioma growth in pregnancy. Open Med (Wars). 2017;12:195–200. https://doi.org/10.1515/med-2017-0029. Published 2017 Jul 13
5. Garcia PJ, Olutoye OO, Ivey RT, Olutoye OA, Riou B. Case scenario: anesthesia for maternal-fetal surgery: the ex uterointrapartum therapy (EXIT) procedure. Anesthesiology. 2011;114:1446–52.

Tocolytic and Uterotonic Agents

Jeffery Thomas, Hanna Mandell, and Leonard J. Soloniuk

Questions

1. Acute tocolysis is associated with:
   A. Reduced rates of emergency cesarean sections for non-reassuring fetal heart rate (NRFH) tracings
   B. Increased rates of neonatal intensive care unit admissions
   C. Improved short-term fetal outcomes
   D. Shorter time-to-delivery intervals
2. **Nifedipine is a calcium channel blocker used for acute tocolysis that:**
   A. Crosses the placenta
   B. Can only be given IV
   C. Does not have a hemodynamic side effect profile
   D. Is known to precipitate fetal acidemia
3. **Which of the following is a contraindication to the use of an ergot alkaloid?**
   A. Hypotension
   B. Fetal growth restriction
   C. Prior cesarean section
   D. Preeclampsia
4. **Carboprost is a synthetic PGF2a analog with the main adverse effect of:**

J. Thomas
Riverside University Health System, Moreno Valley, CA, USA
e-mail: Je.thomas@ruhealth.org

H. Mandell
Universirty of California Riverside, Riverside, CA, USA
e-mail: hanna.mandell@medsch.ucr.edu

L. J. Soloniuk (✉)
Riverside University Health System, Moreno Valley, CA, USA

Loma Linda University, Loma Linda, CA, USA
e-mail: l.soloniuk@ruhealth.org

A. C. Sinha, I. F. Pasca (eds.), *Peripartum Care of the Pregnant Patient*,
https://doi.org/10.1007/978-3-031-62756-9_22

A. Tachysystole
B. Bronchospasm
C. Tachycardia
D. Hyperpyrexia

5. **Which of these tocolytics is commonly used for external cephalic versions?**
   A. Nicardipine
   B. Indomethacin
   C. Atosiban
   D. Terbutaline
6. **Which is true about the use of calcium channel blockers for external cephalic versions?**
   A. Their application has not been widely studied.
   B. They are superior to the use of betamimetics.
   C. They reduce the likelihood of emergent cesarean sections.
   D. They reduce maternal pain perception during the procedure.
7. **In resource-limited settings where intravenous oxytocin is unavailable, a preferred uterotonic might be:**
   A. IM oxytocin
   B. Oral nifedipine
   C. Inhaled betamimetic
   D. Sublingual misoprostol
8. **Immediately following a cesarean section, what pharmacologic uterotonic is recommended to prevent postpartum hemorrhage?**
   A. Methylergonovine
   B. Carboprost
   C. Oxytocin
   D. Misoprostol
9. **What is the recommended loading dose for oxytocin infusion in a patient undergoing a cesarean section?**
   A. 3–5 IU given IV over 1 min
   B. 3–5 IU given IV over 15 s
   C. 6–8 IU given IV over 1 min
   D. 5 IU given IV over 10 s
10. **If the initial loading and infusion dose of oxytocin for an intrapartum cesarean section does not produce adequate uterine tone, the next best step is to administer:**
    A. Another dose of 10 IU given IV
    B. Another dose of 3 IU given IV
    C. A continuous oxytocin infusion of 3 IU/h
    D. A second-line uterotonic
11. **Magnesium sulfate is a tocolytic agent used for preterm labor contractions. Which of the following is true about magnesium sulfate's mechanism of action?**
    A. It increases intracellular calcium levels, which causes vasodilation.
    B. It is a competitive antagonist that competes with calcium for binding sites in vascular smooth muscle.

C. It decreases the production of prostaglandin I2, which causes decreased platelet aggregation
D. It decreases nitric oxide production.

12. **Which of the following neuromuscular blocking agents does NOT have a duration of action that is potentiated by magnesium sulfate?**
A. Rocuronium
B. Cisatracurium
C. Succinylcholine
D. Vecuronium

13. **Methylergonovine (methylergometrine) is an ergot alkaloid used as a uterotonic agent. Which of the following maternal conditions is a relative contraindication?**
A. Gestational diabetes
B. Preeclampsia
C. Asthma
D. Hyperemesis gravidarum

14. **Which of the following uterotonics must be administered intramuscularly?**
A. Misoprostol
B. Methylergonovine (methylergometrine)
C. Carboprost
D. Nifedipine

15. **What is the first-line pharmacologic treatment for a retained placenta?**
A. Continuous oxytocin infusion
B. Intramuscular oxytocin followed by continuous infusion
C. Manual extraction of the placenta
D. Prostaglandin analog (carboprost, misoprostol)

16. **Which is correct about patients with preeclampsia treated with magnesium undergoing cesarean sections?**
A. They require a lower intraoperative dose of oxytocin to achieve adequate uterine tone.
B. They require a higher intraoperative dose of oxytocin to achieve adequate uterine tone.
C. The use of oxytocin is contraindicated in these patients.
D. Oxytocin should only be administered if the blood pressure is under 140/90.

17. **Which of the following has been shown to reduce blood loss when used in conjunction with oxytocin during cesarean sections?**
A. Carbetocin
B. Carboprost
C. Mifepristone
D. Misoprostol

18. **At high doses, oxytocin can commonly cause which of the following side effects?**
A. Hypotension
B. Hypertension
C. Bradycardia

D. Dyspnea

19. **Administration of which drug in preeclamptic patients undergoing cesarean section with general anesthesia may be administered to mitigate the consequential hypertension after laryngoscopy?**
    A. Hydralazine
    B. Labetalol
    C. Magnesium
    D. Nitroglycerin
20. **Which of the following tocolytic agents specifically inhibits the entry of calcium into uterine smooth muscle by working on T-type calcium channels?**
    A. Terbutaline
    B. Magnesium sulfate
    C. Nifedipine
    D. Nonsteroidal anti-inflammatories

Answers and Explanations

1. **C.** A meta-analysis of randomized controlled trials found that administering tocolytic agents for intrapartum non-reassuring fetal status were effective in improving short-term fetal outcomes, which were defined as Apgar score, umbilical artery pH, and base deficit. Rates of NICU admissions also decreased in response to tocolytic therapy. Tocolytics did not affect the number of cesarean sections performed in response to NRFH, but they did allow an increase in the time-to-delivery interval, as well as an increase in decision-to-delivery intervals [1].
2. **A.** Nifedipine is a vasodilator that decreases the resistance indices of the uterine arteries and the umbilical artery [2]. It also decreases the pulsatility index of the middle cerebral artery and is proven to be a superior tocolytic due to positive effects on both the maternal and fetal vessels [3]. Nifedipine can be administered PO and IV. Because nifedipine vasodilates the maternal and fetal vessels, it is less likely to cause fetal acidemia, which would be seen because of fetal vessel vasoconstriction.
3. **D.** Preeclampsia can lead to reduced blood flow and perfusion to vital organs, including the liver and kidneys. The vasoconstrictive effects of ergot alkaloids can further reduce blood flow to these organs, increasing the risk of organ ischemia and potential organ damage. Methylergonovine sustains uterine contractions via activation of adrenergic, dopaminergic, and serotonergic receptors [4]. In patients with either preeclampsia and/or hypertension, other uterotonic agents with a more favorable safety profile, such as oxytocin or prostaglandin analogs, are preferred [4].
4. **B.** Carboprost can precipitate bronchospasm, particularly in asthmatic patients, by stimulating smooth muscle contraction [4]. It is given intramuscularly at a dose of 250 mcg and cannot be administered intravenously [5]. Tachysystole is

not an adverse effect, as carboprost does not affect the rate at which the myometrium contracts. It does not act on beta-adrenergic receptors in the cardiac myocytes and therefore is unlikely to cause tachycardia. Hyperpyrexia is more common following the administration of misoprostol, another prostaglandin analog that similarly induces uterine contractions [4].

5. **D.** Terbutaline is a beta-2 receptor agonist that inhibits endometrial contraction via relaxation of the myometrial smooth muscle cells [6]. In cases of fetal malpresentation that require an external cephalic version (ECV), a tocolytic is typically administered to relax the uterus [7]. Nifedipine, which also causes smooth muscle relaxation of the myometrium by inhibiting calcium influx, has not been adequately studied to establish effectiveness in decreasing the rate of emergency cesarean sections and in increasing ECV success rates when compared to terbutaline [7]. Indomethacin is not as effective as terbutaline, and atosiban is an oxytocin receptor antagonist that does not directly inhibit myometrial contraction.
6. **A.** Calcium channel blockers, such as nifedipine, have been studied as effective tocolytic agents for preterm labor [3, 8]. Their use as tocolytic agents for external cephalic versions lacks sufficient evidence to compare them to terbutaline, which is a betamimetic agent. Calcium channel blockers do not have any consistent correlation to emergent cesarean sections following external cephalic versions, nor do they act on nociceptors to reduce pain perception during the version [7].
7. **A.** Oxytocin receptors are expressed throughout the body, and as pregnancy progresses, the number of oxytocin receptors in the uterus is upregulated [4]. Administration of oxytocin as a uterotonic both directly contracts the myometrium and stimulates the synthesis of prostaglandin PGF2a within the endometrium [4]. Since oxytocin is the preferred uterotonic agent, it may be administered intramuscularly [9]. IM oxytocin has an onset of action within 3–7 min and exerts its effects for 30–60 min.
8. **C.** Oxytocin is the preferred uterotonic that is typically administered in the immediate postpartum period. It directly stimulates contraction of the myometrium and synthesis of prostaglandins in the endometrium [9]. Methylergonovine is an ergot alkaloid that stimulates uterine contractions via activation of adrenergic, dopaminergic, and serotonergic receptors [1]. This is a second-line treatment option for postpartum hemorrhage prevention [4]. Carboprost is a synthetic prostaglandin analog (PGF2a), although it is avoided in patients with asthma due to the possible adverse effect of bronchospasm [5]. Misoprostol is another prostaglandin analog (PGE1) , and its most notable side effect is hyperpyrexia [4]. Prostaglandin analogues stimulate myometrial contraction by activating EP1, EP3, FP, and TP receptors in the myometrium, and they are often used as a second-line treatment [4].
9. **A**. The recommended loading dose for oxytocin infusion in a patient undergoing a cesarean section can vary depending on institutional protocols and the specific clinical situation. However, a common loading dose for oxytocin in this context is typically around 3–5 international units (IU) administered

intravenously (IV) over 1 mi. This is then followed by an infusion dose, commonly set to a rate of 20–40 milliunits per minute (mU/min). This equates to 1.2–2.4 international units (IU) per hour [10]. The goal of the oxytocin infusion is to maintain uterine contractions to control bleeding, especially in response to uterine atony, during and after the cesarean section [11].

10. **B.** Two additional doses of oxytocin can be administered IV following an unsuccessful response to an initial loading dose [4, 10]. A continuous infusion dose is recommended after a trial of two additional 3 IU doses, and administering a second-line uterotonic is the next recommendation if the infusion intervention remains unsuccessful [10].
11. **B**. Magnesium sulfate is a calcium receptor antagonist that vasodilates uterine arteries by competing with calcium for binding sites in vascular smooth muscle cells. It decreases intracellular calcium levels, thus causing vasodilation. The production of prostaglandin I2 is increased in response to magnesium sulfate and decreased platelet aggregation. The increased production of nitric oxide is an additional mechanism of action of magnesium sulfate that ultimately causes vasodilation [12, 13].
12. **C.** Magnesium can be safely used for rapid sequence intubation that involves the administration of succinylcholine. It prolongs the effects of rocuronium, cisatracurium, and vecuronium by suppressing acetylcholine release at the presynaptic membrane, thereby further decreasing the amount of acetylcholine in the neuromuscular junction. These nondepolarizing neuromuscular blockers must be titrated appropriately using a twitch monitor to determine the depth of paralysis [13, 14].
13. **B.** The use of methylergonovine (methylergometrine) as a tocolytic is relatively contraindicated for patients with preeclampsia, gestational hypertension, and preexisting hypertension. Gestational diabetes, asthma, and a history of hyperemesis gravidarum are not contraindications [5].
14. **C.** Carboprost is a uterotonic agent that must be given intramuscularly, not intravenously. Misoprostol can be administered intrauterine, orally, sublingually, vaginally, and rectally. Methylergonovine (methylergometrine) can be given either intramuscularly or intravenously. Nifedipine is not a uterotonic; it is a tocolytic that is administered either orally or intravenously [5].
15. **A**. The first-line pharmacologic treatment for a retained placenta is a continuous infusion of oxytocin. Intramuscular oxytocin can be used prophylactically to prevent postpartum hemorrhage, but it does not supersede the effectiveness of a continuous infusion in the setting of a retained placenta. Oxytocin is preferred because it increases the overall uterine tone, as well as produces powerful phasic contractions. Manual extraction can be performed under anesthesia with agents such as fentanyl, midazolam, and ketamine. Prostaglandin analogs such as carboprost and misoprostol increase contraction strength for a duration of approximately 90 min, but their role as uterotonics is less effective than oxytocin in this scenario [11].
16. **B.** Patients with preeclampsia undergoing magnesium therapy require a higher intraoperative dose of oxytocin during cesarean sections. A prospective study

found that the effective dose in 90% of the population (ED90) of oxytocin was significantly higher in preeclamptic patients receiving magnesium sulfate in comparison to normotensive patients not receiving magnesium sulfate [15]. Oxytocin is not contraindicated in preeclampsia, as it is the recommended treatment for postpartum hemorrhage prevention. Additionally, oxytocin can be administered to patients with hypertension.

17. **D**. Intrauterine misoprostol has been studied as an adjunct treatment for postpartum hemorrhage when given in conjunction with oxytocin. A 2022 study examined different dosages of misoprostol as an additional uterotonic given during cesarean sections, and researchers found that 400 mcg, 600 mcg, and 800 mcg yielded a decreased incidence of postpartum hemorrhage [16]. 400 mcg was determined to be the preferred dose, as it minimized side effects and proved to be equally as effective at preventing bleeding when compared to higher dosages. Carbetocin is an oxytocin analog that is not used in the United States, and carboprost and mifepristone are two uterotonics that are second-line treatments for postpartum hemorrhage.
18. **A.** Oxytocin promotes systemic vasodilation of smooth muscle cells, leading to hypotension if administered in high doses as a uterotonic agent [17]. It can also cause reflex tachycardia [17]. Hypertension, bradycardia, and dyspnea are not likely side effects of an oxytocin infusion.
19. **C.** Administering a bolus of magnesium sulfate after induction has been shown to reduce the resulting hypertension in patients with preeclampsia undergoing cesarean sections under general anesthesia. If the patient has received magnesium preoperatively, the loading dose is a bolus of 30 mg/kg. Patients who are magnesium naive should receive a bolus of 45 mg/kg [18].
20. **C.** Calcium channel blockers, such as nifedipine, specifically work on T-type calcium channels by inhibiting the entry of calcium into uterine smooth muscle. Terbutaline is a beta-adrenergic agonist that increases cyclic AMP (cAMP) to cause smooth muscle relaxation. They do not specifically inhibit calcium entry. Magnesium sulfate inhibits the entry of calcium into uterine smooth muscle, but its mechanism of action is not through T-type calcium channels. Nonsteroidal anti-inflammatories, like indomethacin, inhibit cyclooxygenases and prostaglandin production but do not directly affect calcium channels [19]. They are also contraindicated in the third trimester of pregnancy [20].

References

1. Xodo S, de Heus R, Berghella V, Londero AP. Acute tocolysis for intrapartum nonreassuring fetal status: how often does it prevent cesarean delivery? A systematic review and meta-analysis of randomized controlled trials. Am J Obstet Gynecol MFM. 2022;4(5):100639. https://doi.org/10.1016/j.ajogmf.2022.100639.
2. Güden M, Akkurt MÖ, Eriş Yalçın S, Coşkun B, Akkurt I, Yavuz A, Yirci B, Kandemir NÖ. A comparison of the effects of the most commonly used tocolytic agents on maternal and fetal blood flow. Turk J Obstet Gynecol. 2016;13(2):85–9. https://doi.org/10.4274/tjod.25993.

3. Grzesiak M, Ahmed RB, Wilczynski J. 48-hours administration of nifedipine in spontaneous preterm labor—Doppler blood flow assessment of placental and fetal circulation. Neuro Endocrinol Lett. 2013;34(7):687–92.
4. Heesen M, Carvalho B, Carvalho JCA, Duvekot JJ, Dyer RA, Lucas DN, McDonnell N, Orbach-Zinger S, Kinsella SM. International consensus statement on the use of uterotonic agents during caesarean section. Anaesthesia. 2019;74(10):1305–19. https://doi.org/10.1111/anae.14757.
5. https://anesthesia.ucsf.edu/sites/anesthesia.ucsf.edu/files/wysiwyg/Obstetric_Anesthesia_Pocket_Guide_2020.pdf.
6. Fernandez C, Bloom S, Smulian J, Ananth C, Wendel G. A randomized placebo-controlled evaluation of terbutaline for external cephalic version. Obstetr Gynecol. 1997;90(5):775–9. https://doi.org/10.1016/S0029-7844(97)00440-7.
7. Collaris R, Tan P. Oral nifepidine versus subcutaneous terbutaline tocolysis for external cephalic version: a double-blind randomised trial. BJOG: Int J Obstetr Gynaecol. 2008;116(1):74–81. https://doi.org/10.1111/j.1471-0528.2008.01991.
8. Flenady V, Wojcieszek AM, Papatsonis DN, Stock OM, Murray L, Jardine LA, Carbonne B. Calcium channel blockers for inhibiting preterm labour and birth. Cochrane Database Syst Rev. 2014;2014(6):CD002255. https://doi.org/10.1002/14651858.CD002255.pub2.
9. Adnan N, Conlan-Trant R, McCormick C, Boland F, Murphy DJ. Intramuscular versus intravenous oxytocin to prevent postpartum haemorrhage at vaginal delivery: randomised controlled trial. BMJ. 2018;362:k3546. https://doi.org/10.1136/bmj.k3546. PMID: 30181338; PMCID: PMC6122278.
10. Sumikura H, Inada E. Uterotonics and tocolytics for anesthesiologists. Curr Opin Anaesthesiol. 2016;29(3):282–7. https://doi.org/10.1097/ACO.0000000000000332.
11. Weeks AD. The retained placenta. Afr Health Sci. 2001;1(1):36–41. PMID: 12789132; PMCID: PMC2704447
12. Crowther CA, Brown J, McKinlay CJ, et al. Magnesium sulphate for preventing preterm birth in threatened preterm labour. Cochrane Database Syst Rev. 2014;(8):CD001060.
13. Euser AG, Cipolla MJ. Magnesium sulfate for the treatment of eclampsia: a brief review. Stroke. 2009;40(4):1169–75.
14. Lu JF, Nightingale CH. Magnesium sulfate in eclampsia and pre-eclampsia: pharmacokinetic principles. Clin Pharmacokinet. 2000;38(4):305–14.
15. Tyagi A, Mohan A, Singh Y, Luthra A, Garg D, Malhotra RK. Effective dose of prophylactic oxytocin infusion during cesarean delivery in 90% population of nonlaboring patients with preeclampsia receiving magnesium sulfate therapy and normotensives: an up-down sequential allocation dose-response study. Anesth Analg. 2022;134(2):303–11. https://doi.org/10.1213/ANE.0000000000005701.
16. Sringamwong W, Saokaew S, Mongkhon P. Optimal dose of misoprostol combined with oxytocin for preventing postpartum hemorrhage in cesarean section: a randomised controlled trial. Ann Med Surg (Lond). 2022;78:103931. https://doi.org/10.1016/j.amsu.2022.103931.
17. https://www.openanesthesia.org/keywords/uterotonic-agents-symptoms/.
18. https://www.openanesthesia.org/keywords/magnesium-in-pregnancy/.
19. Mayer C, Apodaca-Ramos I. Tocolysis. [Updated 2022 Sep 22]. In: StatPearls. Treasure Island, FL: StatPearls Publishing. p. 2023. Available from: https://www.ncbi.nlm.nih.gov/books/NBK562212.
20. Koren G, Florescu A, Moldovan Costei A, Boskovic R, Moretti ME. Nonsteroidal antiinflammatory drugs during third trimester and the risk of premature closure of the ductus arteriosus: a meta-analysis. Ann Pharmacother. 2006;40(5):824–9.

Hypertensive Disorders of Pregnancy

Alicia Cryer, Avery Lahodny, and Sarah Smithson

Questions

1. **Which antihypertensive would be preferred if a patient has a persistent severe range blood pressure and no peripheral IV?**
   A. Labetalol 20 mg IV
   B. Labetalol 200 mg orally
   C. Nifedipine IR 10 mg orally
   D. Hydralazine 25 mg orally
2. **What is the preferred medication used prophylactically as a continuous infusion to decrease the risk of the patient subsequently developing eclampsia when diagnosed with preeclampsia with severe features?**
   A. Phenytoin
   B. Magnesium
   C. Nimodipine
   D. Phenobarbital
3. **Which of the following antihypertensive medications are <u>not</u> used for urgent blood pressure control in pregnancy?**
   A. Labetalol
   B. Hydralazine
   C. Nifedipine
   D. Sodium nitroprusside

A. Cryer
University of Pennsylvania at Chester County Hospital, West Chester, PA, USA
e-mail: A.Cryer@ruhealth.org

A. Lahodny · S. Smithson (✉)
Riverside University Health System, Moreno Valley, CA, USA

Loma Linda University, Loma Linda, CA, USA
e-mail: s.smithson@ruhealth.org

A. C. Sinha, I. F. Pasca (eds.), *Peripartum Care of the Pregnant Patient*,
https://doi.org/10.1007/978-3-031-62756-9_23

4. **Magnesium sulfate is used in obstetrics for which indication(s)?**
   A. Fetal neuroprotection
   B. Preterm contractions
   C. Seizure prophylaxis in the setting of preeclampsia with severe features
   D. Treatment for hypertension
   E. A and C only
5. **A patient with a history of which of the following should be started on low-dose aspirin prophylactically for preeclampsia?**
   A. Multifetal gestation
   B. Systemic lupus erythematosus
   C. Chronic hypertension
   D. Type I or II diabetes
   E. All the above
6. **Ideally, when should patients start low-dose aspirin for the prevention of preeclampsia?**
   A. Prior to conception
   B. 12–16 weeks
   C. 28–32 weeks
   D. after 36 weeks
7. **The patient was a 27 y/o G2P1001 who was induced for preeclampsia with severe features at 36 weeks. She received 24 h of postpartum magnesium. On postpartum day 2, the patient was asymptomatic, and her blood pressure was in the normal range. She was discharged on no antihypertensive medications. When should she be seen again for a postpartum blood pressure check?**
   A. Within 12 h discharge
   B. 3–10 days postpartum
   C. 2 weeks postpartum
   D. 6 weeks postpartum
8. **A patient is administered 10 mg of oral nifedipine (immediate release) for sustained severe range blood pressures at 38 weeks. How soon would the blood pressure respond?**
   A. 1–2 min
   B. 20 min
   C. 5–10 min
   D. 60 min
9. **The patient is status post a vaginal delivery at 39 weeks. The neonate weighed 5150 g. During labor, she was treated multiple times for elevated blood pressure with IV labetalol. She was started on magnesium sulfate for seizure prophylaxis. Following delivery of the placenta, the obstetrician notes continued bleeding from uterine atony. Estimated blood loss is 600 ml. Which uterotonic drug is <u>contraindicated</u> in this patient?**
   A. Methergine
   B. Hemabate
   C. Pitocin

D. Misoprostol
E. Tranexamic acid

10. **Which of the following is not a consideration when choosing labetalol as the antihypertensive agent for urgent blood pressure control?**
    A. Asthma
    B. Bradycardia
    C. Heart block
    D. Tachycardia
11. **For a laboring patient, the decision has been made to perform a cesarean delivery for arrest of dilation at 34 weeks following the induction of labor for preeclampsia with severe features. Magnesium sulfate has already been administered for 8 h for seizure prophylaxis. How should magnesium sulfate be managed through delivery and postpartum?**
    A. Magnesium sulfate should be continued through delivery and for 24 h postpartum.
    B. Magnesium sulfate should be paused when cesarean delivery begins and restarted when the uterus is closed and continued for 24 h postpartum.
    C. Magnesium sulfate should be paused when cesarean delivery begins and restarted when the patient has reached the post anesthesia care unit and then continued for 24 h postpartum.
    D. Magnesium sulfate should be discontinued preoperatively.
12. **Which of the following medications is not routinely used for urgent control of high range blood pressures in the setting of preeclampsia?**
    A. Labetalol 20 mg IV
    B. Hydralazine 5 mg IV
    C. Lisinopril 5 mg
    D. Nifedipine 20 mg orally
13. **A 36 y/o G3P2002 presents for her prenatal visit at 18 weeks. She was found to have mild range blood pressure. She also had mild range blood pressures at her first visit at 12 weeks. She denied a history of hypertensive disorders of pregnancy, and she denied hypertension outside of pregnancy. She has never been on an antihypertensive medication. Urine dip in the office is negative for protein. She meets criteria for which of the following diagnosis(es)?**
    A. Gestational hypertension
    B. Preeclampsia without severe features
    C. Chronic hypertension
    D. Both A and C
14. **What blood pressure cutoff is considered a severe range in pregnancy and warrants immediate treatment if sustained after 15 min?**
    A. >150 mmHG SBP or > 100 mmHG DBP
    B. >150 mmHG SBP or >110 mmHG DBP
    C. >160 mmHG SBP or > 110 mmHG DBP
    D. >160 mmHG SBP or > 100 mmHG DBP

15. **Which of the following is <u>not a contraindication</u> to continuous infusion of magnesium?**
    A. Myasthenia gravis
    B. Hypokalemia
    C. Severe renal failure
    D. Cardiac ischemia
16. **If intravenous access is not yet established, what is the appropriate magnesium sulfate dose for the treatment of eclampsia?**
    A. 4 g intramuscular
    B. 16 g intramuscular
    C. 10 g intramuscular
    D. 2 g intraosseous
17. **Which of the following is the preferred treatment for magnesium toxicity?**
    A. Calcium gluconate 1 g IV
    B. Calcium chloride 3 g IV
    C. Protamine sulfate 1.5 mg IV
    D. Vitamin K 2 mg IV
18. **True or false: Concurrent administration of nifedipine and magnesium sulfate should be avoided given the increased risk of hypotension and neuromuscular blockade.**
    A. True
    B. False
19. **What is the desired therapeutic range of magnesium?**
    A. 4.8–9.6 mg/dL (4–8 mEq/L)
    B. 1.5–3.4 mg/dL (1–3 mEq/L)
    C. 10.2–12.5 mg/dL (8–10 mEq/L)
    D. 25.3–30.3 mg/dL (21–25 mEq/L)
20. **Which of the following is considered an appropriate treatment or management for parturients who suffer from pulmonary edema?**
    A. Carbamazepine
    B. Furosemide
    C. Perform chest X-ray every 2 h until resolution
    D. Goal of urine output greater than 20 mL/kg per hour
21. **True or false: Nonsteroidal anti-inflammatory drugs (NSAIDs) should be avoided in the postpartum period in patients with preeclampsia, as they are associated with an increase in blood pressure.**
    A. True
    B. False

Answers and Explanations

1. **C.** Answer choice A is inappropriate, as the patient does not have intravenous access established. Both oral labetalol and oral hydralazine have peak levels at least 1 h or more after administration, while oral immediate-release nifedipine is noted to work within 20 min. A systolic blood pressure greater than 160

mmHg and diastolic blood pressure greater than 110 mmHg increase the risk of maternal hemorrhagic stroke. Severe range systolic blood pressures are the most associated with stroke compared to severe range diastolic blood pressure or acuteness of elevation [1–3].

2. **B.** If the patient does not have any contraindications to magnesium sulfate administration, this is the preferred prophylaxis and treatment for eclampsia [1].
3. **D.** Sodium nitroprusside is the preferred treatment for hypertensive emergencies outside of pregnancy. Intravenous labetalol and hydralazine are well-studied for immediate treatment of severe range blood pressures in pregnancy. The starting dose of IV labetalol is 10–20 mg with guidelines to repeat blood pressure 10 min after administration. The preferred initial dose for IV hydralazine is 5–10 mg with guidelines to repeat blood pressure 20 min after administration. Nifedipine IR is an appropriate treatment and preferred when peripheral intravenous access has not yet been established [4, 5].
4. **E.** Magnesium sulfate halves the risk of eclampsia according to the findings of the *Magpie trial*, and it should be initiated for seizure prophylaxis in patients with preeclampsia with severe features [1, 4]. Magnesium sulfate also has fetal neuroprotective effects, such as reducing the incidence and severity of cerebral palsy. It is initiated for women before an anticipated preterm delivery prior to 32 weeks [6]. It is no longer used as a tocolytic, nor is it reliable as an antihypertensive.
5. **E.** Women who present with any of the high-risk factors for preeclampsia should be given low-dose aspirin for the duration of their pregnancy for preeclampsia prophylaxis. High-risk factors include a history of preeclampsia, multifetal gestation, chronic hypertension, type 1 or 2 diabetes, renal disease, and autoimmune disease. Additionally, patients with two or more moderate risk factors should also be prescribed low-dose aspirin. Moderate risk factors include nulliparity, obesity (BMI>30), family history of preeclampsia, advanced maternal age (age>35 by pregnancy due date), previous adverse pregnancy outcome, low socioeconomic status, and African American race [7].
6. **B**. There is the most significant risk reduction in severe preeclampsia when low-dose aspirin is started between 12 and 16 weeks of gestation [7].
7. **B.** Blood pressure evaluation is recommended between 3 and 10 days postpartum for women with a hypertensive disorder of pregnancy. This evaluation is critical, as greater than one-half of postpartum strokes occur within 10 days postpartum [8].
8. **B.** The onset of action for immediate release of oral nifedipine is 20 min. The onset of action for IV labetalol is 1–2 min. The onset of action for hydralazine (IV or IM) is 10–20 min [3].
9. **A**. Methergine is contraindicated for women with hypertension. Hemabate, pitocin, misoprostol are all uterotonic drugs that could be used in this scenario. Tranexamic acid is an antifibrinolytic agent also used routinely in the treatment of postpartum hemorrhage and may also be considered [9].

10. **D.** Labetalol is relatively contraindicated in a patient with a history of asthma due to risk for broncospasm. Other contraindications for labetalol include bradycardia with HR <50 bpm and heart block due to blocking beta-1 receptors in the heart [4].
11. **A.** Magnesium sulfate is given for seizure prophylaxis, and it should be continued through delivery and for 24 h postpartum for the most effective reduction in seizure incidence [4, 5].
12. **C.** Lisinopril is not an antihypertensive of choice for urgent treatment of severe range blood pressure. Angiotensin-converting enzyme inhibitors are generally avoided in pregnancy. In first-trimester exposure, there is concern for congenital fetal renal dysgenesis and calvarial hypoplasia. Use later in pregnancy is associated with risk for fetal growth restriction. Postpartum ACE inhibitors may be considered in low doses in breastfeeding patients but should be discontinued prior to conception of a future pregnancy [3].
13. **C.** Mild range blood pressures prior to 20 weeks are consistent with a diagnosis of chronic hypertension. Although this increases her risk of superimposed preeclampsia later in pregnancy (diagnosed after 20 weeks), she does not currently meet criteria [3].
14. **C.** A systolic blood pressure greater than 160 mmHg and diastolic blood pressure greater than 110 mmHg increase the risk of maternal hemorrhagic stroke. High-range systolic blood pressures are the most associated with stroke compared to severe range diastolic blood pressure or acuteness of elevation [1].
15. **B.** Hypocalcemia, not hypokalemia, is a contraindication to magnesium sulfate administration. Magnesium sulfate relaxes smooth muscles and results in blockade of calcium transport across cells [1].
16. **C.** Magnesium sulfate 10 g IM, 5 g IM in each buttock, is the initial treatment for eclampsia when no IV is established and there are no contraindications. Magnesium sulfate IM 4 g is subtherapeutic, while magnesium sulfate IM 16 g IM is considered supratherapeutic. Magnesium sulfate is not administered intraosseously [10, 11].
17. **A.** Calcium gluconate IV 1 g is the preferred treatment for magnesium toxicity reversal. Calcium chloride IV (1 g) can also be used. Protamine sulfate and vitamin K are the appropriate treatments for heparin reversal and warfarin reversal, respectively [11].
18. **B.** Retrospective studies have not demonstrated concern for neuromuscular blockade or severe hypotension despite concurrent administration of these calcium antagonists [12].
19. **A.** Answer choice (**B**) is subtherapeutic range and places the patient at increased risk of eclampsia. Answer choice C is the toxicity level associated with respiratory distress. Answer choice (**D**) is the level at which cardiac arrest can occur [13, 14].
20. **B.** Furosemide is a diuretic and should be administered to assist with the resolution of pulmonary edema. Carbmazepine can worsen pulmonary edema. Serial chest X-rays are not indicated in the setting of pulmonary edema. Patient respiratory status and improvement of pulmonary edema can be monitored with

physician exam, oxygen requirements, and urine output greater than 25–30 mL/kg/h.

21. **A.** NSAIDs remain the preferred medication over opioids in the postpartum period. Despite the decrease in prostaglandins resulting in sodium retention and vasoconstriction, NSAIDs have not been found to significantly increase blood pressure even in women with preeclampsia with severe features [15, 16].

References

1. Gestational Hypertension and Preeclampsia. ACOG Practice Bulletin Summary, Number 222. Obstet Gynecol. 2020;135(6):1492–5.
2. Tita AT, Szychowski JM, Boggess K, Dugoff L, Sibai B, Lawrence K, et al. Treatment for mild chronic hypertension during pregnancy. Chronic Hypertension and Pregnancy (CHAP) Trial Consortium. N Engl J Med. 2022; https://doi.org/10.1056/NEJMoa2201295. Published online April 2
3. American College of Obstetricians and Gynecologists' Committee on Practice Bulletins—Obstetrics. ACOG Practice Bulletin No. 203: chronic hypertension in pregnancy. Obstet Gynecol. 2019;133(1):e26–50.
4. Chestnut DH, et al. Hypertensive disorders. In: Chestnut's obstetric anesthesia: principles and practice. Philadelphia, PA: Elsevier; 2020.
5. Altman D, Carroli G, Duley L, Farrell B, Moodley J, Neilson J, Smith D, Magpie Trial Collaboration Group. Do women with preeclampsia, and their babies, benefit from magnesium sulphate? The Magpie Trial: a randomized placebo-controlled trial. Lancet. 2002;359(9321):1877–90. https://doi.org/10.1016/s0140-6736(02)08778-0.
6. Rouse DJ, Hirtz DG, Thom E, et al. A randomized, controlled trial of magnesium sulfate for the prevention of cerebral palsy. N Engl J Med. 2008;359(9):895–905.
7. ACOG Committee Opinion No. 743: Low-dose aspirin use during pregnancy. Obstet Gynecol. 2018;132(1): e44–e52.
8. Optimizing Postpartum Care. ACOG Committee Opinion No. 736. American College of Obstetricians and Gynecologists. Obstet Gynecol. 2018;131:e140–50.
9. Committee on Practice Bulletins-Obstetrics. Practice Bulletin No. 183: postpartum hemorrhage. Obstet Gynecol. 2017;130(4):e168–86.
10. Lockwood CJ, Moore T, et al. Pregnancy-related hypertension. In: Creasy and Resnik's maternal-fetal medicine: principles and practice. Elsevier; 2019.
11. Saha PK, Kaur J, Goel P, Kataria S, Tandon R, Saha L. Safety and efficacy of low dose intramuscular magnesium sulphate ($MgSO_4$) compared to intravenous regimen for treatment of eclampsia. J Obstet Gynecol Res. 2017;43(10):1543–9.
12. Magee LA, Miremadi S, Li J, Cheng C, Ensom MH, Carleton B, Côté AM, von Dadelszen P. Therapy with both magnesium sulfate and nifedipine does not increase the risk of serious magnesium-related maternal side effects in women with preeclampsia. Am J Obstet Gynecol. 2005;193(1):153–63.
13. Sibai BM. Magnesium sulfate prophylaxis in preeclampsia: Lessons learned from recent trials. Am J Obstet Gynecol. 2004;190(6):1520–6.
14. Okusanya BO, Oladapo OT, Long Q, Lumbiganon P, Carroli G, Qureshi Z, Duley L, Souza JP, Gülmezoglu AM. Clinical pharmacokinetic properties of magnesium sulphate in women with preeclampsia and eclampsia. BJOG. 2016;123(3):356–66.
15. Blue NR, Murray-Krezan C, Drake-Lavelle S, Weinberg D, Holbrook BD, Katukuri VR, et al. Effect of ibuprofen vs acetaminophen on postpartum hypertension in preeclampsia

with severe features: a double-masked, randomized controlled trial. Am J Obstet Gynecol. 2018;218(616):e1–8.
16. Wasden SW, Ragsdale ES, Chasen ST, Skupski DW. Impact of nonsteroidal anti-inflammatory drugs on hypertensive disorders of pregnancy. Pregnancy Hypertens. 2014;4:259–63.

Further Reading

American College of Obstetricians and Gynecologists' Committee on Practice Bulletins—Obstetrics. ACOG Practice Bulletin No. 203: chronic hypertension in pregnancy. Obstet Gynecol. 2019;133(1):e26–50.

Lockwood CJ, Moore T, et al. Pregnancy-related hypertension. In: Creasy and Resnik's maternal-fetal medicine: principles and practice. Elsevier; 2019.

Analgesics

Kenneth Nguyen and Leonard J. Soloniuk

Questions

1. **Which of the following is responsible for the indirect excitatory transmission of pain in the spinal cord?**
   A. Release of CGRP
   B. Substance P secretion
   C. Glial cyclooxygenase activation
   D. Release of glutamate
2. **Which of the following spinal cord levels is associated with pain during the first stage of labor?**
   A. T7–T12
   B. T10–L1
   C. L2–L5
   D. S2–S4
3. **A 36-year-old female G3P0020 at 38 weeks and 2 days gestational age with a history of polysubstance abuse in remission and scoliosis presents for induction of labor and requests epidural analgesia for labor. One minute after the epidural was placed and the lidocaine test dose was administered, the patient complained of restlessness and difficulty speaking and began to lose consciousness. Her heart rate fell from 78 to 46, and her blood**

K. Nguyen
Riverside University Health System, Moreno Valley, CA, USA
e-mail: Ke.Nguyen@ruhealth.org

L. J. Soloniuk (✉)
Riverside University Health System, Moreno Valley, CA, USA

Loma Linda University, Loma Linda, CA, USA
e-mail: l.soloniuk@ruhealth.org

A. C. Sinha, I. F. Pasca (eds.), *Peripartum Care of the Pregnant Patient*,
https://doi.org/10.1007/978-3-031-62756-9_24

pressure slightly increased from 110 systolic to 120 systolic. Pulse oximetry showed 98%. What is the next best step in management?

A. Provide positive pressure ventilation.
B. Administer epinephrine 200 mcg iv.
C. Administer a bolus dose of 20% iv lipid emulsion.
D. Administer midazolam.

4. **A healthy 28-year-old G1P1 presented to the labor and delivery ward 6 h after an uncomplicated cesarean delivery of a healthy baby. The patient complained of abdominal pain around the surgical site. Physical exam shows an unremarkable surgical site without swelling, redness, or bleeding. Ibuprofen was recommended for her pain. The patient states that she is concerned that ibuprofen will affect her baby through her breast milk. What is the most appropriate response:**

A. Nonsteroidal anti-inflammatory drugs (NSAIDs) have a significant transfer in breast milk, but since the baby is healthy, she should proceed with ibuprofen.
B. NSAIDs have limited transfer in breast milk, so proceed with ibuprofen.
C. NSAIDs do not provide significant pain control when compared to opioids, so they are superfluous.
D. Administer an NSAID in an IV formulation.

5. **You receive a call about a patient in the obstetrics ward who reports back pain. The patient is a healthy 32-year-old G3P3003 who had an uncomplicated vaginal delivery one day prior with epidural analgesia. Epidural removal was atraumatic with the catheter tip intact and occurred approximately 30 min after delivery. The patient also notes that she has pain in her right leg but not her left leg. The patient reports that she has back pain, worse on her left side, which is exacerbated by coughing. Upon observation, the patient was afebrile and had minimal tenderness and no redness, swelling, or purulence near the epidural insertion site. There is generalized left low extremity weakness and decreased deep tendon reflexes. What is the next best step in management?**

A. Reassure patient and reevaluate in 6 h.
B. Start antibiotics.
C. MRI scan of the lumbar spine.
D. Order multimodal therapy for pain control, including heat and cold and physiotherapy.

6. **What statement is most correct?**

A. Tramadol is associated with spontaneous abortion and major congenital malformations.
B. Neonatal abstinence syndrome is more severe in neonates exposed to methadone maintenance therapy than in those exposed to heroin.
C. Newborn APGAR scores in infants born to mothers using nitrous oxide were significantly depressed from those whose mother did not use nitrous oxide.
D. Sevoflurane does not have analgesic properties at sub-anesthetic concentrations.

7. **The patient is a 37-year-old female, G4P3003, with a history of moderate asthma, two previous cesarean sections, previous postpartum hemorrhage, and postpartum depression complicated by manic episodes who presents for scheduled repeat cesarean section. Prior to the procedure, an epidural was placed for analgesia without any complications. Prior to uterine incision, the patient becomes very anxious and states that she has an increasing amount of abdominal discomfort. Which of the following is the best next step?**
   A. Ketamine 10 mg iv bolus repeated as needed.
   B. Low-dose remifentanil infusion.
   C. Morphine 3 mg iv bolus, repeated as needed.
8. **The patient is a 32-year-old female, G2P1001, undergoing repeat cesarean section under neuraxial anesthesia. The patient states she has had severe postoperative nausea and vomiting with hydromorphone. Spinal anesthesia was successfully performed with 12.5 mg of bupivacaine and 150 mcg of morphine with appropriate sensory levels achieved. The patient continues to have stable vital signs. However, the patient began to have uncontrollable shivering. What is the best action that could have been done to prevent shivering?**
   A. Intrathecal dexmedetomidine 2.5 mcg
   B. Intravenous meperidine 0.3 mg/kg
   C. Intrathecal fentanyl 17 mcg
   D. Intravenous ondansetron 4 mg
9. **Which of the statements regarding labor analgesia is TRUE?**
   A. In the second stage of labor, larger nerve fibers require higher concentrations and/or larger volumes of local anesthetics.
   B. Paracervical block can provide significant pain relief for the labor with fewer fetal complications than epidural analgesia.
   C. Intrathecal administration of morphine produces reliable analgesia during the second stage of labor.
   D. Ropivacaine has more cardiotoxic and arrhythmogenic effects than bupivacaine.
10. **The patient is a 31-year-old G2P1001 at 39 weeks and 2 days gestation with complaints of mild back pain during the current pregnancy. She is admitted to labor and delivery for induction of labor. The patient would like options for nonopioid and nonpharmacologic therapies for her back pain. Which of the following statements is TRUE regarding intradermal water injections?**
   A. The injections are placed over the anterior superior iliac spine (ASIS) and adjacent to the ASIS.
   B. The injections are placed over the posterior superior iliac spine (PSIS) and adjacent to the PSIS.
   C. The injections are placed paramedian between the umbilicus and symphysis pubis.
   D. The injections are placed lateral to the labia majora bilaterally.

11. **Which of the following statements is TRUE regarding systemic analgesics for laboring patients?**
    A. In nulliparous patients administered patient-controlled analgesia (PCA), nalbuphine provides analgesia equivalent to meperidine.
    B. In early labor, patients receiving morphine 2 mg intravenously (iv) were found to have significantly less pain than patients administered acetaminophen.
    C. Nitrous oxide crosses the placenta but has been associated with no changes in fetal APGAR scores.
12. **A patient who is a 32-yo G2P1 at 39 weeks gestation and with no major past medical history presents for repeat cesarean section. Five minutes after spinal analgesia with morphine, fentanyl, and bupivacaine, the patient started to have severe itching around her neck and upper extremities. Which of the following is the <u>least</u> appropriate treatment option for this patient's symptoms?**
    A. Nalbuphine
    B. Acetaminophen
    C. Ondansetron
    D. Tenoxicam
13. **Via which of the following adrenergic receptors does clonidine exert its effects on labor analgesia?**
    A. Alpha-1
    B. Alpha-2
    C. Beta-1
    D. Beta-2
14. **Which of the following is <u>not</u> a systemic effect of labor pain?**
    A. Decrease in uteroplacental perfusion
    B. Increase in gastric acidity
    C. Fetal hypoxemia
    D. Increase in bladder motility
15. **What is the incidence of perineal pain 8 weeks after delivery?**
    A. 7%
    B. 15%
    C. 45%
    D. 90%
16. **A healthy 24-year-old parturient at 17 weeks gestation presented to the hospital for laparoscopic cholecystectomy. Your institution's ERAS (Enhanced Recovery After Surgery) protocol for surgery recommends multiple medications, including duloxetine, acetaminophen, celecoxib, and pregabalin. Which of the following medications would be MOST appropriate to use?**
    A. Duloxetine
    B. Acetaminophen
    C. Celecoxib
    D. Pregabalin

17. **After an uncomplicated vaginal delivery 2 weeks prior, a previously healthy 30-yo G2P2 presented to the hospital for laparoscopic appendectomy. Prior to her procedure, the patient is concerned regarding analgesics and transfer to breast milk. Which of the following is the LEAST appropriate for pain management for this patient?**
    A. Ibuprofen
    B. Hydrocodone
    C. Acetaminophen
    D. Codeine
18. **Nalbuphine is used in obstetric anesthesia for the treatment of shivering, pruritus, and analgesia. It is active at both the mu-opioid receptor and the kappa-opioid receptor. Which of the following statements about nalbuphine is correct:**
    A. Nalbuphine is a mixed mu agonist/antagonist (partial agonist) and a partial kappa agonist.
    B. Nalbuphine is a weak mu antagonist and a kappa agonist.
    C. Nalbuphine is a partial mu agonist and a kappa antagonist.
    D. Nalbuphine is a mu agonist and an NMDA receptor antagonist.
    E. Nalbuphine is a mu agonist and also blocks serotonin and norepinephrine reuptake.
19. **A parturient has a contraindication to neuraxial anesthesia, and you are asked to provide monitored anesthesia care with conscious sedation during her vaginal delivery. Which of the following treatments would be most likely to cause amnesia?**
    A. Nalbuphine 5–10 mg iv every 5 min as needed.
    B. Hydromorphone 0.2 mg iv every 5 min as needed.
    C. Inhaled nitrous oxide 50%.
    D. Ketamine 10–20 mg iv every 5 min as needed.
    E. Dexmedetomidine 2 mcg iv every 5 min as needed.

Answers and Explanations

1. **C**. Noxious stimuli and inflammation occur in the spinal cord during labor and childbirth. Activation of cyclooxygenase in glial cells results in the synthesis of prostaglandins, which play a significant role in the mediation of pain sensitization. This is an indirect mechanism of acute pain processes and transmission during childbirth (**C**). The role of intrathecal NSAIDs, such as ketorolac, is currently under investigation. Nociception results in the release of multiple molecules in the spinal cord that affect pain transmission. These include substance P, calcitonin gene-related peptide, and glutamate, which play a direct role in nociception (**A**, **B**, **D**) [1–3].
2. **B**. Transmission of pain during the first stage of labor occurs at spinal cord levels T10–L1 (**B**). Transmission of pain during the second stage of labor occurs at spinal cord levels S2–S4 (**D**) [1].

3. **C**. With symptoms of restlessness, speech difficulties, and loss of consciousness, this patient is most likely to experience unintentional intravascular local anesthetic systemic toxicity (LAST). LAST is a serious complication that can occur during the administration of epidural anesthesia. Anesthesia providers must be aware of the signs and symptoms that also include dizziness, tinnitus, and perioral paresthesia. Steps in the management of LAST include:
   - Calling for help
   - Positioning patient with left uterine displacement
   - Administration of lipid emulsion
   - Preparation for emergency delivery
   - Maintaining airway, ventilation, oxygenation
   - Benzodiazepines for seizures

   The patient is still oxygenating adequately (**A**), so this is not the most important next step. Patients experiencing LAST are sensitive to the effects of epinephrine and doses used should be less than 1 mcg/kg. Moreover, there is not yet an indication for epinephrine (**B**). Early and rapid administration of lipid emulsion is the key to successful resuscitation of patients with LAST (**C**). The patient is not seizing, so there is no indication for midazolam (**D**) [1].
4. **B**. NSAIDs have limited transfer to breast milk (**A**). Nonsteroidal anti-inflammatory drugs have limited transfer in breast milk. Investigations have shown that less than 1 mg of ibuprofen was found in breast milk after an oral dose of 400 mg. Ibuprofen is also an approved therapeutic drug for children. NSAIDs would be contraindicated if the baby had a cardiac anomaly with dependence on a patent ductus arteriosus. Since the baby is healthy, ibuprofen is compatible with breastfeeding (**B**). NSAIDs can provide significant pain relief and preclude the need for opioid therapy (**C**). Route of administration will not affect toxicity [1–3].
5. **C**. The patient had signs of a possible epidural hematoma and needed immediate (**A**) evaluation. Starting antibiotics (**B**) would be indicated treatment for epidural abscess. However, the clinical picture of epidural abscess is more insidious than what is presented. Patients with an epidural abscess present with a backache and inflammation near the catheter insertion site, along with signs of infection such as fever, malaise, and diaphoresis. MRI is indicated for early diagnosis (**C**). An epidural hematoma presents within 24–48 h of catheter placement with acute constant back pain, exacerbated by percussion or maneuvers that increase spinal pressure such as sneezing, coughing, or straining. The most common sign of hematoma is lower extremity weakness. Due to possible rapid progression to permanent dysfunction, obtaining an MRI for the lumbar spine is the correct answer choice. Treatment for epidural hematoma requires neurosurgical consultation for possible decompression surgery (**D**). Multimodal pain control may be useful for symptomatic pain control, but evaluating the patient for an epidural abscess is more important [4].
6. **B**. Tramadol is a commonly prescribed opioid with mu receptor binding and inhibition of serotonin reuptake. Tramadol's active metabolite, O-desmethyltramadol, does cross the placenta. Tramadol exposure in pregnancy is not associated with an increase in spontaneous abortion or major

congenital malformations (**A**). Neonatal abstinence syndrome is secondary to chronic opioid exposure in utero followed by cessation. Sudden cessation leads to a surge in norepinephrine levels. Symptoms include hyperirritability and sleep deprivation. Methadone and buprenorphine are standard therapies for opioid use disorder. Methadone is associated with more severe neonatal abstinence syndrome than heroin (**B**). Nitrous oxide can be used for analgesia in laboring patients and is not associated with a difference in neonatal APGAR scores (**C**). Inhaled analgesia, such as with sevoflurane, is effective in reducing pain intensity and in giving pain relief in labor (**D**) [5–10].

7. **B**. Although ketamine can provide profound analgesia, it is relatively contraindicated (**A**) in this patient due to a history of postpartum depression with manic episodes. In addition, there is insufficient data about the safety of ketamine with lactation. Patients undergoing repeat cesarean sections may experience more discomfort during peritoneal traction and longer surgery duration. Continuous intravenous infusion (**B**) of low-dose remifentanil has been shown to significantly improve the parturient experience in terms of analgesia and sedation, without noticeable neonatal or maternal adverse effects. Morphine may not be the best choice (**C**), as the patient has a history of moderate asthma prior to delivery and may be sensitive to the histamine release of morphine [11].
8. **C**. The incidence of shivering with spinal anesthesia has been shown to be over 50%. Although the mechanism of shivering is unclear, it is possibly due to vasodilation from the sympathectomy associated with spinal anesthesia. Shivering can lead to interference with surgery and EKG monitoring and increase metabolic demand/oxygen consumption. Intrathecal dexmedetomidine at 5 mcg (**A**) is an effective dose for the prevention of postoperative nausea and vomiting (PONV) and postoperative shivering. It may also prolong motor and sensory block along with increasing the risk of hypotension after spinal anesthesia. It has not been studied at a dose of 2.5 mcg. Although meperidine (**B**) has been shown to effectively prevent shivering, this patient's history of severe PONV with opioids makes it a less appropriate option. Intrathecal fentanyl (**C**) reduces intraoperative shivering. Intravenous ondansetron (**D**) has been shown to prevent shivering under neuraxial anesthesia, but at a dose of 8 mg [12].
9. **A**. The second stage of labor is characterized by pain secondary to stretching of the pelvic floor and vagina (**A**). These somatic nerve fibers enter the spinal cord between S2-S4 and are larger than thoracolumbar nerve roots. To block these fibers, a higher concentration or a larger volume of local anesthetic is needed. However, the risk of hemodynamic/respiratory compromise or dense motor blockade leads to decreased expulsive efforts. Paracervical block (**B**) provides effective analgesia for the first stage of labor but is associated with a high incidence of fetal bradycardia. Intrathecal morphine 0.5 to 2 mg (**C**) provides reliable analgesia during the first stage of labor and less reliably in the second stage of labor. Ropivacaine is less cardiotoxic and arrhythmogenic than bupivacaine (**D**) [13, 14].
10. **B**. Intradermal water injections are a non-opioid treatment option for analgesia during labor. Four injections are placed: Two injections were administered over each posterior superior iliac spine, and two injections were administered 1 cm

medial and 3 cm caudal to the posterior superior iliac spines. The injections are initially painful for the first 20–30 min, but as the pain subsides from the injection, so does the lower back pain [15].

11. **C**. Administered by PCA to nulliparous women, nalbuphine provides better analgesia than meperidine (**A**). A randomized control trial showed that morphine 2mg IV (**B**) had no observed difference in pain compared to acetaminophen. Nitrous oxide does cross the placenta (**C**) and does not affect APGAR scores, fetal heart rate (FHR), or umbilical cord gas measurements. Nitrous oxide has been used since the early 1800s for labor analgesia. Compared to other inhalational agents, it is tasteless and nonirritating. Nitrous oxide does not interfere with uterine contractility. Its administration can be limited by the capacity of the hospital ventilation system in rooms to minimize the exposure to waste gasses. The most common side effects include nausea, vomiting, and drowsiness [16].
12. **B**. Pruritus is a possible side effect of intrathecal and epidural opioids. The incidence is over 80% in parturients receiving neuraxial opioids. Although the mechanism of itching is unknown, many studies have been performed on the treatment of pruritis. All the above drugs have evidence in the treatment of opioid-induced pruritus except for acetaminophen [16].
13. **B**. Clonidine is an alpha-2 agonist and is an adjuvant medication for labor analgesia. Intrathecal clonidine inhibits neurotransmitter release in the dorsal horn of the spinal cord [17, 18].
14. **D**. Labor pain can cause an increase in catecholamine release. Increased levels of catecholamines lead to increased peripheral vascular resistance, eventually resulting in decreased uteroplacental perfusion (**A**). Labor pain can increase gastrin release, causing a resultant increase in gastric acidity (**B**). When laboring patients feel intermittent pain, they often go through cycles of hyperventilation and hypoventilation. During these periods of hypoventilation, maternal and fetal hypoxemia can occur (**C**). Laboring patients experience decompensated bladder motility (**D**) [19].
15. **A**. The incidence of perineal pain 8 weeks after delivery is 7%. Within the first 72 h after childbirth, 90% of women report perineal pain [20].
16. **B**. Prior to 2015, the United States Food and Drug Administration (FDA) categorized the risk of medications during pregnancy as A, B, C, D, and X.

    A: No risk in human studies (studies in pregnant women have not demonstrated a risk to the fetus during the first trimester).

    B: No risk in animal studies (there are no adequate studies in humans, but animal studies did not demonstrate a risk to the fetus).

    C: Risk cannot be ruled out. There are no satisfactory studies in pregnant women, but animal studies have demonstrated a risk to the fetus; the potential benefits of the drug may outweigh the risks.

    D: Evidence of risk (studies in pregnant women have demonstrated a risk to the fetus; potential benefits of the drug may outweigh the risks).

X: Contraindicated (studies in pregnant women have demonstrated a risk to the fetus, and/or human or animal studies have shown fetal abnormalities; risks of the drug outweigh the potential benefits).

Duloxetine (**A**) was Category C. Low-quality evidence shows an increased risk of major birth defects with duloxetine. Although the risk of a short exposure to duloxetine is very small, the evidence for the inclusion of duloxetine in an ERAS protocol is limited, and the benefits do not outweigh the risks. Acetaminophen (**B**) is safe in pregnancy and can be safely used for postoperative analgesia. There has been extensive experience over decades with acetaminophen in pregnancy. There have been no identified risks of an increase in major birth defects, miscarriage, or adverse outcomes. Acetaminophen was a category B medication. Celecoxib (**C**) is a Category C medication. Nonsteroidal anti-inflammatory drugs (NSAIDs) are associated with birth defects, oligohydramnios, fetal renal injury, and intrauterine constriction of the ductus arteriosus. Pregabalin (**D**), like other antiepileptic medications, may cause fetal harm [21, 22].

17. **D**. Breast-feeding has many benefits, such as development of the immune system, decreased risk of infection, and aiding cognitive development. Some common maternal concerns that lead to the decision to not breastfeed include the use of analgesics, especially opioids, and the potential effects on their newborns. Ibuprofen (**A**) is generally considered safe for use during lactation. However, if the infant has a cardiac anomaly with dependence on a patent ductus arteriosus, NSAIDs are contraindicated. Hydrocodone (**B**) is generally considered safe for use during lactation. Acetaminophen (**C**) is considered safe for use during lactation, with the infant exposed to less than 2% of the maternal dose. Codeine (**D**) is NOT considered safe for use during lactation. Codeine is a prodrug that is converted to morphine and codeine-6-glucuronide by the CYP2D6 and UBT2B7 enzymes, respectively, and can be transferred through breast milk. Due to the polymorphism of these enzymes, people can range from poor to ultrafast metabolizers of codeine. Mothers who are ultrafast metabolizers may expose their infants to toxic levels of these metabolites and cause respiratory depression and death. Codeine is not recommended during breastfeeding due to the unknown status of the mother's metabolism [22–24].
18. **A**. Nalbuphine (**A**) is a mu-opioid receptor mixed agonist/antagonist (partial agonist) and kappa agonist. Its use can precipitate acute withdrawal in opioid-tolerant patients. Partial mu agonist medications are associated with a lower risk of respiratory depression. Pentazocine is an example of a weak mu antagonist and a kappa agonist (**B**). Butorphanol is an example of a partial mu agonist and a kappa antagonist (**C**). Buprenorphine is an example of a partial mu agonist and a kappa antagonist (**C**). Methadone is an example of a mu agonist and a NMDA-receptor antagonist (**D**). Tramadol is a mu agonist that also blocks serotonin and norepinephrine (noradrenalin) reuptake (**E**) [25].
19. **D**. Amnesia with ketamine is common, unlike the other agents listed at the specified dosages [26].

References

1. Chestnut DH, Wong CA, Tsen LC, Kee WD, Beilin Y, Mhyre J. Chapter 20: The pain of childbirth and its effect on the mother and fetus. In: Chestnut's obstetric anesthesia: principles and practice. Elsevier; 2020. p. 430–2.
2. Hata AN, Breyer RM. Pharmacology and signaling of prostaglandin receptors: multiple roles in inflammation and immune modulation. Pharmacol Ther. 2004;103(2):147–66. https://doi.org/10.1016/j.pharmthera.2004.06.003.
3. Eisenach JC, Curry R, Hood DD, Yaksh TL. Phase I safety assessment of intrathecal ketorolac. Pain. 2002;99(3):599–604. https://doi.org/10.1016/S0304-3959(02)00208-7.
4. Operater. Diagnosis and management of spinal and peripheral nerve hematoma. NYSORA; 2022. Retrieved 1 Mar 2023, from https://www.nysora.com/topics/complications/diagnosis-management-spinal-peripheral-nerve-hematoma/
5. Sørensen AMS, Noergaard MM, Gotfredsen DR, Kjærbye-Thygesen A, Jimenez-Solem E, Askaa B, Poulsen HE, Horwitz H, Andersen JT. Exposure to tramadol during early pregnancy and risk of spontaneous abortion or major congenital malformations. Obstet Gynecol. 2022;139(4):545–53. https://doi.org/10.1097/AOG.0000000000004714.
6. Johnson K, Greenough A, Gerada C. Maternal drug use and length of neonatal unit stay. Addiction. 2003;98(6):785–9. https://doi.org/10.1046/j.1360-0443.2003.00391.x.
7. Kandall SR, Albin S, Gartner LM, Lee KS, Eidelman A, Lowinson J. The narcotic-dependent mother: fetal and neonatal consequences. Early Hum Dev. 1977;1(2):159–69. https://doi.org/10.1016/0378-3782(77)90017-2.
8. Anbalagan S, Mendez MD. Neonatal Abstinence syndrome. [Updated 2023 Mar 6]. In: StatPearls. Treasure Island, FL: StatPearls Publishing. p. 2023. Available from: https://www.ncbi.nlm.nih.gov/books/NBK551498/.
9. Likis FE, Andrews JC, Collins MR, Lewis RM, Seroogy JJ, Starr SA, Walden RR, McPheeters ML. Nitrous oxide for the management of labor pain: a systematic review. Anesth Analg. 2014;118(1):153–67. https://doi.org/10.1213/ANE.0b013e3182a7f73c. Erratum in: Anesth Analg. 2014 Apr;118(4):885
10. Klomp T, van Poppel M, Jones L, Lazet J, Di Nisio M, Lagro-Janssen AL. Inhaled analgesia for pain management in labor. Cochrane Database Syst Rev. 2012;(9):CD009351. https://doi.org/10.1002/14651858.CD009351.pub2.
11. Yan W, Xiong Y, Yao Y, Zhang FJ, Yu LN, Yan M. Continuous intravenous infusion of remifentanil improves the experience of parturient undergoing repeated cesarean section under epidural anesthesia, a prospective, randomized study. BMC Anesthesiol. 2019;19(1):243. https://doi.org/10.1186/s12871-019-0900-x.
12. Liu J, Wang Y, Ma W. Shivering prevention and treatment during cesarean delivery under neuraxial anesthesia: a systematic review. Minerva Anestesiol. 2018;84(12):1393–405. https://doi.org/10.23736/S0375-9393.18.12478-3.
13. Galindo A, Hernandez J, Benavides O, Ortegon de Munoz S, Bonica JJ. Quality of spinal extradural anaesthesia: the influence of spinal nerve root diameter. Br J Anaesth. 1975;47(1):41–7. https://doi.org/10.1093/bja/47.1.41. PMID: 1148074.
14. Baraka A, Noueihid R, Hajj S. Intrathecal injection of morphine for obstetric analgesia. Anesthesiology. 1981;54(2):136–40. https://doi.org/10.1097/00000542-198102000-00007.
15. Saxena KN, Nischal H, Batra S. Intracutaneous injections of sterile water over the secrum for labor analgesia. Indian J Anaesth. 2009;53(2):169–73.
16. Kumar K, Singh SI. Neuraxial opioid-induced pruritus: an update. J Anesthesiol Clin Pharmacol. 2013;29(3):303–7. https://doi.org/10.4103/0970-9185.117045.
17. Lee LH, Irwin MG, Lim J, Wong CK. The effect of celecoxib on intrathecal morphine-induced pruritus in patients undergoing Cesarean section. Anesthesia. 2004;59(9):876–80. https://doi.org/10.1111/j.1365-2044.2004.03797.x.

18. Colbert S, O'Hanlon DM, Chambers F, Moriarty DC. The effect of intravenous tenoxicam on pruritus in patients receiving epidural fentanyl. Anesthesia. 1999;54(1):76–80. https://doi.org/10.1046/j.1365-2044.1999.00610.x.
19. Tamdee D, Charuluxananan S, Punjasawadwong Y, Tawichasri C, Patumanond J, Sriprajittichai P. A randomized controlled trial of pentazocine versus ondansetron for the treatment of intrathecal morphine-induced pruritus in patients undergoing cesarean delivery. Anesth Analg. 2009;109(5):1606–11. https://doi.org/10.1213/ANE.0b013e3181b72e93.
20. East CE, Sherburn M, Nagle C, Said J, Forster D. Perineal pain following childbirth: prevalence, effects on postnatal recovery and analgesia usage. Midwifery. 2012;28(1):93–7. https://doi.org/10.1016/j.midw.2010.11.009.
21. Richardson JL, Damkier P, Diav-Citrin O, George N, Greenall AJ, Oliver AM, Stephens S, Hodson KK. A critical appraisal of controlled studies investigating malformation risks following pregabalin use in early pregnancy. Br J Clin Pharmacol. 2023;89(2):630–40. https://doi.org/10.1111/bcp.15607.
22. Kramer MS, Aboud F, Mironova E, Vanilovich I, Platt RW, Matush L, Igumnov S, Fombonne E, Bogdanovich N, Ducruet T, Collet JP, Chalmers B, Hodnett E, Davidovsky S, Skugarevsky O, Trofimovich O, Kozlova L, Shapiro S, Promotion of Breastfeeding Intervention Trial (PROBIT) Study Group. Breastfeeding and child cognitive development: new evidence from a large, randomized trial. Arch Gen Psychiatry. 2008;65(5):578–84. https://doi.org/10.1001/archpsyc.65.5.578.
23. Chantry CJ, Howard CR, Auinger P. Full breastfeeding duration and associated decrease in respiratory tract infection in US children. Pediatrics. 2006;117(2):425–32. https://doi.org/10.1542/peds.2004-2283.
24. Nishimura T, Suzue J, Kaji H. Breastfeeding reduces the severity of respiratory syncytial virus infection among young infants: a multicenter prospective study. Pediatr Int. 2009;51(6):812–6. https://doi.org/10.1111/j.1442-200X.2009.02877.x.
25. Kaski SW, White AN, Gross JD, Siderovski DP. Potential for Kappa-opioid receptor agonists to engineer nonaddictive analgesics: a narrative review. Anesth Analg. 2021;132(2):406–19. https://doi.org/10.1213/ANE.0000000000005309.
26. Lim G, Bader AM. Chapter 22: Systemic analgesia: parenteral and inhalational agents. In: Chestnut's obstetric anesthesia principles and practice. 6th ed. Elsevier; 2020: 453-473

Adjuvants in Neuraxial Anesthesia

Yudhyavir Singh

Questions

1. **The first opioid used intrathecally was:**
   A. Morphine
   B. Fentanyl
   C. Diamorphine
   D. Sufentanil
2. **Intrathecal opioids produces analgesia by**
   A. Direct action on the dorsal horn of the spinal cord
   B. Modulating descending inhibitory pain pathways
   C. Diffusion of small amounts of opioid into the epidural space results in systemic absorption leading to centrally mediated analgesia
   D. All the above
3. **All drugs are recommended for intrathecal use, except:**
   A. Fentanyl
   B. Sufentanil
   C. Morphine
   D. Pethidine
4. **Intrathecal dose range of fentanyl is:**
   A. 10–25 μg
   B. 2.5–15 μg
   C. 10–50 μg
   D. 10–100 μg
5. **Late respiratory depression is caused by which of the following epidural opioids?**
   A. Fentanyl
   B. Morphine

Y. Singh (✉)
AIIMS, New Delhi, India

A. C. Sinha, I. F. Pasca (eds.), *Peripartum Care of the Pregnant Patient*,
https://doi.org/10.1007/978-3-031-62756-9_25

C. Pethidine
D. Sufentanil

6. **All are true regarding delayed respiratory depression, except:**
A. Usually develop between 6 and 12 h.
B. Occurs after intrathecal administration of morphine.
C. Results due to cephalad migration of opioid.
D. It commonly occurs with lipophilic opioids.

7. **Adrenaline as adjuvant in neuraxial anesthesia do NOT:**
A. Cause venoconstriction reducing the clearance of local anesthetics and opioids.
B. Prolong labor.
C. Directly enhance analgesia by alpha-2 agonism.
D. Adrenaline prolonged the duration of blockade more with lidocaine as compared to bupivacaine.

8. **Sodium bicarbonate is used to alkalinize local anesthetic solutions for the neuraxial blockade. Which of the following statements is NOT true?**
A. Alkalinization of LA results improved depth of block.
B. Alkalinization of LA results in an increase in the unionized fraction of drugs.
C. Alkalinization of LA results in decreased lipid solubility.
D. Alkalinization of LA speeds the onset of the epidural blockade.

9. **Most common side effect with neuraxial opioid is:**
A. Pruritus
B. Nausea and vomiting
C. Urinary retention
D. Constipation

10. **Non-opioid spinal additives have limited data for clinical use, except:**
A. Clonidine
B. Dexmedetomidine
C. Midazolam
D. Magnesium

11. **Treatment of pruritus includes all the following, except:**
A. Naloxone
B. Propofol
C. Serotonin (5HT3) antagonists
D. Dexamethasone

12. **Transcutaneous carbon dioxide monitoring has been recently recommended for:**
A. Intrathecal fentanyl
B. Intrathecal morphine
C. Intrathecal pethidine
D. Epidural morphine

13. **Which spinal adjuvant is a good substitute in obstetric patients with allergies to LAs?**
A. Meperidine
B. Fentanyl

C. Morphine
D. Neostigmine

14. **Regarding shivering which of the following statements is NOT true:**
A. Shivering is one of the common complications of neuraxial obstetric anesthesia.
B. Intraoperative body heat and fluid loss, response to pain, or excitement of the sympathetic nervous system are risk factors.
C. Adjuvants like pethidine, fentanyl, dexmedetomidine, and sufentanil in neuraxial anesthesia have no effect on perioperative shivering.
D. Opioids have a hyperthermic effect through the activation of μ-receptors, which is the anti-shivering mechanism of opioids.

15. **When used in neuraxial anesthesia, ketamine blocks:**
A. Mu-opioid receptors in the brainstem
B. NMDA receptors on secondary afferent neurons in the spinal cord's dorsal horn
C. Serotonin transmission
D. Modulating descending stimulatory pathways

16. **The most potent agents for counteracting pruritus without reversing the analgesic effects are:**
A. Naloxone and naltrexone
B. Employing high dose histamine-1 receptor agonists
C. Increasing the dosage of opioid medications
D. Avoiding any interventions due to the non-responsiveness of pruritus to treatment

17. **Epidural dexamethasone may be associated with an increase in all of the following, except:**
A. Blood glucose levels
B. Adhesive arachnoiditis
C. Maternal hypothermia
D. Nausea and vomiting

18. **All are true regarding neostigmine as a labor analgesia, except:**
A. It acts by inhibiting acetylcholinesterase and thus increasing the concentration of acetylcholine which binds muscarinic and nicotinic receptors in the dorsal horn of the spinal cord.
B. Intrathecal neostigmine is associated with severe nausea and vomiting.
C. Epidural neostigmine is associated with respiratory depression and pruritus.
D. Neostigmine relieves somatic pain better than visceral pain.

19. **In labor analgesia, the use of clonidine as an adjuvant is not associated with:**
A. Sedation
B. Hypotension
C. Bradycardia
D. Respiratory depression

20. **Neurotoxicity or neurological deficit is associated with which of following spinal additives:**
A. Midazolam
B. Ketamine

C. Neostigmine
D. Clonidine

21. **Protracted vomiting can be caused by:**
    A. Intrathecal neostigmine
    B. Epidural neostigmine
    C. Intrathecal morphine
    D. Epidural morphine

Answers and Explanations

1. **A.** The first opioid to be used intrathecally was morphine with the initial clinical study published in 1979. Opioids are the most common and the earliest used local anesthetic adjuvants [1].
2. **D**. Neuraxial opioid analgesia is primarily mediated by binding pre and post-synaptic mu-opioid receptors in the substantia gelatinosa of the dorsal horn of the spinal cord. Intrathecal opioids potentially act as ligands on opioid receptors in three different areas to produce analgesia. Firstly, they act directly on the dorsal horn of the spinal cord (their main site of action). Secondly, they modulate descending inhibitory pain pathways when transported supra-spinally through bulk CSF flow. Thirdly a small amount of opioid diffuses into the epidural space with subsequent systemic absorption resulting in centrally mediated analgesia (minor effect) [2, 3].
3. **D**. Pethidine has an active metabolite (norpethidine), which in high concentrations may cause seizures and hallucinations. Pethidine differs from other opioids in that it exhibits local anesthetic properties (motor and sensory fiber block). An intrathecal dose of 1mg/kg produces surgical anesthesia; however, the incidence of adverse outcomes is high, and its use by this method is not recommended. Epidural pethidine is effective in treating postoperative analgesia after cesarean delivery and may be administered as a patient-controlled epidural analgesia technique. Moreover, the incidence of adverse effects is epidurally less [2, 3].
4. **A**. The appropriate dose depends on the type of opioid (potency, efficacy, lipid solubility), indication for use, addition of other adjuvants, patient factors, and route of administration as shown in Table 1. Intrathecal drugs have direct access to the central nervous system (CNS) and need relatively small doses for

Table 1 Opioid dosing [2, 4, 5]

Opioid	Intrathecal dose	Epidural dose
Fentanyl	10–25 μg	50–100 μg
Sufentanil	2–10 μg	10–50 μg
Morphine	50–300 μg	2–5 mg
Diamorphine	300–400 μg	2–3 mg
Pethidine	Not recommended	25–50 mg

analgesic effect compared to epidural dosing. Intrathecal doses are approximately one-tenth of the epidural dose [2–5].

5. **B**. Respiratory depression is potentially the most serious adverse effect caused by neuraxial opioids. Early respiratory depression generally develops within 2 h of epidural administration of lipophilic opioids such as sufentanil and fentanyl. Delayed respiratory depression usually develops between 6 and 12 h after intrathecal administration of poorly lipid soluble opioids such as morphine. It is due to cephalad migration of the opioid in the CSF which reaches opioid receptors in the respiratory center. It is uncommon with lipophilic opioids because they rapidly penetrate the spinal cord, leaving minimal free opioid in the CSF [4, 5].
6. **D**. Delayed respiratory depression usually occurs between 6 and 12 h after intrathecal injection of poorly lipid soluble opioids such as morphine. It is due to the cephalad migration of the opioid in the CSF, which reaches opioid receptors in the respiratory center. It is uncommon with lipophilic opioids because they rapidly penetrate the spinal cord, leaving only minimal free opioid in the CSF [4, 5].
7. **B**. Adrenaline is the most used vasoconstrictor adjunct for local anesthetics. It is also an alpha-2 receptor agonist and has its own analgesic effect mediated in the spinal cord. It acts by decreasing the vascular absorption of local anesthetic to maintain a higher concentration at the nerve root increasing the density of motor block and thus prolonging the duration of blockade. This results in possible slowing of labor through β2-agonism. The delayed vascular absorption reduces systemic plasma levels of local anesthetics and therefore the risk of systemic local anesthetic toxicity. Bupivacaine is highly lipid soluble and binds more avidly to the tissue leading to less systemic absorption as compared to less lipid soluble agents like lidocaine. The addition of adrenaline to bupivacaine for use in the epidural space decreases systemic absorption by around 10–20% and is less effective at prolonging the duration of blockade when compared to lidocaine [2, 6].
8. **C**. Sodium bicarbonate can be used to speed the onset of action of epidural lidocaine. Lidocaine is a weak base. Alkalinization of a lidocaine solution results in a more rapid onset of neural blockade (reduced latency), improved depth of block, and an increase in the spread of epidural blockade. This is particularly suitable for epidural anesthesia in the obstetric area when urgent cesarean delivery is required. The unionized form of lidocaine is lipid soluble and can easily diffuse across the lipid phase of the neural membrane. The more alkaline the solution, the greater the unionized fraction of lidocaine. The addition of sodium bicarbonate 8.4% to lidocaine increases the pH, thereby increasing the unionized fraction. This allows a greater proportion of local anesthetic to diffuse across the neural membrane. This local anesthetic diffuses into the spinal nerves in the epidural space as well as aid diffusion through the dura and arachnoid to reach the subarachnoid space, thus speeding the onset of the block by between 2 and 5 min [2, 6].

9. **A**. Pruritus is the most common adverse effect of neuraxial opioids and it manifests within the first few hours of administration. It is usually localized to the face, neck, and thorax. The major side effects of neuraxial opioids are nausea and vomiting, urinary retention, respiratory depression, and constipation. Other adverse effects include sedation, gastrointestinal dysfunction, sexual dysfunction, ocular dysfunction and thermoregulatory dysfunction, CNS excitation, and viral reactivation (herpes simplex labialis virus) [7].
10. **A**. Non-opioid spinal adjuvants with limited data include midazolam, magnesium, ketamine, neostigmine, and dexmedetomidine. Most of them have limited evidence except clonidine, which prolongs the anesthetic block and enhances postoperative analgesia with minimal side effects, although with limited approval for epidural and intrathecal use in obstetric patients [2, 4].
11. **D**. The mechanism for pruritus is not fully understood but is believed to be mediated by the migration of opioids that binds to opioid receptors in the trigeminal nucleus. It occurs more with poorly lipid-soluble agents like intrathecal morphine than fentanyl (almost 70% incidence of pruritus with intrathecal morphine compared to 10% with fentanyl). Histamine-1 receptor antagonists were also found to be helpful even though the pruritus is not mediated by histamine release. Opioid receptor antagonists such as naloxone are most effective in managing pruritus but may decrease analgesic effects. Propofol has been used to treat and prevent pruritus. It exerts its antipruritic action through the inhibition of the posterior horn transmission in the spinal cord [4, 7].
12. **B.** Neuraxial opioids as adjuvants required monitoring of all patients. The monitoring includes clinical surveillance, pulse oximetry, and transcutaneous carbon dioxide monitoring [8–11].
13. **A**. Meperidine is a synthetic opioid agonist and is the only opioid that has significant local anesthetic activity in the dose range normally used for analgesia. It is hydrolyzed in the liver to petidinic acid and is also demethylated to norpetidine, a neurotoxic metabolite. In obstetric patients, meperidine has been used as a spinal adjuvant, as a single agent for epidural or spinal for labor pain, and for anesthesia-analgesia in cesarean delivery. As a sole drug in the spinal for cesarean section, meperidine had been used with good results. Meperidine is a good substitute in patients with allergies to local anesthetics [7–9].
14. **C.** Shivering is one of the common complications of obstetric anesthesia. Patients with shivering often suffer from uncontrolled muscular activity. The risk factors for shivering in patients undergoing cesarean sections may be intraoperative body heat and fluid loss, response to pain, or due to excitement of the sympathetic nervous system. The incidence of shivering during cesarean section is very high; therefore, it is an indispensable part of obstetric anesthesia to prevent this side effect. Adjuvants like pethidine, fentanyl, dexmedetomidine, and sufentanil have preventive effects on perioperative shivering during cesarean sections. Of this, pethidine, fentanyl, and sufentanil are opioids, and according to the research, opioids have a hyperthermic effect through the activation of μ-receptor, which might be the anti-shivering effect. Moreover, compared with

the other two opioids, pethidine has a better preventive effect on shivering [12–14].

15. **B.** When utilized in neuraxial anesthesia, ketamine acts by blocking NMDA receptors located on secondary afferent neurons in the dorsal horn of the spinal cord. This mechanism reduces the transmission of nociceptive information along the spinal pathways. At elevated doses, ketamine can also exert additional, minor analgesic effects by binding to opioid receptors and modulating descending inhibitory pathways through the inhibition of neurotransmitter reuptake [9].
16. **A**. While the pruritus is not driven by histamine release, the use of histamine-1 receptor antagonists (like chlorpheniramine) can offer relief, although they might induce sedation. For managing this issue, low doses of opioid receptor antagonists like naloxone have proven useful. Naloxone (at doses of <2 mcg/kg/h) and naltrexone (at doses of 6–9 mg) are the most potent agents for counteracting pruritus without reversing the analgesic effects [2, 4, 7].
17. **D.** Maternal inflammation, even if not originating from an infection, plays a role in the occurrence of elevated temperatures linked to epidural procedures during labor. The use of epidural dexamethasone has the potential to mitigate such temperature increases and could potentially serve as a preventive measure for epidural-related fever. However, larger-scale investigations are necessary to substantiate this theory and to ascertain the optimal dosage for achieving this intended outcome. Epidural dexamethasone alleviates maternal temperature elevation after epidural analgesia and is associated with decreased nausea and vomiting. This effect can be attributed to the decrease in IL-6 levels [6].
18. **C**. Neostigmine acts by inhibiting acetyl-cholinesterase and preventing the breakdown of acetylcholine. It increases the concentration of acetylcholine, which binds to muscarinic and nicotinic receptors in the dorsal horn of the spinal cord and thus provides analgesia with no motor or sympathetic blockade. It is most useful as an adjunct rather than a sole anesthetic agent. The intrathecal neostigmine enhances analgesia from systemically and neuraxially administered opioids and alpha-2 adrenoceptor agonists but a high incidence of severe nausea and vomiting precludes its use by this route. However, epidural neostigmine is not associated with an increased risk of nausea and vomiting. Also, it does not cause respiratory depression or pruritus either alone or in combination with neuraxial opioids [2, 4, 11].
19. **D**. Clonidine is a centrally acting partial alpha-2 adrenoceptor agonist. Its analgesic effect is mediated by binding on the postsynaptic alpha-2 receptors (G-protein coupled inhibitory receptors) in the dorsal horn of the spinal cord, resulting in decreased nociceptive transmission. Clonidine is a useful adjunct for labor epidural analgesia. Numerous obstetric studies have shown that for cesarean delivery with spinal anesthesia, intrathecal clonidine 30–60μg increases the duration of sensory block, but it does not affect proprioception or produce motor blockade. Sedation, hypotension, and bradycardia are the main side effects of neuraxial clonidine. Changes in blood pressure are dose-dependent. Clonidine does not cause respiratory depression or increase the risk

of nausea, vomiting, urinary retention, or pruritus when combined with neuraxial opioids [2, 5, 15].

20. **A.** Midazolam is a benzodiazepine acting on GABA-A receptors. GABA-A receptors are ligand-gated receptors located throughout the CNS and GABA is mainly an inhibitory neurotransmitter of the CNS. These GABA-A receptors are located densely on the dorsal horn of the spinal cord. Benzodiazepines produce their analgesic effect by increasing the inhibition of nociceptive neurons in this area. Both intrathecal and epidural midazolam prolong the duration of anesthesia, decrease postoperative analgesic requirements, and reduce the incidence of nausea and vomiting, but the studies are limited for obstetric intrathecal use. Intrathecal midazolam is associated with neurotoxicity resulting in neurological deficits in animal studies [2, 4].
21. **A.** The incidence of nausea and vomiting associated with neuraxial opioid is between 20% and 50%. It is more common in females with intrathecal morphine, and it is dose-dependent. Intrathecal neostigmine is associated with protracted nausea and vomiting, which is difficult to treat [5].

References

1. Wang JK, Naus LA, Thomas JE. Pain relief by intrathecal applied morphine in man. Anaesthesiology. 1979;50:149–51.
2. Kangure N. Adjuvant agents in neuraxial blockade. Anaesthesia tutorial of the week 230. http://e-safe-anaesthesia.org/e_library/03/Neuraxial_adjuvants_TOTW_230_2011.pdf.
3. Clark, Vicki, Marc Van de Velde, Roshan Fernando, editors. Oxford textbook of obstetric anaesthesia; 2016.
4. Goma HM, Flores-Carrillo JC, Whizar-Lugo VM. Spinal additives in subarachnoid anaesthesia for cesarean section. In: Topics in spinal anaesthesia. InTech; 2014. https://doi.org/10.5772/58851.
5. Warren DT, Liu SS. Chapter 8: Analgesic adjuvants in neuraxial anesthesia. In: Hadzic A, editor. NYSORA textbook of regional anesthesia and acute pain management. McGraw Hill; 2007.
6. Swain A, Nag DS, Sahu S, Samaddar DP. Adjuvants to local anesthetics: current understanding and future trends. World J Clin Cases. 2017;5(8):307–23. https://doi.org/10.12998/wjcc.v5.i8.307.
7. Saiah M, Borgeat A, Wilder-Smith OH, Rifat K, Suter PM. Epidural-morphine-induced pruritus: propofol versus naloxone. Anesth Analg. 1994;78(6):1110–3.
8. Cheun JK, Kim AR. Intrathecal meperidine as the sole agent for cesarean section. J Korean Med Sci. 1989;4:135–8.
9. Yu SC, Ngan Kee WD, Kwan AS. Addition of meperidine to bupivacaine for spinal anaesthesia for caesarean section. Br J Anaesth. 2002;88:379–83.
10. Nguyen Thi TV, Orliaguet G, Ngû TH, Bonnet F. Spinal anesthesia with meperidine as the sole agent for cesarean delivery. Reg Anesth. 1994;19:386–9.
11. American Society of Anesthesiologists Task Force on Neuraxial Opioids, Horlocker TT, Burton AW, Connis RT, Hughes SC, Nickinovich DG, Palmer CM, Pollock JE, Rathmell JP, Rosenquist RW, Swisher JL, Wu CL. Practice guidelines for the prevention, detection, and management of respiratory depression associated with neuraxial opioid administration. Anesthesiology. 2009;110(2):218–30.

12. De Witte J, Sessler DI. Perioperative shivering: physiology and pharmacology. Anesthesiology. 2002;96(2):467–84. https://doi.org/10.1097/00000542-200202000-00036.
13. Ikeda T, Kurz A, Sessler DI, Go J, Kurz M, Belani K, Larson M, Bjorksten AR, Dechert M, Christensen R. The effect of opioids on thermoregulatory responses in humans and the special antishivering action of meperidine. Ann N Y Acad Sci. 1997;813:792–8.
14. Zhang YW, Zhang J, Hu JQ, Wen CL, Dai SY, Yang DF, Li LF, Wu QB. Neuraxial adjuvants for prevention of perioperative shivering during cesarean section: a network meta-analysis following the PRISMA guidelines. World J Clin Cases. 2019;7(16):2287–301.
15. Mehta N, Aasima tu Nisa Qazi S. Adjuvant drugs to local anesthetics. In: Topics in local anesthetics. IntechOpen; 2020. https://doi.org/10.5772/intechopen.91980.

General Anesthesia

Nisha Branch and Jack Peace

Questions

1. **During morning rounds, the obstetric team informs you of a 33-year-old gravida 1 para 0 patient being admitted for an elective cesarean delivery at 39 weeks and 0 days' gestation. The obstetric team requests that the case be done with neuraxial anesthesia to allow her husband in the room and expects the procedure to be short. They remind you that there are four additional cesarean deliveries scheduled that day. During your preoperative evaluation, the patient reports a past medical history of asthma and migraine headaches without aura. She notes some worsening shortness of breath over the last month. On exam, you note a midsystolic ejection murmur radiating to the carotids, pulmonary rales, and marked bilateral lower extremity edema. You decide that after some additional testing the procedure should not be done under spinal or general anesthesia but rather with a carefully dosed epidural and continuous hemodynamic monitoring because:**
   A. The patient's lower extremity edema may make positioning for spinal anesthesia challenging
   B. General anesthesia with sevoflurane is well tolerated in pregnancy and will allow faster delivery of the fetus, so the other cases can proceed on time
   C. Husbands usually prefer to stay in the waiting room until the baby is born
   D. Pregnant patients with severe/symptomatic aortic stenosis have the best postpartum outcomes when their hemodynamics can be closely managed/adjusted during delivery
2. **A 26-year-old gravida 1 para 0 patient is undergoing an urgent cesarean delivery for fetal heart rate tracing. During the procedure, you begin to**

N. Branch · J. Peace (✉)
Lewis Katz School of Medicine at Temple University, Philadelphia, PA, USA
e-mail: Nisha.Branch@tuhs.temple.edu; jack.peace@tuhs.temple.edu

A. C. Sinha, I. F. Pasca (eds.), *Peripartum Care of the Pregnant Patient*,
https://doi.org/10.1007/978-3-031-62756-9_26

administer nitrous oxide in response to a request from the patient for anxiolysis. What effect would you expect as a result?

A. Uterine relaxation
B. No significant effect on uterine tone
C. Uterine relaxation and vasoconstriction of uterine arteries
D. Vasodilation of uterine arteries

3. **A 32-year-old gravida 2 para 1 patient at term gestation is undergoing an elective repeat cesarean delivery under general anesthesia after refusing spinal anesthesia. The patient's history included gastroesophageal reflux, obesity with a BMI of 32 kg/m^2, and a reported history of intraoperative awareness during a laparoscopic appendectomy 2 years prior. After an uneventful induction, the patient was maintained with sevoflurane at a mean alveolar concentration (MAC) of 1.0 and an FiO_2 of 75% throughout the surgery. Which of the following complications is most likely to develop?**
   A. Intraoperative awareness
   B. Postpartum hemorrhage due to decreased uterine tone
   C. Elevated intraoperative blood pressure
   D. Maternal hypoxia
4. **A 33-year-old gravida 2 para 1 patient at term gestation is in the second stage of labor after a prolonged induction of labor. Despite no medical contraindications, the patient declined epidural anesthesia for the management of labor pain on admission. Prolonged late decelerations are noted on fetal heart rate tracing, and the decision is made to perform an emergent cesarean delivery. The patient denied any significant past medical history and had an uncomplicated labor epidural for a vaginal delivery 2 years prior. What is the next best step in her anesthetic care?**
   A. Offer the patient the choice of an epidural or spinal for anesthesia during the cesarean delivery.
   B. Perform a combined spinal-epidural (CSE) technique since she has no contraindications to neuraxial anesthesia.
   C. Proceed with general endotracheal anesthesia using sevoflurane and nitrous oxide.
   D. Proceed with monitored anesthesia care and a physiologic airway to expedite delivery of the baby.
5. **Which is most true regarding inhalational volatile anesthetics?**
   A. They freely cross the placenta and cause minimal effects on the fetus if delivery occurs within 10 min of induction and $\leq$ 1.0 minimum alveolar concentration (MAC) is maintained.
   B. They cannot cross the placenta but affect uterine tone via active transport.
   C. They can only cross the placenta at high concentrations (MAC > 1.0) via bulk flow.
   D. They freely cross the placenta via pinocytosis and can be detected in fetal circulation.
6. **A 27-year-old gravida 4 para 2 patient whose past medical history is significant only for a body mass index (BMI) of 41 kg/m^2 is undergoing an**

emergent cesarean delivery under general anesthesia for fetal bradycardia. During rapid sequence induction, intubation was noted to be difficult due to impaired visualization secondary to oropharyngeal edema, but intubation was successful on the first attempt. She is maintained with isoflurane at a minimum alveolar concentration (MAC) of 0.5 immediately following induction until delivery occurs 20 min later. The remainder of the procedure was completed without complications. Based on the above scenario, which of the following postoperative findings is this patient high risk for developing?

A. Intraoperative awareness
B. Urinary retention
C. Corneal abrasion
D. Postoperative laryngospasm

7. **A 31-year-old gravida 1 para 0 patient at 39 weeks' gestation needs to undergo a cesarean delivery for failure to progress after induction of labor. The patient's past medical history was significant for childhood asthma and immune thrombocytopenic purpura (ITP), with a current platelet count of 43,000. You proceed with general endotracheal anesthesia and after an uncomplicated induction and initial maintenance with sevoflurane at a minimum alveolar concentration (MAC) of 1.2. The fetal scalp electrode is left in place, and the tracing shows fetal bradycardia. What physiologic change of pregnancy most likely contributed to this complication?**
   A. Decreased blood flow through the placenta due to hypotension from volatile anesthetic and lack of placental autoregulation
   B. Decreased functional residual capacity (FRC) at term which resulted in hypocapnia after intubation
   C. Increased blood flow through the placenta due to increased circulating maternal blood volume overwhelming the fetal cardiovascular system
   D. Soluble sevoflurane diffusing through the uterus resulting in fetal bradycardia
8. **A 27-year-old gravida 1 para 0 patient at 13 weeks' gestation presents with anorexia and abdominal pain that was initially periumbilical and is now sharp and localized to the right lower quadrant. She also reported two episodes of emesis in the last 4 h. After surgical evaluation and workup, she was diagnosed with acute appendicitis, and the surgeon recommended laparoscopic appendectomy. Which of the following is the best management approach?**
   A. Due to her pregnancy, surgery should be avoided, and appendicitis should be managed medically to avoid fetal exposure to anesthetics.
   B. Acute appendicitis in pregnancy is a surgical emergency, and the patient should undergo laparoscopic appendectomy under general endotracheal anesthesia.
   C. Due to this stage of fetal development, the patient should proceed with surgery under spinal anesthesia to avoid teratogenic effects of volatile anesthetics.

D. Due to her pregnant state, surgery should be postponed until the third trimester, and the patient's symptoms should be temporized with medical management to avoid fetal exposure to volatile anesthetics.

9. **You are setting up the operating room for your shift when the obstetric team brings in a 25-year-old gravida 2 para 1 patient at 37 weeks' gestation with symptoms concerning placental abruption and requests anesthesia for emergent cesarean delivery. Fetal heart rate tracing reveals multiple prolonged decelerations. The only information you're able to obtain is that she denies any significant medical problems, medication, or food allergies and last ate 7.5 h ago. Which of the following is the next best step in her anesthetic management?**
   A. Discuss the risks and benefits of each epidural, spinal, and general anesthesia for cesarean delivery.
   B. Obtain verbal consent and proceed with combined spinal-epidural (CSE) technique.
   C. Obtain written consent and proceed with general endotracheal anesthesia using succinylcholine for induction and total intravenous anesthesia (propofol and remifentanil) for maintenance.
   D. Obtain verbal consent and proceed with spinal anesthesia using bupivacaine, fentanyl, and morphine.
   E. Obtain verbal consent as time allows and proceed with general endotracheal anesthesia using propofol and succinylcholine for induction and sevoflurane and nitrous oxide for maintenance.

10. **A 43-year-old gravida 4 para 0 at 39 weeks' gestation has been laboring for 22 h after induction of labor for preeclampsia without severe features. She failed epidural anesthesia earlier in her course and declined a repeated attempt. She is now complaining of a headache with blurred vision, and her blood pressure is 191/111. Her most recent labs show a creatinine of 1.2 mg/dL (from 0.7 mg/dL previously) and a platelet count of 101,000 (from 107,000 previously). The decision is made to proceed with cesarean delivery. What is the best approach to her anesthetic management?**
    A. Avoid spinal anesthesia due to her decreased platelet count, but attempt a repeat epidural anesthetic.
    B. Proceed with general endotracheal anesthesia using propofol and succinylcholine for induction and sevoflurane and nitrous oxide for maintenance.
    C. Proceed with spinal anesthesia, assuming the patient consents.
    D. Avoid spinal anesthesia due to her prior failed epidural.

Two-part question (please answer questions 11–12 based on the information below)

39-year-old gravida 3 para 2 patient required a cesarean delivery for failed induction in the setting of preeclampsia with severe features. Her last recorded blood pressure was 162/107 mmHg, and her most recent platelet count was 49,000. You decide to proceed with general anesthesia using propofol and succinylcholine for induction and isoflurane and nitrous oxide for maintenance.

11. **What additional medication would be most beneficial in this patient if given after induction?**
    A. IV nitroglycerin titrated to maintain blood pressure within 20% of baseline
    B. Ondansetron to prevent nausea during induction
    C. Glycopyrrolate to prevent bradycardia
    D. Famotidine to increase gastric pH
12. **What is the mechanism of action of nitroglycerin on uterine tone for this patient?**
    A. It is converted to oxygen (O_2) and carbon dioxide (CO_2), which relax uterine smooth muscle.
    B. It is converted to nitrogen (N_2) and carbon dioxide (CO_2), which relax uterine smooth muscle.
    C. It is converted to nitric oxide (NO), which then stimulates the enzyme guanylate cyclase in uterine smooth muscle.
    D. It exerts its relaxant effects directly on vascular uterine muscle.
13. **When combined with 50% nitrous oxide, which concentration of sevoflurane is most likely to prevent maternal intraoperative awareness and minimize neonatal effects during cesarean delivery?**
    A. 0.4%
    B. 0.8%
    C. 1.0%
    D. 1.5%
14. **A 26-year-old gravida 1 para 0 patient is undergoing emergent cesarean delivery under general anesthesia with 0.5% isoflurane and 50% nitrous oxide. It has been more than 4 min since hysterotomy, and the obstetrician asks you to "increase the gas" because they need more uterine relaxation to deliver the baby. You respond by saying:**
    A. Yes, I'll increase the nitrous oxide concentration
    B. Yes, I'll increase the isoflurane concentration
    C. No, but I will switch to 0.5% sevoflurane instead
    D. Instead, I'll administer sublingual nitroglycerin to temporarily relax the uterus
15. **What differences in 1-min and 5-min Apgar scores would you expect from a baby delivered by cesarean under general anesthesia compared to a baby delivered by cesarean under spinal anesthesia?**
    A. 1 min, decreased; 5 min, decreased
    B. 1 min, increased; 5 min, decreased
    C. 1 min, no difference; 5 min, no difference
    D. 1 min, decreased; 5 min, no difference
16. **A 23-year-old gravida 1 para 0 patient at term is undergoing a cesarean delivery under general anesthesia using sevoflurane. Given the changes in physiology during pregnancy, what is the expected change in the blood-gas solubility for this patient?**
    A. Increased by 10%
    B. Decreased by 10%

C. Increased by approximately 20%
D. No difference

17. **Which of the following is a generally accepted approach to minimum alveolar concentration (MAC) limits for pregnant patients undergoing cesarean delivery under general endotracheal anesthesia?**

	Prior to delivery	Following delivery
A.	Halogenated agent up to 1 MAC in 50% FiO_2	Halogenated agent up to 0.75 MAC with nitrous oxide up to 70% in oxygen
B.	Halogenated agent up to 1.5 MAC in 50% FiO_2	Halogenated agent up to 0.4 MAC with nitrous oxide up to 70% in oxygen
C.	Halogenated agent up to 1 MAC with nitrous oxide up to 70% concentration	Halogenated agent up to 0.75 MAC with nitrous oxide 75% in oxygen
D.	Halogenated agent up to 1.5 MAC with nitrous oxide up to 70% concentration	Halogenated agent up to 0.75 MAC and discontinue nitrous oxide administration

18. **Comparing pregnancy at term to the nonpregnant state, what is the physiologic change in anesthetic requirements for volatile halogenated agents?**
    A. Decreased by 60%
    B. Decreased by 30%
    C. Increased by 60%
    D. Increased by 30%
19. **A pregnant patient is undergoing emergent cesarean delivery for uterine rupture under general endotracheal anesthesia with desflurane. The baby has been delivered, and the surgeon is having trouble controlling the bleeding. Oxytocin administration was initiated within 1 min of delivery. What anesthetic adjustment can be made to decrease blood loss?**
    A. Increase desflurane to achieve minimum alveolar concentration (MAC) > 1.0.
    B. Decrease desflurane to achieve MAC = 1.0.
    C. Decrease desflurane to achieve MAC < 0.75.
    D. Increase desflurane to achieve MAC > 1.25.
20. **Which of the following is a common indication for the use of general anesthesia with volatile anesthetics on labor and delivery?**
    A. Category I fetal heart rate tracing
    B. Repair of a 1 cm vaginal laceration
    C. Manual extraction of retained placenta
    D. Early decelerations

Answers and Explanations

1. **D**. This patient's presentation is concerning for a diagnosis of aortic stenosis (AS), which is a relative contraindication to spinal anesthesia [1]. There are several absolute and relative contraindications to spinal anesthesia, including AS, severe hypovolemia, refusal of regional anesthesia, severe coagulopathy, and in some instances, extensive spinal surgery. AS is poorly tolerated in

pregnancy, and if known prior to pregnancy, this condition is usually a contraindication to becoming pregnant. In patients who may have been previously asymptomatic and undiagnosed, management of the parturient can be challenging. Those with severe symptomatic AS need a proper workup before proceeding with surgery. This may include an echocardiogram, electrocardiogram, additional laboratory testing, and a cardiology consult. In this case, a patient with severe symptomatic AS will likely not tolerate the abrupt hemodynamic changes associated with the functional sympathectomy that occurs with spinal anesthesia, making this approach inadvisable in this patient. An epidural catheter that is gradually dosed with close monitoring of hemodynamics can mitigate the impact of a sympathectomy and may represent an anesthetic option for this case. While general anesthesia may be well tolerated in pregnancy and provides rapid and predictable hemodynamic effects, the speed of surgery and additional cases should not be prioritized over individual patient care needs (**B**). General anesthesia is not without risks, which include fetal depression, uterine relaxation, pulmonary aspiration, and inability to ventilate/intubate due to pregnancy-induced airway changes. Support persons provide a means of "verbal anesthesia" and can be a helpful source of reassurance during a very stressful time for the patient (**C**) [2]. Lower extremity edema is not a contraindication to neuraxial anesthesia (**A**).

2. **B**. Nitrous oxide has not been proven to exert any significant effect on uterine tone and is not the standard treatment intraoperatively to address increased uterine tone (**A**) [3]. Nitrous oxide (commonly known as laughing gas) is relatively inexpensive, odorless, and colorless and is in the gaseous phase at ambient temperatures. It is an NMDA receptor antagonist and is often used either during labor or cesarean delivery for its hypnotic effects. A minimum alveolar concentration (MAC) of nitrous oxide of 1.0 requires a concentration of 104%, and therefore, an MAC of 1.0 cannot be achieved at normal atmospheric pressures. There is some concern that nitrous oxide has teratogenic effects, and as a result, its use is frequently avoided in the first and second trimester [4]. Nitrous oxide has a minimal effect on uterine blood flow (**C**, **D**).
3. **B**. Postpartum hemorrhage is a concern in all patients undergoing cesarean delivery under general anesthesia. The most common cause of severe postpartum hemorrhage is uterine atony, and all inhaled halogenated volatile anesthetics cause dose-dependent uterine relaxation. Augmentation of uterine contractions with oxytocin administered immediately after delivery is common practice but may not be sufficient to eliminate the risk of uterine atony caused by halogenated anesthetic agents. While intraoperative awareness is a concern in patients undergoing cesarean delivery under general anesthesia, awareness is uncommon at a minimum alveolar concentration (MAC) of 1.0 (**A**). One strategy to minimize the risk of both intraoperative awareness and iatrogenic uterine atony is to maintain a MAC of 1.0 using volatile anesthetic agents until delivery; then after delivery, decrease halogenated agents to a MAC of 0.5–0.75, and use other agents to increase the depth of anesthesia and minimize risk of recall (e.g., midazolam, nitrous oxide, propofol) [5]. Patients may experience a

transient increase in blood pressure immediately following intubation; however, at an MAC of 1.0, this is unlikely to persist throughout the surgery (**C**). This patient was maintained with an FiO2 of 75%, which is unlikely to result in maternal hypoxia (**D**).

4. **C**. In this patient, expedient delivery is paramount. Prolonged late decelerations are considered an obstetric emergency. Due to the rapid and predictable onset of commonly used agents, general anesthesia is the preferred anesthetic modality for emergent cesarean delivery. Preparing the patient for surgical incision and for the administration of general anesthesia should be performed simultaneously. Ideally, induction of anesthesia should proceed as soon as the obstetric team is ready to make a surgical incision to minimize fetal exposure to anesthetic agents (effects are generally minimal if delivery occurs within 10 min). If this procedure was less urgent, it would be appropriate to have a discussion with the patient again regarding anesthetic options (**A**). Given that this is a primary cesarean delivery, the duration of surgery is less of a concern, and a spinal anesthetic alone may be faster to perform and have fewer risks than a combined spinal-epidural (CSE) technique (**B**). Monitored anesthesia care is not among the standard modalities for cesarean delivery, particularly for an emergent case (**D**). Laboring and pregnant patients are at high risk for aspiration, and the administration of medications that can blunt airway protective reflexes in the absence of a protected airway is usually avoided.
5. **A**. Inhaled anesthetic agents cross the placenta via diffusion due to their low molecular weight. Inhalational volatile anesthetics at high doses (minimum alveolar concentration [MAC] > 1.0) can result in uterine relaxation, and at an MAC $\geq$ 2.0, they can also interfere with the action of oxytocin. Fatty acids, amino acids, vitamins, and calcium are transported across the placenta via active transport (**B**). Bulk flow refers to the movement of water due to differences in osmotic and hydrostatic pressure (**C**). Intravenous anesthetics cross the placenta and can be detected in fetal circulation. Opiates such as remifentanil cross the placenta and can result in respiratory depression in the infant, although the clinical effect of these compounds on newborn respiratory status is controversial. Large molecules, such as immunoglobulins, are transported by pinocytosis (**D**).
6. **A**. Intraoperative awareness is of significant concern in cesarean deliveries conducted under general anesthesia [6]. The fact that this patient was maintained on a minimum alveolar concentration (MAC) of 0.5 prior to delivery increases her risk of intraoperative awareness. Strategies to reduce the risk of intraoperative awareness during emergent cesarean delivery include maintaining MAC at 1.0 prior to fetal delivery, using amnestic intravenous agents (e.g., midazolam) following delivery, and avoiding neuromuscular blocking agents. Urinary retention is always a possibility after general anesthesia; however, younger women are usually at lower risk for this complication. Foley catheters are often maintained following a cesarean delivery and are generally removed after the effects of any anesthetic agents have worn off (**B**). Corneal abrasion is always a possibility with any general anesthetic, especially in an urgent or emergent setting.

However, in this scenario, this is less of a concern compared with the potential for intraoperative awareness (**C**). Despite the oropharyngeal edema noted during intubation, this does not increase her risk for postoperative laryngospasm (**D**), although she should be monitored for signs of postoperative airway obstruction.

7. **A**. At term, placental autoregulation is decreased; therefore, blood flow is directly proportional to maternal blood pressure [4]. Volatile inhaled anesthetics result in systemic vasodilation, decreased uterine tone, and fetal depression, especially at higher doses. These effects can be minimized by maintaining a minimum alveolar concentration (MAC) of no greater than 1.0 up until delivery (ideally not to exceed 10 min) and then decreasing the volatile agent to an MAC of 0.75. At higher MAC values, the patient is more likely to experience decreased systemic vascular resistance (SVR) and hypotension, causing decreased preload. While plasma volume is increased at term, in the setting of hypotension and decreased SVR, it is far more likely that the placenta (and thereby the fetus) experiences inadequate rather than excess blood flow and gas exchange (**C**). The physiologic decrease in functional residual capacity (FRC) at term highlights the importance of denitrogenation prior to induction. This can be aided by using head straps to secure the circuit mask while applying monitors and asking the patient to take deep breaths (vital capacity) for as long as time permits. This minimizes the risk of hypoxia or hypercapnia between induction and intubation. If there is difficulty with intubation, this is likely to result in hypercapnia, not hypocapnia (**B**). Sevoflurane usually does not have a significant effect on fetal heart rate. Moreover, inhaled anesthetics diffuse across the placenta and not the uterus (**D**).
8. **B**. General endotracheal anesthesia is the most appropriate choice for laparoscopic surgery, either in pregnancy or the nonpregnant state. Elective surgery should be avoided during pregnancy; necessary surgery, however, should not be withheld because of concerns of fetal anesthetic exposure concerns (**A**, **C**) [7]. While the FDA has issued a black box warning regarding the effects of commonly used anesthetic agents in pregnancy and infancy, no study has shown detrimental effects of a single anesthetic using modern agents on fetal development [8, 9]. NSAIDs can result in premature closure of the ductus arteriosus and should be avoided in pregnancy. The effects of sugammadex on pregnancy and fetal development are unknown, but due to its ability to sequester progesterone, its use is best avoided in early pregnancy [10]. It is generally not feasible to perform laparoscopic surgery under neuraxial anesthesia (**D**). Spinal or epidural anesthesia, however, is a reasonable choice for an open appendectomy. It may be reasonable to offer neuraxial anesthesia for open appendectomy in the appropriate circumstances.
9. **E**. Placental abruption is an obstetric emergency and is often associated with fetal distress. In some situations, the need for emergent cesarean delivery precludes a full discussion of the risks and benefits of anesthetic options (**A**). While written consent is an optimal way to document a discussion of risks and benefits, the needs of the patient(s) must take precedence. In this situation, the fetus

is showing signs of distress, and the surgical team is requesting emergent surgery, making written consent an inappropriate delay in care (**C**). Placental abruption can be associated with either occult or overt bleeding, which may result in coagulopathy. In the absence of laboratory studies demonstrating normal coagulation parameters, performing neuraxial anesthesia in patients with placental abruption may put patients at risk for spinal-epidural hematoma (**B**, **D**). Given the need for emergent delivery, proceeding with verbal consent (if possible) and general endotracheal anesthesia is the most appropriate anesthetic option.

10. **C**. Patients diagnosed with preeclampsia with severe features may have a combination of conditions that impact the anesthetic plan. Preeclampsia is more common in patients with existing/prepregnancy hypertension, extremes of maternal age, obesity, history of chronic kidney disease, and multiple gestations, among others. Preeclampsia can be associated with thrombocytopenia. Depending on the urgency of the delivery, neuraxial anesthesia is an appropriate management technique that can minimize the risk of significant hypo- or hypertension in these patients. This patient's blood pressure was significantly elevated, and laryngoscopy could result in a marked increase in blood pressure and heart rate from baseline, which is a concern when providing general anesthesia (**B**) [11]. The patient's platelet count, while low, does not preclude neuraxial anesthesia (**A**, **C**) [12]. While a failed epidural may mean that a subsequent attempt at a spinal may be difficult or unsuccessful, it is not an absolute contraindication to subsequent attempts at neuraxial anesthesia. High spinal is a concern following failed epidural, as epidurally administered medications may compress the thecal sac, causing unexpected cephalad spread of spinal anesthetic agents. In the event of a failed epidural, a period of at least 30 min is recommended between cessation of epidural medication administration and spinal anesthesia to minimize the risk of high spinal (**D**).
11. **A**. In this patient, her platelet count puts her at high risk for bleeding following neuraxial anesthesia, making general anesthesia a safer choice [12]. Laryngoscopy and endotracheal intubation are associated with marked increases in blood pressure and heart rate. In an already hypertensive patient, it is essential to prevent significant elevations in blood pressure, as this could increase the risk for maternal complications (e.g., stroke, myocardial infarction, etc.) [11]. Titration of nitroglycerin immediately prior to induction or with induction medications is an appropriate approach to providing general endotracheal in a patient with preeclampsia with severe features. Intraoperatively, nitroglycerin or other antihypertensive agents can be given if needed after the airway is secured. Ondansetron is beneficial to prevent nausea in awake patients undergoing cesarean delivery but does not prevent vomiting during induction, especially if administered immediately prior to induction. It is reasonable to administer ondansetron for prophylaxis of postoperative nausea and vomiting (**B**). Glycopyrrolate can be used to prevent bradycardia associated with treatment of postspinal hypotension with phenylephrine, and some recommend its use as prophylaxis for nausea in this setting as well. However, with general

anesthesia using inhaled anesthetics, this is not required immediately prior to induction (**C**). Famotidine has an onset of action between 15 and 30 min and therefore is most useful in minimizing the effect of an aspiration event if administered at least 30 min prior to induction (**D**). In elective cases, there should be adequate time to give this medication preoperatively; however, in an urgent or emergent situation, there are other medications that would be of greater benefit. Oral sodium citrate is a nonparticulate antacid that can be given prior to induction to immediately increase gastric pH.

12. **C**. Nitroglycerin is a nitrate that is converted to nitric oxide (NO), which is the intermediate compound common to all nitrates. NO then stimulates the enzyme guanylate cyclase by activating cyclic guanosine 3',5'-monophosphate (cGMP). This activation results in the release of calcium ions and subsequent relaxation of uterine smooth muscle [13]. There are several effective routes of administration for the use of nitroglycerin for uterine relaxation, including sublingual, intrabuccal, and intravenous (IV). IV administration allows for an immediate dose-dependent effect lasting several minutes, whereas the sublingual route lasts 1–5 min. When used for uterine relaxation, no route of administration has been shown to be superior to others [14].
13. **D**. Patients undergoing cesarean delivery under general anesthesia are at high risk for intraoperative awareness [6]. The bispectral index (BIS) is a useful tool that can estimate the depth of anesthesia and minimize the risk of intraoperative awareness. BIS values below 60 are associated with a high probability of unconsciousness. A study utilizing BIS monitoring found that a combination of sevoflurane 1.5% and nitrous oxide 50% in oxygen was able to maintain a BIS value < 60 more reliably than a combination of sevoflurane 1.0% and nitrous oxide 50% in oxygen [15].
14. **D**. Sublingual and intravenous nitroglycerin are convenient means of providing temporary relaxation during cesarean delivery to aid with difficult fetal extraction [13]. Nitroglycerin has a short half-life, lowering the risk for iatrogenic uterine atony following delivery of the fetus. Intramuscular terbutaline, a beta-agonist, has a slower onset and longer half-life, making its use in this situation less optimal. Nitrous oxide does not produce uterine relaxation (**A**). Increasing the concentration of halogenated agent is suboptimal because it could contribute to fetal depression or uterine atony following delivery (**B**). Sevoflurane (0.5%) is a relatively low anesthetic dose and may increase the risk for intraoperative awareness and would likely provide less uterine relaxation than 0.5% isoflurane.
15. **C**. Few modern studies have compared the effect of modern anesthetic agents on neonatal Apgar scores. In randomized controlled trials comparing general anesthesia and spinal anesthesia, there was no difference in 1- and 5-min Apgar scores [14, 16]. When general anesthesia was compared to epidural anesthesia, however, there were higher 1- and 5-min Apgar scores in the epidural group. The physiologic basis for this difference is unclear, although changing practices in the use of anesthetic agents and hemodynamic management of postspinal hypotension may play a role. Differences among specific induction agents and

their impact on Apgar scores do exist in the literature. Most textbooks still recommend a dose of thiopental of 4–5 mg/kg for the induction of general anesthesia for cesarean delivery, as it is associated with fewer fetal depressant effects than propofol [3]. Studies comparing thiopental to propofol have demonstrated greater neonatal depression in infants exposed to propofol, although no studies have compared these induction agents directly to regional anesthesia [17, 18]. Thiopental is no longer available in the USA, and propofol has become the new standard induction agent when general anesthesia is needed [19]. Few studies have examined the effects of inhaled anesthetics on Apgar scores [20]. On the other hand, studies have shown a difference in neonatal outcome when time from incision to delivery is minimized, whether regional or general anesthesia is used [21]. As the use of general anesthesia is reserved for cases in which regional anesthesia is contraindicated, minimizing fetal exposure is more likely to be of greater importance than the choice of anesthetic agent for induction or maintenance.

16. **D**. Several physiologic changes of pregnancy affect the behavior of sevoflurane. Changes in the respiratory system, including a decrease in functional residual capacity and an increase in tidal volume and respiratory rate, impact the rate of onset of general anesthetics. Changes in the sensitivity to halogenated agents during pregnancy reduce anesthetic requirements by 25–40% [22]. However, none of these changes are known to impact the blood-gas solubility of inhaled volatile anesthetics (**A**, **B**, **C**).
17. **A**. The use of general anesthesia for cesarean delivery is usually reserved for emergent cases or those for which regional anesthesia is contraindicated. General anesthetic agents can freely cross the placenta, can result in fetal depression, and can impact uterine tone. Given these effects, a reasonable strategy is to maintain approximately 1.0 minimum alveolar concentration (MAC), regardless of the volatile agent used, until delivery of the infant. MAC values should generally not exceed 1.0, as these values are associated with maternal hypotension that can impact fetal blood flow. Once the infant is delivered, the halogenated agent should be reduced to an MAC of 0.5–0.75 to minimize the potential for uterine atony. Nitrous oxide (up to 70%) can be added to a halogenated volatile anesthetic (resulting in a combined MAC value of approximately 1.0) until the end of case (**B**). Ideally, nitrous oxide should not be administered until after delivery of the infant to minimize the potential for fetal sedation or hypoxemia (**C**, **D**). Following delivery, the nitrous oxide concentration should not exceed 70% to minimize the risk for maternal hypoxemia (**C**). Bispectral index (BIS) monitoring can be used to titrate general anesthetic agents to minimize the risk for intraoperative awareness.
18. **B**. Pregnant patients are more sensitive to inhalational anesthetic agents and have a physiologic decrease in minimum alveolar concentration (MAC) of approximately 25–40% [22]. This can be seen as early as the first trimester. Multiple theories exist to explain this change, including higher circulating levels of progesterone (which has sedating effects) or endogenous endorphins.

19. **C**. Halogenated anesthetic agents are associated with uterine atony, which is a major contributor to postpartum hemorrhage. This is especially true with anesthetic concentrations greater than or equal to 1.0 MAC (**A**, **B**, **D**). If halogenated anesthetic agents are used during cesarean delivery, it is reasonable to reduce anesthetic concentrations to less than 0.75 MAC after delivery to minimize the risk of iatrogenic uterine atony. Given that intraoperative awareness is a concern during obstetric surgery, supplementation with intravenous amnestic agents (e.g., midazolam) is reasonable. If uterine atony persists with the use of halogenated anesthetics, total intravenous anesthesia (TIVA) can be used.
20. **C**. General anesthesia with volatile anesthetic agents has a variety of uses in labor and delivery. Generally, volatile anesthesia is reserved for emergent situations where neuraxial anesthesia is not an appropriate option. Small vaginal lacerations sustained during delivery can often be repaired under preexisting epidural anesthesia or local anesthesia (**B**). Manual extraction of a retained placenta, however, can be significantly more painful, making volatile anesthetics an appropriate choice. In addition to providing hypnosis, halogenated volatile anesthetics can provide uterine relaxation, facilitating placental extraction (**C**). Category I fetal heart rate tracing indicates a healthy fetus and is not an indication for delivery (**D**). Early decelerations are a normal finding on fetal heart rate tracing that occur because of fetal head compression and are not an indication for delivery (**A**).

References

1. Lewey J, Andrade L, Levine LD. Valvular heart disease in pregnancy. Cardiol Clin. 2021;39(1):151–61. https://doi.org/10.1016/j.ccl.2020.09.010.
2. ACOG: A Partner's Guide to Pregnancy. https://www.acog.org/womens-health/faqs/a--partners-guide-to-pregnancy; 2023. Accessed February 2023.
3. Chestnut D, Wong C, Tsen L, Ngan Kee W, Beilin Y, Mhyre J, et al. Chestnut's obstetric anesthesia: principles and practice. 5th ed. New York, NY: Elsevier Health Sciences; 2014.
4. Lim G, Facco FL, Nathan N, Waters JH, Wong CA, Eltzschig HK. A review of the impact of obstetric anesthesia on maternal and neonatal outcomes. Anesthesiology. 2018;129(1):192–215. https://doi.org/10.1097/aln.0000000000002182.
5. Butterworth JF, Mackey DC, Wasnick JD. Morgan and Mikhail's clinical anesthesiology. 7th ed. McGraw-Hill Education; 2022.
6. Pandit JJ, Andrade J, Bogod DG, Hitchman JM, Jonker WR, Lucas N, et al. The 5th National Audit Project (NAP5) on accidental awareness during general anesthesia: summary of main findings and risk factors. Anesthesia. 2014;69(10):1089–101. https://doi.org/10.1111/anae.12826.
7. American College of Obstetricians and Gynecologists. ACOG Committee Opinion No. 775: nonobstetric surgery during pregnancy. Obstet Gynecol. 2019;133(4)
8. ASA Response to the FDA Med Watch Warning. https://www.asahq.org/advocacy-and-asapac/fda-and-washington-alerts/washington-alerts/2016/12/asa-response-to-the-fda-med-watch; 2016. Accessed 1 Mar 2023.

9. Ing C, Warner DO, Sun LS, Flick RP, Davidson AJ, Vutskits L, et al. Anesthesia and developing brains: unanswered questions and proposed paths forward. Anesthesiology. 2022;136(3):500–12. https://doi.org/10.1097/aln.0000000000004116.
10. Willett B, Togioka Bensadigh, Hofer Zakowski. Society for obstetric anesthesia and perinatology statement on Sugammadex during pregnancy and lactation; 2019.
11. Huang CJ, Fan YC, Tsai PS. Differential impacts of modes of anesthesia on the risk of stroke among preeclamptic women who undergo Cesarean delivery: a population-based study. Br J Anaesth. 2010;105(6):818–26. https://doi.org/10.1093/bja/aeq266.
12. Bauer ME, Arendt K, Beilin Y, Gernsheimer T, Perez Botero J, James AH, et al. The society for obstetric anesthesia and perinatology interdisciplinary consensus statement on neuraxial procedures in obstetric patients with thrombocytopenia. Anesth Analg. 2021;132(6):1531–44. https://doi.org/10.1213/ane.0000000000005355.
13. Axemo P, Fu X, Lindberg B, Ulmsten U, Wessén A. Intravenous nitroglycerin for rapid uterine relaxation. Acta Obstet Gynecol Scand. 1998;77(1):50–3. https://doi.org/10.1034/j.1600-0412.1998.770111.x.
14. Apfelbaum JL, Hawkins JL, Agarkar M, Bucklin BA, Connis RT, Gambling DR, Mhyre J, Nickinovich DG, Sherman H, Tsen LC, Yaghmour ET. Practice guidelines for obstetric anesthesia: an updated report by the American Society of Anesthesiologists Task Force on Obstetric Anesthesia and the Society for Obstetric Anesthesia and Perinatology. Anesthesiology. 2016;124(2):270–300. https://doi.org/10.1097/aln.0000000000000935.
15. Chin KJ, Yeo SW. Bispectral index values at sevoflurane concentrations of 1% and 1.5% in lower segment cesarean delivery. Anesth Analg. 2004;98(4):1140–4. https://doi.org/10.1213/01.Ane.0000103186.64302.38.
16. Dick W, Traub E, Kraus H, Töllner U, Burghard R, Muck J. General anesthesia versus epidural anesthesia for primary cesarean section—a comparative study. Eur J Anesthesiol. 1992;9(1):15–21.
17. Celleno D, Capogna G, Tomassetti M, Costantino P, Di Feo G, Nisini R. Neurobehavioral effects of propofol on the neonate following elective cesarean section. Br J Anaesth. 1989;62(6):649–54. https://doi.org/10.1093/bja/62.6.649.
18. Capogna G, Celleno D, Sebastiani M, Muratori F, Costantino P, Cipriani G, et al. Propofol and thiopentone for cesarean section revisited: maternal effects and neonatal outcome. Int J Obstet Anesth. 1991;1(1):19–23. https://doi.org/10.1016/0959-289x(91)90025-l.
19. Devroe S, Van de Velde M, Rex S. General anesthesia for cesarean section. Curr Opin Anesthesiol. 2015;28(3):240–6. https://doi.org/10.1097/aco.0000000000000185.
20. Toscano A, Pancaro C, Giovannoni S, Minelli G, Baldi C, Guerrieri G, et al. Sevoflurane analgesia in obstetrics: a pilot study. Int J Obstet Anesth. 2003;12(2):79–82. https://doi.org/10.1016/s0959-289x(02)00195-4.
21. Khaw KS, Ngan Kee WD, Lee A, Wang CC, Wong AS, Ng F, et al. Supplementary oxygen for elective Cesarean section under spinal anesthesia: useful in prolonged uterine incision-to-delivery interval? Br J Anaesth. 2004;92(4):518–22. https://doi.org/10.1093/bja/aeh092.
22. Palahniuk RJ, Shnider SM, Eger EI 2nd. Pregnancy decreases the requirement for inhaled anesthetic agents. Anesthesiology. 1974;41(1):82–3. https://doi.org/10.1097/00000542-197407000-00021.

Further Reading

Chestnut D, Wong C, Tsen L, Ngan Kee W, Beilin Y, Mhyre J, et al. Chestnut's obstetric anesthesia: principles and practice. 5th ed. New York, NY: Elsevier Health Sciences; 2014.

Devroe S, Van de Velde M, Rex S. General anesthesia for cesarean section. Curr Opin Anesthesiol. 2015;28(3):240–6. https://doi.org/10.1097/aco.0000000000000185.

Inhaled Anaesthetics

Sunanda Gupta, Seema Partani, and Akshay Toshniwal

Questions

1. **All the following statements are correct for nitrous oxide <u>except</u>:**
   A. Quick onset and requires short time to achieve peak effects
   B. Once discontinued, more than 90% metabolism occurs within 45 s
   C. Weak analgesic effect mediated through N-methyl-D-aspartate (NMDA) antagonism
   D. Minimal side effects when used at <50% concentration
2. **Which of the following characteristics of Entonox is <u>incorrect</u>?**
   A. Maximal effects achieved within 15 s
   B. Consists of equal volumes (50:50) of nitrous oxide and oxygen
   C. Crosses the placenta readily
   D. Rapidly excreted by neonatal lungs after delivery
3. **Nitrous oxide interferes with nucleic acid synthesis by inhibiting:**
   A. Methionine synthase
   B. Methyltransferase
   C. Homocysteine
   D. Methylenetetrahydrofolate reductase

S. Gupta
Anaesthesiology, Geetanjali Medical University, Udaipur, Rajasthan, India

S. Partani
Partani ENT Hospital, Udaipur, Rajasthan, India

A. Toshniwal (✉)
Department of Anaesthesiology, Geetanjali Medical College and Hospital, Geetanjali University, Udaipur, Rajasthan, India

A. C. Sinha, I. F. Pasca (eds.), *Peripartum Care of the Pregnant Patient*,
https://doi.org/10.1007/978-3-031-62756-9_27

4. **The following factors facilitate rapid transfer of inhalational agents across the placenta except:**
   A. Low molecular weight
   B. High lipid solubility
   C. Co-administration of opioids
   D. Prolonged induction to delivery interval
5. **Placental transfer of which of the following inhalational agents does not occur?**
   A. Nitrous oxide
   B. Desflurane
   C. Isoflurane
   D. Sevoflurane
6. **Possible pathophysiology for teratogenicity by exposure to inhalational anesthetics in pregnancy may:**
   A. Increase neuronal cell death
   B. Decrease neural stem cell migration
   C. Alter cytoskeletal structure of neuronal glial cells
   D. All the above
7. **First use of inhalational agents for pain relief was done by:**
   A. Sir James Young Thompson, in 1814
   B. Sir James Young Thompson, in 1847
   C. John Snow in 1814
   D. Joseph Priestley, in 1847
8. **Regarding intraoperative awareness during general anesthesia for cesarean section, the correct statement is:**
   A. Increased time duration between IV induction and onset of inhalational agents increases the chances of intraoperative awareness
   B. End-tidal vapor concentration monitoring may help to prevent awareness
   C. Target bispectral index (BIS) value of <60 helps to minimize awareness
   D. All the above statements are correct
9. **Which of the following inhalational agents has lowest fetal/maternal (F/M) ratio?**
   A. Enflurane
   B. Isoflurane
   C. Sevoflurane
   D. Nitrous oxide
10. **Minimal alveolar concentration (MAC) during pregnancy is approximately decreased by:**
    A. 15%
    B. 30%
    C. 45%
    D. 60%

11. **Effects of prolonged administration of high concentrations of inhalational anesthetics may result in all except:**
    A. Neonatal flaccidity
    B. Cardiorespiratory depression
    C. Depressed neonate not responding to assisted ventilation
    D. Increased maternal blood loss
12. **Regarding use of Entonox in labor analgesia, the incorrect statement is:**
    A. Entonox provides labor pain relief in 50% of mothers
    B. 50% nitrous oxide with oxygen provides labor analgesia by decreasing the
    C. magnitude of uterine contractions
    D. All apparatuses must be checked regularly to avoid inhalation of 100% oxygen first followed by nitrous oxide
    E. Adequate scavenging systems are required to prevent environmental pollution
13. **Which of the following inhalational agents should be <u>avoided</u> in hypertensive disorders of pregnancy?**
    A. Desflurane
    B. Isoflurane
    C. Sevoflurane
    D. Enflurane
14. **Which of the following statements is <u>false</u> about the use of inhalational anesthetic agents in obstetrics?**
    A. These agents produce dose-dependent decreases in uterine smooth muscle contractility.
    B. Limiting the volatile agent concentration (<0.5 MAC) limits the intrapartum fetal exposure and increases postpartum uterine relaxation.
    C. Higher MAC (1.5–2) can provide uterine relaxation during obstetric maneuvers.
    D. Uterine relaxation produced by volatile anesthetics may cause greater blood loss than in patients receiving nitrous oxide-barbiturate-opioid anesthesia.
15. **Regarding placental transfer of volatile anesthetic agents, the following statements are true except:**
    A. Volatile agents readily cross the placenta and are transferred to the fetus.
    B. Fetal concentration depends on maternal plasma concentrations and duration of exposure.
    C. Volatile agents are not excreted rapidly by neonatal lungs after delivery.
    D. Entonox may cause placental vasoconstriction leading to impaired fetal oxygenation. So statement C is incorrect.
16. **The beneficial effects of volatile anesthetic agents when used in low concentration (<1 MAC) with 50% nitrous oxide in obstetrics include all <u>except</u>:**
    A. Reduce the incidence of maternal recall
    B. Provide uterine relaxation for obstetric maneuvers
    C. Ideal for maintenance of general anesthesia during cesarean section
    D. Enhance the uteroplacental blood flow which is compromised by nitrous oxide

17. **A 50:50 mixture of nitrous oxide/oxygen (Entonox) is prepared by:**
    A. Poynting effect
    B. Lamination
    C. Second gas effect
    D. Concentration effect
18. **Rapid uptake of inhalational anesthetic agents occurs because of:**
    A. Decrease in FRC by 20% at term
    B. Minute ventilation increasing by 50%
    C. Increase in metabolic demands of the feto-placental unit
    D. All the above
19. **Maintaining pseudocritical temperature of Entonox is important because:**
    A. It reduces the teratogenic effects of N_2O
    B. It acts synergistically, with $GABA_A$ modulators, to increase amnesia and hypnosis
    C. It prevents hypoxic consequences to the patients
    D. It decreases its ozone depletion potential
20. **Inhalational anesthetics mediate their effects by the following mechanisms of actions:**
    (i) Inhibition of glutamate receptors
    (ii) Inhibition of NMDA receptors
    (iii) Inhibition of glycine receptors
    A. (i) and (ii) are true.
    B. (ii) and (iii) are true.
    C. (i) and (iii) are true.
    D. All are true.

Answers and Explanations

1. **B.** Since nitrous oxide has low blood-gas partition coefficient (0.47), it has faster onset of action; hence it requires a short time to achieve its peak effect (**A**). It has antagonistic effects on NMDA receptors, thus providing weak analgesic effects (**C**) [1]. When N_2O is used in >50% concentration, its analgesic efficacy is improved; however side effects like maternal sedation are more pronounced along with decreased inspired concentration of maternal oxygen (**D**) [1]. Ninety-nine percent of N_2O is exhaled unchanged and <1% undergoes metabolism (**B**) [1].
2. **A.** Entonox, not available for use in the USA, is used in many countries for labor analgesia and consists of a cylinder with equal volume [50:50] of nitrous oxide and oxygen (**B**) [1]. Its use is limited in the USA due to exposure of healthcare staff to nitrous oxide. It readily crosses the placenta (**C**) [1]. It is relatively insoluble and is rapidly excreted by neonatal lungs after delivery (**D**) [1]. About 45 seconds is required to achieve maximal analgesic effect (**A**) [1].

3. **A.** Enzyme methionine synthase converts homocysteine to methionine which is an important factor of nucleic acid synthesis. N_2O inhibits methionine synthase, thus interfering with nucleic acid synthesis [2, 3].
4. **C.** The low molecular weight and high lipid solubility facilitate rapid transfer of inhalational anesthetic to the placenta. A prolonged induction to delivery interval leads to greater transfer of these agents to the placenta (**A**, **B**, **D**) [4]. Co-administration of opioids does not affect the placental transfer.
5. **B.** Nitrous oxide rapidly crosses the placenta within 3 min [5] as it has a fetal/maternal (F/M) ratio of 0.83 (**A**). Isoflurane [6] and sevoflurane [7] also cross the placenta with F/M ratio of 0.71 and 0.38, respectively (**C**, **D**). However, there is no published data regarding placental transfer of desflurane.
6. **D.** Exposure to inhalational anesthetics in the period of high synaptogenesis results in an increase in neuronal cell death and decrease in neural stem cell migration, and there may be alteration in cytoskeletal structure of neuronal glial cells (**A**, **B**, **C**) [8]. All the above options are correct.
7. **B.** In 1847, Sir James Young Simpson used chloroform for the first time for relief of labor pain [9].
8. **D.** Prolonged time duration between intravenous induction agents and achieving adequate inhalational agent vapor tension influence the incidence of awareness (**A**). Achieving adequate vapor concentration during maintenance of general anesthesia is a key factor to avoid intraoperative awareness; hence end-tidal vapor concentration monitoring may help to prevent awareness (**B**) [10]. For adequate depth of anesthesia during GA, BIS value should be <60 (**C**) [11]. So all the above statements are correct.
9. **C.** Enflurane has an F/M ratio of 0.6. Isoflurane [6] has an F/M ratio of 0.71. Sevoflurane [7] has an F/M ratio of 0.38. Nitrous oxide [5] has an F/M ratio of 0.83.
10. **B.** MAC is reduced in pregnancy by 30% and returns to normal within 12–72 h after delivery [12].
11. **C.** Inhaled anaesthetic agents, in high concentration cross the placental barrier, causing neonatal flaccidity, hypotonia, cardiovascular depression, and uterine atony resulting in increased maternal blood loss (**A**, **B**, **D**) [7]. However, a neonate with respiratory depression, due to inhalational agents, usually responds to assisted ventilation which facilitates exhalation of these agents (**C**) [7].
12. **B.** It has been reported that Entonox provides effective labor analgesia in 50% of mothers (**A**) [13, 14]. Entonox has a pseudocritical temperature of -6°C at a cylinder pressure of 137 bar (13,700 kPa) and is therefore a compressed gas during storage at room temperature. It must not be stored below its pseudocritical temperature, or it will separate under a process called "lamination." At lower temperatures the gases of Entonox get separated, so the apparatus must be checked regularly (**B**) [15]. N_2O provides pain relief by NMDA antagonism and does not interfere with uterine activity (**C**). Adequate scavenging is important, while using inhalational anesthetics, to prevent environmental pollution and health hazards to healthcare personnel (**D**).

13. **A.** Since desflurane causes sympathetic stimulation during rapid increases in inspired concentration, it should be avoided in hypertensive disorders of pregnancy [16].
14. **B.** Volatile anesthetics provide dose-dependent decrease in uterine smooth muscle contractility and blood flow. The effects are modest at 0.5 MAC and become substantial at > 1 MAC. Nitrous oxide does not alter uterine contractility in doses that are used to provide analgesia during vaginal delivery [12].
15. **A**. Volatile anesthetics are lipophilic and have low molecular weight; hence they readily cross the placenta and are transferred to the fetus. Fetal concentration depends on maternal plasma concentrations and duration of exposure (**A**, **B**). They are readily excreted by neonatal lungs once neonatal respiration is established (**C**) [1]. Maternal hyperventilation is associated with the use of Entonox which may cause placental vasoconstriction leading to impaired fetal oxygenation (**D**) [1]. So statement (**C**) is incorrect.
16. **B.** Volatile anesthetics when used in low concentration (<1 MAC) combined with 50% N_2O ensure amnesia [7] (**A**), so ideal for maintenance of general anesthesia during cesarean delivery (**C**) but do not cause adequate uterine relaxation for obstetric maneuvers (**B**). Inhalational anesthetics when used in combination with nitrous oxide counteract the vasoconstrictive effect of nitrous oxide (**D**).
17. **A**. Poynting effect occurs when gaseous oxygen is bubbled through liquid nitrous oxide. It increases the vapor pressure of the mixture to form a gas at pressures which far exceed those capable of liquid nitrous oxide alone [15]. At cylinder pressure of 137 bar (13,700 kPa), Entonox has a pseudocritical temperature of −6 °C and is therefore a compressed gas during storage at room temperature. When stored at temperature less than pseudocritical temperature, it separates into oxygen gas above a layer of liquid nitrous oxide, the process known as lamination [15]. The speed of onset of other volatile agents is increased by nitrous oxide and is known as the second gas effect [15]. Higher concentrations of nitrous oxide help to increase the concentration of other volatile agents, and this is known as concentration effect [15].
18. **D**. FRC at term decreases by 20% due to upward displacement of diaphragm by the gravid uterus. The minute ventilation at term is increased by 50% [17]. Increased maternal resting metabolic rate and increased metabolic demands of the feto-placental unit cause an increase in oxygen consumption by 60% [17]. All these factors contribute to increased uptake of inhalational agents in obstetric patients.
19. **C.** Entonox has a pseudocritical temperature of −6 °C and is therefore a compressed gas during storage at room temperature [16]. When stored at temperature less than pseudocritical temperature, it separates into oxygen gas above a layer of liquid nitrous oxide, the process known as lamination [16]. This results in delivery of pure oxygen first followed by delivery of concentrated nitrous oxide resulting in hypoxic consequences to the patient [16].
20. **A.** Glutamate and NMDA are excitatory neurotransmitters in CNS, and their receptors are inhibited by inhaled anesthetics, [12] whereas glycine is an inhibitory neurotransmitter in the spinal cord, and glycine receptors are potentiated by volatile anesthetic agents [12].

References

1. Monteiro R, Salman M, Malhotra S, et al. Analgesia, anaesthesia and pregnancy—a practical guide, vol. 4. Cambridge University Press; 2019. p. 70–1.
2. Brodsky JB, Cohen EN. Adverse effects of nitrous oxide. Med Toxicol. 1986;1(5):362–74.
3. Fujinaga M, Baden JM, Yhap EO, et al. Reproductive and teratogenic effects of nitrous oxide, isoflurane, and their combination in Sprague-Dawley rats. Anesthesiology. 1987;67(6):960–4.
4. Lumley J, Walker A, Marum J, Wood C. Time: an important variable at Caesarean section. J Obstet Gynaecol Br Commonw. 1970;77:10–23.
5. Marx GF, Joshi CW, Orkin LR. Placental transmission of nitrous oxide. Anesthesiology. 1970;32:429–32.
6. Dwyer R, Fee JP, Moore J. Uptake of halothane and isoflurane by mother and baby during caesarean section. Br J Anaesth. 1995;74:379–83.
7. Farragher R, Maharaj CH, Higgins BD, et al. Sevoflurane and the feto-placental vasculature: the role of nitric oxide and vasoactive eicosanoids. Anesth Analg. 2008;107:171–7.
8. Dahl V, Spreng U. Anaesthesia for Non-Obstetric Surgery. In: Clark V, De Velde MV, Fernando R, editors. Oxford textbook of obstetric anaesthesia. United Kingdom: Oxford Publications; 2016. p. 159–60.
9. Browne I, Deighan M. Non neuraxial labour analgesia. In: Santos A, Epstein JN, Chaudhary K, editors. Obstetric anaesthesia. USA: McGraw Hill Education; 2015. p. 171.
10. Lewy DM, Saule L. General anaesthesia for Cesarean delivery. In: Clark V, De Velde MV, Fernando R, editors. Oxford textbook of obstetric anaesthesia. UK: Oxford Publications; 2016. p. 343.
11. Chin KJ, Yeo SW. A BIS-guided study of sevoflurane requirements for adequate depth of anaesthesia in Caesarean section. Anaesthesia. 2004;59:1064–8.
12. Flood P, Rathmell JP, Shafer S. Inhaled anaesthetics. In: Stoeltings pharmacology and physiology in anaesthetic practice, vol. 5; 2017. p. 98–159.
13. Rosen M. Recent advances in pain relief in childbirth. I. Inhalation and systemic analgesia. Br J Anaesth. 1971;43:837–48.
14. Marx GF, Katsnelson T. The introduction of nitrous oxide analgesia into obstetrics. Obstet Gynecol. 1992;80:715–8.
15. Brown SM, Sneyd JR. Nitrous oxide in modern anaesthetic practice. BJA Educ. 2016;16(3):87–91.
16. Ebert TJ, Muzi M. Sympathetic hyperactivity during desflurane anesthesia in healthy volunteers. A comparison with isoflurane. Anesthesiology. 1993;79:444–53.
17. Delgado C, Ring L, Mushambi MC. General anaesthesia in obstetrics. BJA Educ. 2020;20(6):201–7.

Further Reading

Chestnut DH, Wong CA, Tsen LC, Ngan Kee WD, Beilin Y, Mhyre J. Chestnut's obstetric anesthesia: principles and practice. 6th Edition; 2019.

Intravenous Anesthetic Agents in Obstetric Patients

Shilpa Kasodekar and Aparajita Nathroy

Questions

1. **What is/are the pharmacological factor/factors that affects/affect drug delivery across the placenta?**
   A. Concentration gradient across the placenta
   B. Lipid solubility
   C. Drug molecular weight
   D. All the above
2. **What is/are the placental factor/factors that affects/affect drug delivery?**
   A. Placental drug transporters
   B. pH of the maternal and fetal blood
   C. Surface area (number of microvilli per cm^2)
   D. All the above
3. **Most of the drugs cross the placenta by:**
   A. Passive or facilitated diffusion
   B. Active diffusion
   C. Both active and passive diffusion
   D. Receptor-mediated endocytosis
4. **Drugs that cross the placenta via passive or facilitated diffusion include all the following except:**
   A. Midazolam
   B. Acetaminophen
   C. Norepinephrine

S. Kasodekar (✉) · A. Nathroy
PD Hinduja Hospital and Medical Research Centre, Khar, Mumbai, India

A. C. Sinha, I. F. Pasca (eds.), *Peripartum Care of the Pregnant Patient*,
https://doi.org/10.1007/978-3-031-62756-9_28

D. Glucocorticoids

5. **Which of the following statements is <u>false</u>?**
   A. Medications that cannot easily cross the blood-brain barrier have difficulty crossing the placental barrier.
   B. Most sedative and anaesthetic medications can cross the placenta with relative ease, the exception being agents that are hydrophilic, highly ionized, or large in molecular size.
   C. Uterine tight junctions, being like that of the blood-brain barrier, facilitate the crossing of large molecules, such as with heparin.
   D. Hydrophilic and ionized neuromuscular blocking agents generally neither cross the placenta nor the blood-brain barrier.
6. **Which of the following statements about benzodiazepines is <u>false</u>?**
   A. Benzodiazepines are lipid soluble and cross the placenta at a greater rate during the later stages of pregnancy.
   B. Benzodiazepines can safely be taken during the third trimester as it does not impose any risk to the fetus.
   C. Benzodiazepine use is not recommended in the third trimester near anticipated delivery, as it has shown associations with hypotonia or "floppy infant syndrome," lethargy, hypothermia, respiratory depression, and feeding difficulties after delivery.
   D. There has been an increased use of prescription benzodiazepines for the treatment of anxiety, depression, and, in the later stages of pregnancy, insomnia.
7. **What mechanism prevents the passage of depolarizing and nondepolarizing muscle relaxants across the placental barrier into the developing fetus?**
   A. High degree of protein binding
   B. Ionized or highly charged molecules
   C. Rapid active transport removal from fetal circulation
   D. "Tight junctions" within the placenta
8. **Which medication/medications has/have been used for treatment of nausea and vomiting in pregnancy?**
   A. Ondansetron
   B. Dimenhydrinate
   C. Doxylamine
   D. All the above
9. **Opioids were considered under which category in FDA Pregnancy?**
   A. Category C medication
   B. Category B medication
   C. Category D medication
   D. Category A medication
10. **Which of the following drugs crosses the placenta?**
   A. Heparin
   B. Glycopyrrolate
   C. Neostigmine
   D. Rocuronium

11. **All the statements are correct, <u>except</u>:**
    A. Atropine crosses the placenta and causes fetal tachycardia
    B. It is advisable to avoid nitrous oxide exposure in pregnant patients with methylenetetrahydrofolate reductase deficiency
    C. Volatile anesthetics cause uterine smooth muscle relaxation
    D. Ketamine has been designated FDA Pregnancy Category C medication
12. **Which of the following drugs causes premature closure of the PDA in pregnancy?**
    A. NSAIDS
    B. Thiazide
    C. ACE inhibitor
    D. Beta-blocker

Answers and Explanations

1. **D**. Throughout the pregnancy the placental exchange is a dynamic circulatory process. The main determinants of drug transfer are highly influenced by the structural components that comprise the placental lining and the drug's individual pharmacologic profile.
2. **D**. Placental exchange is a dynamic circulatory process throughout pregnancy. The determinants of drug transfer depend on the structural components that comprise the placental lining and the drug's nonpharmacological profile (Table 1) [1]. The outer lining of the uterus is composed of fatty, fibrous connective tissue called the perimetrium, made of an outer syncytiotrophoblast and an inner cytotrophoblast layer. The main fundamental unit of the placental lining is made of fetal vascular projections called the chorionic villi. The outer syncytiotrophoblast layer of villi is directly in contact with maternal circulation and serves as the rate-limiting step for placental drug transfer [1]. In addition to the lipophilic outer membrane, the inner uterine endometrial lining is composed of tight junctions that provide a selective barrier, comparable with the blood-brain barrier. The endometrial lining undergoes constant remodeling throughout gestation, with dramatic changes in thickness, surface area, and concentration of transporter proteins. The original thickness of the placental lining decreases nearly

Table 1 Factors affecting drug delivery across the placenta

Placental factors	Pharmacologic factors
Metabolism	Concentration gradient across placenta
Placental drug transporters	Lipid solubility
pH of maternal and fetal blood	Drug molecular weight
Surface area (number of microvilli per cm^2)	pKa
Thickness	Protein binding
Uteroplacental blood flow	

ten times by the third trimester [2]. With further progression of the pregnancy, the inner cytotrophoblast layer fades, which facilitates rapid drug diffusion to the fetus [1]. The two layers control the exchange of gases, nutrients, hormones, and immune cells via various mechanisms of entry including passive diffusion, facilitated transport, active transport, and receptor-mediated endocytosis.

3. **A**. Most drugs cross the placenta by passive or facilitated diffusion. For instance, midazolam and acetaminophen commonly undergo passive diffusion, which occurs either transcellularly or through water channels within the placental membrane [1]. Drugs such as glucocorticoids and some antimicrobials (e.g., cephalosporins) are structurally like endogenous compounds and rely on facilitated diffusion affected by the number of carrier proteins present and the extent of the concentration gradient. Another mode of drug transfer includes active transport. Unlike passive and facilitated transport, active transport relies on energy in the form of adenosine triphosphate to move drugs such as norepinephrine and dopamine against an unfavorable concentration gradient. Active transporters are found on both sides of the placental membrane and allow bidirectional drug delivery (i.e., from mother to fetus and vice versa). Receptor-mediated endocytosis is much less understood. This mode of transport is believed to take a longer amount of time, as it requires membrane envelopment and release to the other side of the cell.
4. **C**. Most drugs cross the placenta by passive or facilitated diffusion. Midazolam and acetaminophen undergo passive diffusion either transcellularly or through water channels within the placental membrane [1]. Drugs such as glucocorticoids and some antimicrobials (e.g., cephalosporins) are structurally like endogenous compounds and rely on facilitated diffusion affected by the number of carrier proteins present and the extent of the concentration gradient. Another mode of drug transfer includes active transport. Unlike passive and facilitated transport, active transport relies on energy in the form of adenosine triphosphate to move drugs such as norepinephrine and dopamine against an unfavorable concentration gradient. Active transporters are found on both sides of the placental membrane and allow bidirectional drug delivery (i.e., from mother to fetus and vice versa). Receptor-mediated endocytosis is much less understood. This mode of transport is believed to take a longer amount of time, as it requires membrane envelopment and release to the other side of the cell.
5. **C**. Uterine tight junctions, being structurally like the blood-brain barrier, effectively prevent the crossing of large molecules like heparin [3]. Medications that cannot easily cross the blood-brain barrier have difficulty crossing the placental barrier. Thorough understanding of medications and the degree to which the drug may cross the placenta is critical to fetal safety, particularly in the first trimester. Most sedative and anesthetic medications can cross the placenta with relative ease, the noted exception being agents that are hydrophilic, highly ionized, or large in molecular size [1]. Hydrophilic and ionized neuromuscular blocking agents generally neither cross the placenta nor the blood-brain barrier.

Although the blood-brain and placental barriers have obviously different roles within the overall system of the human body, similarities exist at the structural level that may serve to further guide the understanding and management of the parturient undergoing sedation or general anaesthesia.

6. **B.** Benzodiazepines can safely be taken during the third trimester as it does not impose any risk to the fetus. Benzodiazepines are lipid soluble and cross the placenta at a greater rate in the latter stages of pregnancy. Benzodiazepine use is not recommended in the third trimester near anticipated delivery, as it has shown associations with hypotonia or "floppy infant syndrome," lethargy, hypothermia, respiratory depression, and feeding difficulties after delivery. Globally, there has been an increased use of prescription benzodiazepines for the treatment of anxiety, depression, and, in the later stages of pregnancy, insomnia. Gastroesophageal reflux disease is a contributing factor for sleeping difficulties during the third trimester, as the supine position increases discomfort. Women also experience more anxiety in the third trimester and seek prescription benzodiazepines. There is no clear consensus delineating the trimesters in which benzodiazepine exposure could cause fetal harm, and practitioners must take into consideration the risks when weighing benzodiazepine use [4].
7. **B.** The water-soluble and positively charged highly ionized molecules of both depolarizing and nondepolarizing neuromuscular blocking drugs effectively prevent transfer across the placenta when administered in clinically relevant doses [4]. Rocuronium and succinylcholine were designated as FDA Pregnancy Category B and C, respectively, and are not known to induce skeletal muscle weakness or paralysis in the neonate. Pregnancy also leads to a decreased relative concentration of plasma cholinesterase because of increases in plasma volume. This not only affects hepatic clearance rates but also causes variations in the onset and duration of action for neuromuscular blocking drugs. As a result, attentive monitoring of the patient's neuromuscular function and slow judicious use of reversal agents are necessary to prevent rapid increases in circulating acetylcholine, which may cause uterine contractions [5].
8. **D.** Ondansetron was designated FDA Pregnancy Category B and is commonly prescribed to treat pregnancy-related nausea and vomiting related to pregnancy (i.e., "morning sickness") along with antihistamines such as dimenhydrinate and doxylamine [4]. First-generation antihistamines are known to also provide dose-dependent central nervous system depression. Initially, there was concern around the use of ondansetron in the first trimester of pregnancy and its potential teratogenicity. Dexamethasone has commonly been indicated for prophylactic postoperative nausea and vomiting in parturients. Over the years, further research has led to questions regarding the safety of administering dexamethasone in early pregnancy and whether the repeat administration of synthetic glucocorticoids at high doses affects maternal-fetal outcomes related to immunologic disturbances at the maternal-fetal interface. Conversely, the administration of steroids has also been helpful in providing protective effects for the parturient at risk for preterm delivery during the second and early third trimesters [6]. Healthy placental development and uterine remodeling

throughout the trimesters are crucial to fetal development. Immunosuppressive effects of dexamethasone can block placental growth factors, decrease key immune cells, and alter progesterone/estradiol levels, which can shrink the placenta and lead to unfavorable pregnancy outcomes [7].

9. **A**. That is Category C medication. Opioids readily cross the placenta and can be problematic. Maternal use of codeine, oxycodone, and hydrocodone was implicated among the opioids that may contribute to congenital heart defects, neural tube defects, and clubfoot. The possibility of opioid "imprinting" occurring to the fetus when fentanyl crosses into the fetal circulation and amniotic fluid has been suggested [8].
10. **C**. Neostigmine crosses the placenta and fetal bradycardia can occur, while glycopyrrolate does not. Atropine may be preferred to glycopyrrolate to antagonize the muscarinic effects of neostigmine during reversal. Among the anticoagulants heparin does not cross the placenta but warfarin crosses the placenta and is teratogenic. Quaternary ammonium compounds do not cross the placenta in normal clinical dose [9].
11. **D**. Ketamine was not assigned an FDA pregnancy category and still lacks adequate and well-controlled studies on safe use during pregnancy. Atropine crosses the placenta and causes fetal tachycardia. Nitrous oxide depresses the activity of methionine synthetase, an essential enzyme for DNA synthesis, causing a buildup of methylene tetrahydrofolate and homocysteine and leading to a lack of biologically active folate essential to fetal development or increased thrombosis in the parturient [10]. The use of volatile anesthetic agents has been advocated as they relax the uterus, although high concentrations can cause undesirable hypotension.
12. **A**. NSAIDs cause premature ductus arteriosus closure and should be avoided after 28 weeks. ACE inhibitors cause intrauterine growth restriction, oligohydramnios, and renal impairment. Beta-blockers cause intrauterine growth restriction, neonatal hypoglycemia, and bradycardia. Thiazides cause neonatal thrombocytopenia [9].

References

1. Griffiths SK, Campbell JP. Placental structure, function and drug transfer. Contin Educ Anaesth Crit Care Pain. 2015;15(2):84–9. https://doi.org/10.1093/bjaceaccp/mku013.
2. Włoch S, Pałasz A, Kamiński M. Active and passive transport of drugs in the human placenta. Ginekol Pol. 2009;80(10):772–7.
3. North Bristol NHS Trust. Information for pregnant women or women who have given birth who are receiving low molecular weight heparin. 2021. Accessed April 24, 2021. https://www.nbt.nhs.uk/maternity-services/pregnancy/heparin-use-during-pregnancy.
4. Shin J. Anesthetic management of the pregnant patient: Part 2. Anesth Prog. 2021;68(2):119–27. https://doi.org/10.2344/anpr-68-02-12.
5. Bucklin B, Gambling DR, Wlody DJ. A practical approach to obstetric anesthesia. Lippincott Williams & Wilkins; 2009.

6. Østensen M, Khamashta M, Lockshin M, et al. Antiinflammatory and immunosuppressive drugs and reproduction. Arthritis Res Ther. 2006;8(3):209. https://doi.org/10.1186/ar1957.
7. Ahmadabad HN, Jafari SK, Firizi MN, et al. Pregnancy outcomes following the administration of high doses of dexamethasone in early pregnancy. Clin Exp Reprod Med. 2016;43(1):15–25. https://doi.org/10.5653/cerm.2016.43.1.15.
8. Brimdyr K, Cadwell K. A plausible causal relationship between the increased use of fentanyl as an obstetric analgesic and the current opioid epidemic in the US. Med Hypotheses. 2018;119:54–7.
9. Nejdlova M, Johnson T. Anaesthesia for non-obstetric procedures during pregnancy. Contin Educ Anaesth Crit Care Pain J. 2012;12(4):203–6.
10. Fujinaga M. Teratogenicity of nitrous oxide. Best Pract Res Clin Anaesthesiol. 2021;15(3):363–75. https://doi.org/10.1053/bean.2001.0180.

Local Anesthetics and Local Anesthetic Systemic Toxicity (LAST) in Relation to Obstetric Anesthesia

Shashank Paliwal and Anju Grewal

Questions

1. **All are the reasons for a smaller dose requirement of a local anesthetic for neuraxial blockade in pregnant women except:**
   A. Epidural venous engorgement
   B. Enhanced neuronal sensitivity to local anesthetics
   C. A lower pH of CSF
   D. Hormonal and biochemical changes
2. **The half-life of 2-chloroprocaine in maternal plasma is increased due to the following:**
   A. Decrease in pseudocholinesterase activity
   B. Faster absorption of drugs from the injection site
   C. Increased binding proteins
   D. Decreased spread
3. **Which is true about lidocaine in pregnancy?**
   A. The free plasma fraction is increased.
   B. The volume of the central compartment is decreased.
   C. The volume of distribution has decreased.
   D. Urinary excretion is affected in pregnancy.
4. **Which of the following changes can be seen in the metabolism of bupivacaine during pregnancy?**
   A. Higher serum 2,6-pipecoloxylidide (PPX) concentrations
   B. Reduced protein binding during late pregnancy
   C. Lower effective dose

S. Paliwal (✉)
Department of Anaesthesiology, All India Institute of Medical Sciences, Bathinda, Punjab, India

A. Grewal
Department of Anaesthesiology and Critical Care, AIIMS Bathinda, Bathinda, Punjab, India

A. C. Sinha, I. F. Pasca (eds.), *Peripartum Care of the Pregnant Patient*,
https://doi.org/10.1007/978-3-031-62756-9_29

D. Decreased metabolism by hepatic microsomal cytochrome P450
E. All the above

5. **Rank local anesthetics in order of decreasing CNS toxicity**:
   A. Bupivacaine > lidocaine > 2-chloroprocaine > ropivacaine
   B. Bupivacaine > ropivacaine > lidocaine > 2-chloroprocaine
   C. Lidocaine > 2-chloroprocaine > ropivacaine > bupivacaine
   D. 2-Chloroprocaine > ropivacaine > bupivacaine > lidocaine
6. **Which of the following is/are risk factor/factors for local anesthetic toxicity?**
   A. Drugs with a low cardiovascular collapse/central nervous system (CC/CNS) ratio
   B. Pregnancy
   C. Transverse abdominis plane (TAP) block
   D. All the above
7. **Bupivacaine toxicity but not lidocaine toxicity can lead to malignant ventricular arrhythmia because**:
   A. Bupivacaine dissociates from sodium channels at a slow rate during diastole
   B. Bupivacaine has lower lipid solubility
   C. Bupivacaine has a longer duration of action
   D. Bupivacaine has a higher CC/CNS ratio
8. **The most common presenting feature seen in LAST is**:
   A. Cardiovascular collapse
   B. Seizure
   C. Malignant arrhythmia
   D. Apnea
9. **Pregnancy increases the risk of LAST because of**:
   A. Epidural vein distention
   B. Pregnancy-related decreases in protein binding
   C. Altered cardiomyocyte electrophysiology by hormonal effects of progesterone
   D. Increased neuronal susceptibility to local anesthetics
   E. All the above
10. **What percentage of cases of LAST have cardiovascular symptoms in the absence of CNS toxicity?**
    A. 5%
    B. 7%
    C. 11%
    D. 15%
11. **The most frequent ECG abnormality seen in LAST is**:
    A. Bradyarrhythmia
    B. Ventricular tachycardia
    C. ST changes
    D. Ventricular fibrillation
12. **Management of cardiac arrhythmia/arrest includes the following**:
    A. Advanced life support modified for pregnancy.

   B. Lidocaine can be used to treat bupivacaine-induced ventricular arrhythmia.
   C. Epinephrine doses should be > 1 μg/kg.
   D. Vasopressin.
   E. Beta-adrenergic blockers.
13. **The preferred treatment for LA-induced arrhythmia is as follows**:
   A. Lidocaine therapy
   B. Amiodarone
   C. Beta-blocker
   D. Adenosine
14. **Parturients are at a higher risk for refractory cardiac arrest after LAST than nonpregnant patients because of**:
   A. Reduced functional residual capacity
   B. Aortocaval compression
   C. Dilated azygous system
   D. All the above
15. **All measures are used to decrease the incidence of LAST in obstetric patients <u>except</u> for the following**:
   A. The epidural administration of 0.75% bupivacaine was avoided.
   B. Use of levorotatory isomers of bupivacaine.
   C. Fractionation of therapeutic dose.
   D. Intravenous injection of 0.25% bupivacaine.
16. **The preferred drug to suppress seizures in the management of local anesthetic systemic toxicity is as follows**:
   A. Benzodiazepines
   B. Propofol
   C. Magnesium
   D. Thiopentone
17. **All the following are true regarding lipid emulsion therapy for the treatment of LAST except**:
   A. Exogenous lipids create a gradient between tissue and blood
   B. Administration is based on the severity and progression of LAST
   C. Propofol can be used as a substitute for lipid emulsions
   D. The maximum dose is 10 mL/kg over the first 30 min
18. **Allergic reactions due to local anesthetics are associated with**:
   A. Additives and preservatives such as methylparaben and metabisulfite
   B. Response to procedural trauma
   C. Delayed hypersensitivity reaction
   D. History of allergy to latex
   E. All the above
19. **Incidence of local anesthetic systemic toxicity (LAST) per 1000 peripheral nerve blocks is**:
   A. 0.27
   B. 0.50
   C. 1.27
   D. 1.50

20. **Which local anesthetic among the following has the highest CC/CNS ratio?**
    A. Bupivacaine
    B. Lidocaine
    C. Ropivacaine
    D. Etidocaine
21. Measures to prevent local anesthetic systemic toxicity (LAST) in pregnant women include the following except:
    A. Use of the lowest effective dose of local anesthetic (LA)
    B. Ultrasound-guided nerve blockade
    C. Fast bolus injection of LA
    D. Use of the least toxic local anesthetic

Answers and Explanations

1. **C**. In fact, pregnant women have a higher cerebrospinal fluid (CSF) pH. An elevated pH level enhances the ratio of local anesthetic present in its base form and promotes drug diffusion through nerve membranes. The rest of the choices are correct, as epidural venous engorgement increases the spread of the drug, hormonal changes modulate neural blockade susceptibility, and neuronal sensitivity is enhanced in pregnancy [1].
2. **A**. Pregnancy shows a decrease of 30–40% in pseudocholinesterase activity, which is responsible for rapid hydrolysis of 2-chloroprocaine [2]. This leads to its prolonged absorption and effect with a higher risk of systemic toxicity. Choices B and C are incorrect.
3. **A**. There is a decrease in alpha1-acid glycoprotein (AAG), to which lidocaine is predominantly bound in plasma, leading to an increase in the free fraction of the drug [3]. This, in turn, also increases the volume of distribution and volume of concentration of lidocaine. Pregnancy does not affect urinary excretion of lidocaine; it remains unchanged.
4. **E**. 2,6-Pipecoloxylidide (PPX) is produced by dealkylation of bupivacaine in the liver, which is increased in pregnancy due to unclear reasons. Protein binding is reduced in late pregnancy, including albumin and alpha1-acid glycoprotein (AAG), to which bupivacaine extensively binds. Microsomal oxidases are competitively inhibited by progesterone and estrogen. The effective dose (ED50) is reduced (3.96 vs 4.14) in pregnant women for motor block in the case of intrathecal administration [4]. Choices A, B, C, and D are all correct.
5. **B**. CNS toxicity is dependent upon the blood concentration of local anesthetic and its potency. Local anesthetics can be ranked according to the CNS toxicity they can produce with a given amount of mean cumulative dose, in decreasing order as bupivacaine > ropivacaine > lidocaine > 2-chloroprocaine [5].
6. **D**. The risk factors for local anesthetic toxicity are related to the patient, injected drug, and technique used.
   I. The ratio of the drug dose to cause cardiovascular collapse to the dose causing a seizure is called the CC/CNS ratio. A higher ratio is considered safer,

as the early presentation of CNS features can help in diagnosis before cardiovascular collapse.

II. Physiological changes in pregnancy, such as decreased protein binding (increased peak free drug), increased cardiac output (enhanced uptake of drugs at the injected site), rapid absorption, and increased sensitivity to drugs, make parturients more susceptible to LAST.

III. Local anesthetic infiltration technique and the vascularity of the injection site are risk factors for LAST. TAP block involves injection of LA into the intermuscular plane in large quantities (the vascular supply of muscles is very high), which has the potential for higher systemic absorption [6].

7. **A**. Both lidocaine and bupivacaine affect the cardiovascular system by rapidly blocking sodium channels during systole. However, bupivacaine is slower in dissociating during longer diastole, making it more intense and potent in depression of ventricular conduction [7]. Bupivacaine is more lipid soluble, making it easier to cross the blood–brain barrier. It also has a longer duration of action than lidocaine. Bupivacaine has a narrower ratio of dose that can cause cardiovascular collapse to the dose required to cause convulsion, leading to its low safety margin.
8. **B**. Most cases of LAST follow a typical progressive pattern of presentation with a combination of CNS and cardiovascular system. The first and most common signs and symptoms are related to CNS toxicity, primarily in the form of a seizure. Prodromal signs such as perioral paresthesia, agitation, and audiovisual disturbances have also been described as early manifestations in a few patients. One-third of the reported cases progress to involve the cardiovascular system with dysrhythmias, conduction defects, hypotension, and arrest [6].
9. **E**. Obstetric patients are at an increased risk of LAST, and many of them receive regional anesthesia with exposure to local anesthetics. These patients are susceptible to local anesthetics for the following reasons:

   I. Distension of epidural veins leads to an increase in drug absorption and increases the risk of catheter migration in the case of epidural anesthesia.

   II. Increased cardiac output accelerates perfusion at the site of injection, causing more uptake of the drug.

   III. Pregnancy causes a decrease in protein binding in the plasma, increasing the proportion of free drug [8].

   IV. Progesterone and estradiol can lead to alterations in the electrophysiology of cardiomyocytes [9].

   V. Pregnancy may enhance neuronal susceptibility to local anesthetics, decreasing the seizure threshold [10].
10. **C**. LAST may present with a wide spectrum of signs and symptoms, with CNS symptoms being the first and most common to occur before cardiovascular signs. CNS findings may be especially difficult to see if the patient is receiving sedation or general anesthesia. In nearly 11% of cases, cardiovascular symptoms occur without CNS features [11].
11. **A**. Cardiovascular toxicity by local anesthetics commonly presents in the form of arrhythmia, with bradyarrhythmia being the most common. Other

abnormalities include ventricular ectopia, widening of the QRS complex, and conduction defects [11].

12. **A**. In 2010, the American Society of Regional Anesthesia and Pain Medicine (ASRA) published a practice advisory in the form of a checklist for managing local anesthetic systemic toxicity, which was subsequently updated [12]. It includes the following steps (modified for pregnancy):
    1. Call for help.
    2. Manual left uterine displacement was performed.
    3. Initial management:
       (a) Airway management: Ventilate with 100% oxygen.
       (b) Seizure suppression: Benzodiazepines are preferred. Propofol should be avoided if the cardiovascular system is involved.
       (c) Alert the nearest facility with cardiopulmonary bypass capability.
    4. Management of cardiac arrhythmias:
       (a) Basic and advanced cardiac life support (modified for pregnancy).
       (b) Reduce individual epinephrine doses to <1 μg/kg.
       (c) Avoid vasopressin, calcium entry-blocking agents, beta-adrenergic blockers, and local anesthetics.
    5. If clinically unstable or symptoms progressed, a 20% lipid emulsion was infused.
       (a) Administer a bolus of 1.5 mL/kg (lean body mass) intravenously over 1 min (approximately 100 mL).
       (b) A continuous intravenous infusion of 0.25 mL/kg/min (approximately 18 mL/min) was started.
       (c) Repeat the bolus once or twice if cardiovascular collapse persists.
       (d) The infusion rate was doubled to 0.5 mL/kg/min if blood pressure remained low.
       (e) Continue the infusion for at least 10 min after achieving cardiovascular stability.
       (f) The maximum dose is approximately 10 mL/kg over the first 30 min.

13. **B**. Amiodarone is the antiarrhythmic first line of drug for local anesthetic-induced ventricular arrhythmia [6]. Lidocaine therapy will worsen the symptoms and should not be given. Calcium entry-blocking agents, vasopressin, and beta-adrenergic blockers are avoided (refer to answer 12 for the management of LAST).
14. **D**. Obstetric patients are at a higher risk of refractory cardiac arrest due to the following:
    I. Reduced functional residual capacity, which speeds up hypoxemia.
    II. A large uterus compressing the aortocaval leads to inefficient cardiac compression in the supine position.
    III. Engorged dilated epidural vessels cause injected drugs to rapidly reach the heart.
15. **D**. The use of low doses of local anesthetics and incremental injections will decrease the incidence of LAST. Levorotatory isomers such as levobupivacaine and ropivacaine provide a greater safety margin when administered in large

quantities with a higher CC/CNS ratio. They have dose-dependent vasoactive properties, which decrease absorption and prolong duration [6]. Intravascular injection of the drug will increase the risk of toxicity; hence, choice D is the answer.

16. **A**. Benzodiazepines, such as midazolam or diazepam, with strong anticonvulsant properties are preferred for managing seizures in LAST. Propofol and thiopentone are cardiac depressants and should not be given. Refer to answer 12 for the management of LAST.
17. **C**. The rapid administration of lipid emulsion causes a gradient between tissue and blood that draws a high concentration of local anesthetic from the heart or brain into the aqueous plasma. This is called the sink effect [13]. The administration is based upon the severity and stage of LAST. Propofol formulation has inadequate lipid content to cause a gradient and treat LAST. Moreover, it causes cardiac depression, which will aggravate hypotension. Refer to answer 12 for the dosage of lipid emulsion.
18. **E**. Allergic reactions are rare but may be IgE- or non-IgE-mediated reactions due to the presence of additives such as methylparaben, metabisulfite, latex, etc. The symptoms may also be caused by procedural trauma of drug administration, hyperventilation or vasovagal syncope during drug injection, sympathetic stimulation leading to palpitations and tachycardia caused by epinephrine, or edema resulting from the injection procedure itself [14].
19. **A**. Local anesthetic systemic toxicity is a serious and potentially life-threatening occurrence that can occur when local anesthetic techniques are used in different healthcare environments. The utilization of these techniques has become more widespread, and the estimated incidence of LAST is currently 0.03%, equivalent to 0.27 episodes per 1000 peripheral nerve blocks [6].
20. **B**. Levorotatory isomers such as levobupivacaine and ropivacaine have a CC/CNS ratio of 2, ropivacaine of 5, etidocaine of 4.4, and lidocaine of 7.1 [6].
21. **C**. The following measures can be taken to prevent LAST:
    - I. Use the lowest effective dose of local anesthetic.
    - II. Use the least toxic anesthetic such as levobupivacaine.
    - III. Use slow incremental injections.
    - IV. Aspirate the catheter before injecting the drug.
    - V. Use ultrasound-guided blocks to prevent intravascular injection and minimize the amount of drug administered.
    - VI. Maintain continuous vigilance for signs and symptoms of LAST.

References

1. Fagraeus L, Urban BJ, Bromage PR. Spread of epidural analgesia in early pregnancy. Anesthesiology. 1983;58:184–7. https://doi.org/10.1097/00000542-198302000-00015.
2. Kuhnert BR, Kuhnert PM, Philipson EH, et al. The half-life of 2-chloroprocaine. Anesth Analg. 1986;65:273–8.

3. Wood M, Wood AJ. Changes in plasma drug binding and alpha 1-acid glycoprotein in mother and newborn infant. Clin Pharmacol Ther. 1981;29:522–6. https://doi.org/10.1038/clpt.1981.73.
4. Pihlajamäki K, Kanto J, Lindberg R, et al. Extradural administration of bupivacaine: pharmacokinetics and metabolism in pregnant and non-pregnant women. Br J Anaesth. 1990;64:556–62. https://doi.org/10.1093/bja/64.5.556.
5. Scott DB. Evaluation of the toxicity of local anaesthetic agents in man. Br J Anaesth. 1975;47:56–61. https://doi.org/10.1093/bja/47.1.56.
6. El-Boghdadly K, Pawa A, Chin KJ. Local anesthetic systemic toxicity: current perspectives. Local Reg Anesth. 2018;11:35–44. https://doi.org/10.2147/LRA.S154512.
7. Clarkson CW, Hondeghem LM. Mechanism for bupivacaine depression of cardiac conduction: fast block of sodium channels during the action potential with slow recovery from block during diastole. Anesthesiology. 1985;62:396–405.
8. Tsen LC, Tarshis J, Denson DD, et al. Measurements of maternal protein binding of bupivacaine throughout pregnancy. Anesthes Analg. 1999;89:965. https://doi.org/10.1213/00000539-199910000-00027.
9. Moller RA, Datta S, Fox J, et al. Effects of progesterone on the cardiac electrophysiologic action of bupivacaine and lidocaine. Anesthesiology. 1992;76:604–8. https://doi.org/10.1097/00000542-199204000-00018.
10. Butterworth JF, Walker FO, Lysak SZ. Pregnancy increases median nerve susceptibility to lidocaine. Anesthesiology. 1990;72:962–5. https://doi.org/10.1097/00000542-199006000-00002.
11. Di Gregorio G, Neal JM, Rosenquist RW, Weinberg GL. Clinical presentation of local anesthetic systemic toxicity: a review of published cases, 1979 to 2009. Reg Anesth Pain Med. 2010;35:181–7. https://doi.org/10.1097/aap.0b013e3181d2310b.
12. Neal JM, Mulroy MF, Weinberg GL. American Society of Regional Anesthesia and Pain Medicine checklist for managing local anesthetic systemic toxicity: 2012 Version. Reg Anesth Pain Med. 2012;37:16–8. https://doi.org/10.1097/AAP.0b013e31822e0d8a.
13. Bern S, Weinberg G. Local anesthetic toxicity and lipid resuscitation in pregnancy. Curr Opin Anesthesiol. 2011;24:262. https://doi.org/10.1097/ACO.0b013e32834654df.
14. Bhole MV, Manson AL, Seneviratne SL, Misbah SA. IgE-mediated allergy to local anaesthetics: separating fact from perception: a UK perspective. Br J Anaesth. 2012;108:903–11. https://doi.org/10.1093/bja/aes162.

Uterotonics and Antifibrinolytics

Ivan Rybkin

Questions

1. **Maternal hemorrhage is defined as signs or symptoms of hypovolemia within 24 h after birth or as a cumulative blood loss of:**
   A. 500 ml
   B. 750 ml
   C. 1000 ml
   D. 1500 ml
2. **The most common source of postpartum hemorrhage is:**
   A. Uterine artery
   B. Surgical site bleeding (hysterotomy)
   C. Vaginal or cervical laceration
   D. Retained placenta
   E. Coagulation defect
3. **The first-line pharmacologic agent of choice to be used after vaginal or cesarean delivery to prevent postpartum hemorrhage is as follows:**
   A. Carboprost (Hemabate)
   B. Methylergonovine maleate (Methergine)
   C. Oxytocin receptor agonist
   D. Misoprostol
4. **A grand multiparous patient presented with advanced cervical dilation and proceeded with rapid vaginal delivery. After vaginal delivery, uterine atony was diagnosed with significant vaginal bleeding. The patient has no IV access. The next best pharmacologic treatment option is:**
   A. Methergine administered IM
   B. Bimanual uterine massage

I. Rybkin (✉)
Riverside University Health System, Moreno Valley, CA, USA
e-mail: i.rybkin@ruhealth.org

A. C. Sinha, I. F. Pasca (eds.), *Peripartum Care of the Pregnant Patient*,
https://doi.org/10.1007/978-3-031-62756-9_30

   C. Misoprostol administered rectally
   D. Carboprost (Hemabate) administered IM
   E. Oxytocin administered IM
5. **Which of the following uterotonic medications is contraindicated in patients with hypertensive disorder or cardiovascular disease?**
   A. Oxytocin
   B. Methylergonovine maleate (Methergine)
   C. Carboprost (Hemabate)
   D. Misoprostol
6. **Which of the following uterotonic medications is contraindicated in patients with asthma or active pulmonary disease?**
   A. Oxytocin
   B. Methylergonovine maleate (Methergine)
   C. Carboprost (Hemabate)
   D. Misoprostol
7. **How frequently can one administer carboprost (Hemabate) in the setting of postpartum hemorrhage?**
   A. Once
   B. Every 5–15 min
   C. Every 15–90 min
   D. Every 2–4 h
8. **Due to an increased risk of vascular thrombosis in the immediate postpartum period, antifibrinolytic agents such as tranexamic acid should be avoided when managing patients with postpartum hemorrhage. True or False?**
   A. True
   B. False
9. **Tranexamic acid was found to be most effective at preventing postpartum hemorrhage when given within what period from delivery?**
   A. 1–3 h
   B. 3–6 h
   C. 6–12 h
   D. 12–24 h
10. **What is the mechanism of action of tranexamic acid (TXA)?**
   A. It prevents the conversion of prothrombin to thrombin.
   B. It prevents the conversion of plasminogen to plasmin.
   C. It prevents conversion of fibrinogen to fibrin.
   D. It prevents the conversion of fibrin to plasmin.

Answers

1. **C**. The old definition of postpartum hemorrhage differentiated vaginal and cesarean routes of deliveries. Blood loss greater than 500 ml for vaginal delivery (**A**) and 1000 ml for cesarean delivery (**C**) cutoffs was used. Currently, we

use 1000 ml as the definition of postpartum hemorrhage regardless of the route of delivery. In addition, postpartum hemorrhage can also be diagnosed if a patient demonstrates signs or symptoms of hypovolemia within the first 24 h after birth [1].

2. **A**. Uterine atony is responsible for 70–80% of postpartum hemorrhage and should first be evaluated as the cause of postpartum hemorrhage [1]. Answers **B**, **C**, **D**, and **E** are all potential cases of postpartum hemorrhage but are not as common. Careful examination of the vagina and cervix should be performed after atony has been ruled out [1].
3. **C.** Since most cases of postpartum hemorrhage are due to uterine atony, oxytocin receptor agonists are used to rapidly contract the uterus after delivery and prevent hemorrhage. Oxytocin is a rapidly acting agent and is the most appropriate first-line choice. Other agents in answers **A**, **B**, and **D** are also used to manage hemorrhage due to atony; however, they are not the first-line options [1].
4. **E**. A first-line pharmacologic agent of choice due to uterine atony is oxytocin administered as 10 units intramuscularly. It is the most effective of all options and has the fewest side effects.

   Bimanual uterine massage (**B**) is an important step and should be performed, but it is a nonpharmacologic therapy. Other pharmacologic agents (answers **A**, **C**, **D**) are good second-line pharmacologic options [1].
5. **B**. Methergine (methylergonovine maleate) is contraindicated in patients with hypertension, preeclampsia, gestational hypertension, and significant cardiovascular disease, as it can cause worsening of hypertension resulting in cerebrovascular accident or myocardial infarction. Oxytocin (**A**) and misoprostol (**D**) can both be used in patients with hypertensive disorders. Carboprost (**C**) should be used with caution in patients with hypertensive disorders [1].
6. **C**. Carboprost (Hemabate) should be avoided in patients with asthma, as well as active pulmonary or hepatic disease. The use of Hemabate can cause bronchospasm, leading to the deterioration of pulmonary function in these patients. Oxytocin (**A**), Methergine (**B**), and misoprostol (**D**) can all be used in this patient population [1].
7. **C**. Carboprost (Hemabate) can be administered every 15–90 min for up to eight doses. One should be aware that it can cause significant diarrhea, and some providers prefer to administer medications to decrease GI motility. Misoprostol is given once (**A**); methylergonovine (Methergine) is typically administered every 2–4 h (**D**) [1].
8. **B**. This is a false statement. The use of antifibrinolytics such as tranexamic acid (TXA) in the obstetric population is encouraged even in the setting of a hypercoagulable state of pregnancy and the immediate postpartum period. Using TXA significantly reduces mortality from postpartum hemorrhage, as seen in the WOMAN trial [1].
9. **A**. A large, randomized control trial (WOMAN trial) assessed the administration of TXA within 3 h of birth, which significantly reduced mortality (1.2% vs. 1.7%) due to postpartum hemorrhage in women who had received TXA vs the

control group. TXA can also be administered prophylactically to reduce the amount of blood loss during delivery (cesarean or vaginal delivery) [1].

10. **B**. Tranexamic acid works by reversibly binding plasminogen, which prevents the formation of plasmin. Plasmin participates in fibrin degradation and clot dissolution. Administering TXA therefore prevents clot degradation [1].

References

1. Shields LE, Goffman D, Caughey AB. Practice Bulletin No. 183: Postpartum hemorrhage. Obstet Gynecol. 2017:1–19.

Further Reading

Escobar MF, Nassar AH, Theron G, et al. FIGO recommendations on the management of postpartum hemorrhage 2022. Int J Gynaecol Obstet. 2022;157(Suppl. 1):3–50. https://doi.org/10.1002/ijgo.14116.

Gallos ID, Papadopoulou A, Man R, et al. Uterotonic agents for preventing postpartum haemorrhage: a network meta-analysis. Cochrane Database Syst Rev. 2018;12(12):CD011689. https://doi.org/10.1002/14651858.CD011689.pub3.

Sentilhes L, Lasocki S, Ducloy-Bouthors AS, et al. Tranexamic acid for the prevention and treatment of postpartum haemorrhage. Br J Anaesth. 2015;114(4):576–87. https://doi.org/10.1093/bja/aeu448.

ACLS in Pregnancy

Chelsea Lee, Alexandra Vacaru, and John V. Agapian

Questions

1. **Physiological changes during pregnancy include all of the following *except*:**
   A. Functional residual capacity decreases by 10–25% during pregnancy
   B. Increased renal blood flow by 40%
   C. Cardiac output rises 30–50%
   D. Intravascular volume is decreased, and uterine vascular resistance is increased
2. **Chest compressions of the gravid patient should be performed at a rate of:**
   A. At least 100 per minute
   B. 40–50 per minute
   C. 60–80 per minute
   D. Less than 40
3. **Left uterine displacement during CPR ______.**
   A. Has no benefit
   B. Should be continuously performed
   C. Should be performed at the end of the compression cycle
   D. Only recommended when the uterus is easily palpated
4. **When defibrillation is needed, ______.**

C. Lee
Riverside University Health System, Moreno Valley, CA, USA

A. Vacaru
Loma Linda University, Loma Linda, CA, USA

J. V. Agapian (✉)
Riverside University Health System, Moreno Valley, CA, USA

Loma Linda University, Loma Linda, CA, USA

University of California Riverside, Riverside, CA, USA
e-mail: john.agapian@gte.net

A. C. Sinha, I. F. Pasca (eds.), *Peripartum Care of the Pregnant Patient*,
https://doi.org/10.1007/978-3-031-62756-9_31

A. 120–200 J should be used with subsequent energy escalation if not effective
B. Contraindicated in pregnant patient
C. Less energy should be delivered to protect the fetus
D. More energy than normal is required to also benefit the fetus

5. **For shock-resistant ventricular fibrillation, ______.**
   A. Transcutaneous pacing should be initiated
   B. Adenosine should be pushed
   C. Amiodarone should be administered
   D. Vasopressin support should be started
6. **Because of the physiological changes that take place during pregnancy, ______.**
   A. ACLS drug doses are adjusted to a higher dose
   B. Usual ACLS drug dosage is recommended
   C. ACLS drug doses are adjusted to a lower dose
   D. Many of the ACLS drugs are contraindicated
7. **During CPR of the gravid patient, ______.**
   A. Continuous fetal monitoring should be performed
   B. Fetal monitoring is performed between each compression
   C. Fetal monitoring is not recommended
   D. Fetal heart rate monitoring is more important than material heart rate monitoring
8. **Factors that may contribute to aortocaval compression of the gravid uterus include all of the following *except*:**
   A. Lower body mass index
   B. Weight of the amniotic fluid
   C. The number of fetuses
   D. Relationship of the fetus to the woman's anatomy
9. **Perimortem cesarean delivery (PMCD) ______.**
   A. Should only be considered after the patient has been pronounced
   B. May help relieve aortocaval compression when manual LUD was not adequate
   C. Should only be considered if fetal heart tones are still present
   D. Currently not a recommended practice guideline
10. **Perimortem cesarean delivery (PMCD) ______.**
    A. Should be considered after 4 min if ROSC cannot be achieved
    B. Should never be performed
    C. Should be performed only after four rounds of CPR and no ROSC
    D. Should be performed immediately after the airway is established
11. **Up to how many days after delivery or termination of pregnancy is maternal mortality defined as?**
    A. 14 days
    B. 30 days
    C. 42 days
    D. 90 days

12. **Unstable pregnant patients should be managed utilizing all of the following *except*:**
    A. Full left lateral decubitus position placement
    B. Administration of 100% oxygen
    C. Intravenous access below the diaphragm
    D. Addressing precipitating factors
13. **During pregnancy, stroke volume ______.**
    A. Increases by 20–30%
    B. Decreases by 20–30%
    C. Increases by 10–20%
    D. Decreases by 10–20%
14. **For pregnant patients in cardiac arrest, ______.**
    A. Fetal monitors should be attached and used
    B. Magnesium administration should be stopped
    C. Calcium chloride/gluconate should be stopped
    D. Give one breath every 3 s
15. **Using defibrillator pads rather than paddles allows for the following:**
    A. Increased potential for task saturation
    B. Intermittent display of electrical cardiac activity
    C. Fetal monitoring
    D. Ability to be used to both defibrillate and pace

Answers and Explanations

1. **D**. During pregnancy, intravascular volume is increased, and uterine vascular resistance is decreased. Total blood volume, plasma volume, and red blood cell mass increase during pregnancy, with plasma volume increasing more than red blood cell mass. An increase in progesterone, estrogen, and nitric oxide during pregnancy will cause a decrease in systemic vascular resistance during pregnancy [1]. As the fetus grows, the diaphragm is elevated, resulting in a decrease in functional residual capacity by 10–25%. This reduction in FRC with the increase in oxygen consumption during pregnancy leads to the rapid development of hypoxemia during apnea or hypoventilation. In addition, there is an increase in ventilation, causing mild respiratory alkalosis with metabolic compensation [1, 2]. There is an additional task of filtering fetal metabolic byproducts. Therefore, there is an increase in renal blood flow by 40% and glomerular hyperfiltration [1, 3]. Stroke volume and maternal heart rate increase during pregnancy. This results in an increase in cardiac output by 30–50% [4, 5].
2. **A**. Per the American Heart Association, chest compressions on a pregnant patient should be performed at a rate of at least 100 per minute [6].
3. **B**. During pregnancy, lying in the supine positioning results in aortocaval compression. Aortocaval compression should be relieved continuously with manual left uterine displacement during CPR and during postarrest care. For manual

left uterine displacement, the uterus is cupped and elevated upward and to the left [7].

4. **A**. Per ACLS, patients should be defibrillated at 120–200 joules on a biphasic defibrillator when a patient is in ventricular fibrillation or pulseless ventricular tachycardia. These principles are the same in pregnancy. Transthoracic impedance is unchanged during pregnancy, meaning energy requirements during cardiac arrest are also unchanged [8]. Energy from defibrillation does not cause harm to the fetus and is safe in all trimesters [7].
5. **C**. Similar to defibrillation therapy, medical therapy is the same for patients who are pregnant or nonpregnant. In shock-resistant ventricular fibrillation and tachycardia, amiodarone 300 mg should be given. Patients can be given additional 150 mg doses as needed [1]. Two separate randomized control studies performed by Dorian et al. [9] and Kudenchuk et al. [10] have demonstrated better survival rates to a medical center for out-of-hospital cardiac arrest with amiodarone than lidocaine.
6. **B**. Current American Heart Association recommendations are to use same ACLS drug dosages in pregnant patients as in nonpregnant patients [1]. The first randomized study looking at the efficacy of epinephrine with patients undergoing ACLS demonstrated improvement in ROSC with epinephrine, but no overall difference in survival [11]. Per AHA guidelines, 1 mg epinephrine can be given every 3–5 min during cardiac arrest. Vasopressin has also been studied and it has not been demonstrated that it has better outcomes than epinephrine. Per 2010 AHA guidelines, 40 U of vasopressin can be a substitute for the first or second dose of epinephrine. However, vasopressin can induce uterine contractions, and epinephrine is the agent of choice during pregnancy [12].
7. **C**. ACLS guidelines state continuous fetal monitoring should not be used during cardiac arrest [13]. Continuous fetal monitoring would not direct management and may serve as a distraction from appropriate ACLS management [14]. When cardiac arrest is managed with delivery of the fetus, continuous fetal monitoring should be started after ROSC [1].
8. **A**. Aortocaval compression is dependent on uterine weight and the position of the fetus related to woman's anatomy. Uterine weight is affected by weight of the fetus, number of the fetus, and weight of amniotic fluid. BMI does not contribute to uterine weight [1].
9. **B.** Perimortem cesarean delivery (PMCD) is the delivery of the fetus during resuscitation with maternal cardiac arrest. Even when a fetus is not viable, the gravid uterus can cause aortocaval compression depending on the uterine weight, and PMCD should be considered [7].
10. **A**. Per ACLS, if the uterine fundus is at or above the umbilicus and ROSC has not been achieved in 4 min of maternal cardiac arrest, PMCD is recommended. Four minutes is the recommended time because the risk of fetal neurological damage starts at 4–6 min of anoxic cardiac arrest when resuscitative efforts fail [15].
11. **C**. Per AHA, maternal mortality refers to the death of a woman during pregnancy or within 42 days after giving birth or terminating pregnancy. This

definition applies when the cause of death is related to or worsened by the pregnancy or its management [1].

12. **C**. Timely intervention in pregnant patients experiencing instability is crucial in preventing cardiac arrest. It is imperative to optimize maternal hemodynamics, by placing the patient in a full left lateral decubitus position to relieve aortocaval compression, treat hypoxemia, and establish intravenous access *above* the diaphragm to ensure that the intravenously administered therapy is not obstructed by the gravid uterus [1].
13. **A**. Stroke volume refers to the quantity of blood pumped into the aorta during each cardiac cycle. In pregnancy, the blood volume increases. This leads to an increase in the amount of blood returning to the heart (the preload), and the afterload is reduced because of maternal vasodilatation, resulting in a 20–30% increase in the stroke volume [5].
14. **B**. The ACLS In-Hospital Cardiac Arrest in Pregnancy Algorithm recommends detaching or not using fetal monitors for the fetus (**A**). Magnesium administration should be stopped and reversed with calcium chloride/gluconate (**C**). The airway should be supported, and the mother should be provided one breath every 6 s, not 3 s (**D**) [13].
15. **D**. The benefits of using pads rather than paddles allows for the decreased potential for task saturation (it is unnecessary to hold the pads once they are placed), not increased (**A**). There is also a continuous display of electrical cardiac activity, and this may be used to simultaneously defibrillate and pace if the pads are placed both anteriorly and posteriorly (**B**). Fetal monitoring in the setting of maternal cardiac arrest is not advised and may distract the staff and harm management (**C**) [14].

References

1. Jeejeebhoy FM, et al. Cardiac arrest in pregnancy: a scientific statement from the American heart association. Circulation. 2015;132(18):1747–73.
2. Contreras G, et al. Ventilatory drive and respiratory muscle function in pregnancy. Am Rev Respir Dis. 2012.
3. Varga I, et al. Analysis of maternal circulation and renal function in physiologic pregnancies; parallel examinations of the changes in the cardiac output and the glomerular filtration rate. J Matern Fetal Med. 2000;9(2):97–104.
4. San-Frutos L, et al. Hemodynamic changes during pregnancy and postpartum: a prospective study using thoracic electrical bioimpedance. J Matern Fetal Neonatal Med. 2011;24(11):1333–40.
5. Tan EK, Tan EL. Alterations in physiology and anatomy during pregnancy. Best Pract Res Clin Obstet Gynecol. 2013;27(6):791–802.
6. Berg RA, et al. Part 5: adult basic life support: 2010 American Heart Association guidelines for cardiopulmonary resuscitation and emergency cardiovascular care. Circulation. 2010;122(18_suppl_3):S685–705.
7. Vanden Hoek TL, et al. Part 12: cardiac arrest in special situations: 2010 American Heart Association guidelines for cardiopulmonary resuscitation and emergency cardiovascular care. Circulation. 2010;122(18_suppl_3):S829–61.

8. Nanson J, et al. Do physiological changes in pregnancy change defibrillation energy requirements? Br J Anesth. 2001;87(2):237–9.
9. Dorian P, et al. Amiodarone as compared with lidocaine for shock-resistant ventricular fibrillation. N Engl J Med. 2002;346(12):884–90.
10. Kudenchuk PJ, et al. Amiodarone for resuscitation after out-of-hospital cardiac arrest due to ventricular fibrillation. N Engl J Med. 1999;341(12):871–8.
11. Olasveengen TM, et al. Intravenous drug administration during out-of-hospital cardiac arrest: a randomized trial. JAMA. 2009;302(20):2222–9.
12. Bossmar T, et al. Receptors for and myometrial responses to oxytocin and vasopressin in preterm and term human pregnancy: effects of the oxytocin antagonist atosiban. Am J Obstet Gynecol. 1994;171(6):1634–42.
13. ACLS In-Hospital Cardiac Arrest in Pregnancy Algorithm. ACLS Medical Training [cited 2023 05/12/2023]. aclsmedicaltraining.com/acls-in-hospital-cardiac-arrest-in-pregnancy-algorithm/#:~:text=Fetal%20monitoring%20should%20not%20beteam%20should%20conduct%20the%20resuscitation.
14. Lipman S, et al. The Society for Obstetric Anesthesia and Perinatology consensus statement on the management of cardiac arrest in pregnancy. Anesth Analg. 2014;118(5):1003–16.
15. Katz V, Balderston K, DeFreest M. Perimortem cesarean delivery: were our assumptions correct? Am J Obstet Gynecol. 2005;192(6):1916–20.

Massive Maternal Hemorrhage and REBOA

Chelsea Lee and Sara Edwards

Questions

1. **Typical application of REBOA in obstetrics requires placement of the catheter in which location?**
   A. Zone I
   B. External iliac artery
   C. Zone III
   D. Zone II
   E. REBOA catheters are not recommended for obstetrics use
2. **Which of the following anatomic landmarks define zone I for REBOA catheter placement?**
   A. Between the innominate artery and the left subclavian artery
   B. Between the celiac and inferior mesenteric arteries
   C. Between the external and internal iliac arteries
   D. Between the left subclavian and celiac arteries
   E. Between the renal arteries and iliac bifurcation
3. **A 32-year-old female G6P3 at 14 weeks gestation, with a history of hepatitis C and preeclampsia, presented with profuse vaginal hemorrhage. The initial blood pressure was 90/50 with a HR of 120. IV fluids are initiated, and labs are sent. OB is called to evaluate the patient and identify placental abruption with a need for emergent surgical intervention. You are called to preop the patient. Initial labs on POC:**

C. Lee · S. Edwards (✉)
Riverside University Health System, Moreno Valley, CA, USA
e-mail: s.edwards@ruhealth.org

A. C. Sinha, I. F. Pasca (eds.), *Peripartum Care of the Pregnant Patient*,
https://doi.org/10.1007/978-3-031-62756-9_32

Hgb 9.2
Hct 27.6%
INR 4.2
K+ 3.5
pH 7.25

Based on patient presentation and preliminary labs, what resuscitative measures might support this patient intraoperatively?

A. Ongoing crystalloid resuscitation in the setting of hypotension
B. 10 units of O(−) packed red blood cells on call to the OR
C. 10 mg of vitamin K and ongoing crystalloid resuscitation prior to the OR
D. Administer 2 units of fresh frozen plasma now and prepare 4 units of packed red blood cells on call to the OR
E. Wait for the full set of labs to return prior to administration of blood products

4. **Pregnant patients receiving REBOA hemorrhage control during C-section are at what risk of thrombosis compared to other hemorrhaging patients?**
   A. Decreased risk; pregnant patients have larger blood volume and are at increased risk for bleeding
   B. Increased risk; pregnant patients are hypercoagulable
   C. Equivocal risk; no difference has been reported in the risk for thrombosis between pregnant patients and the general population
   D. REBOA catheters are contraindicated for use in pregnant patients
   E. REBOA catheters stop blood flow to the distal vessels and limit the risk for clot formation
5. **With the use of standard thromboelastogram, the American College of Surgeons recommends which triggers for resuscitation?**
   A. Plasma for r-value >9 s
   B. Plasma and/or cryoprecipitate for *k*-time >4 s
   C. Cryoprecipitate and/or plasma for α angle <60 °
   D. Platelets for mA <55 mm
   E. Anti-fibrinolytics for LY30 >7.5%
   F. All of the above
   G. None of the above
6. **Hemorrhage may occur in the peripartum period due to uterine atony. Management strategies include the following:**
   A. Blakemore tube placement
   B. Administration of oxytocin IV 10–40 units per 1000 mL or 10 units IM
   C. The use of 100 mcg IV phenylephrine to promote peripheral vasodilation
   D. Administration of only packed red blood cells and crystalloids
   E. Administration of octreotide 50 mcg and then 50 mcg/h
7. **What is a risk factor for uterine atony?**
   A. Anorexia nervosa
   B. Alcoholism
   C. Rapid labor
   D. Fetus that is small for gestational age
   E. Diabetes mellitus

8. **Optimal administration of blood products is delivered via:**
   A. Triple-lumen central venous catheter
   B. Intraosseous catheter
   C. 22 g peripheral venous catheter
   D. 16 g peripheral venous catheter
   E. Radial artery catheter
9. **A patient undergoes cesarean section. Following delivery, the patient began to experience hemorrhage. She is hypotensive, and massive transfusion is initiated. A hysterectomy is performed. She received 16 units of packed red blood cells, 13 units of fresh frozen plasma, and 2 packs of platelets. Additional cryoprecipitate is administered. The patient continues to bleed and has hypotension despite source control and targeted resuscitation. The cause for these ongoing derangements may be secondary to the following:**
   A. The patient's pH was 7.35
   B. The ionized calcium concentration is 0.7 mmol/L
   C. Base deficit is 2
   D. The axillary temperature is 33.6 °C
   E. A, C, and D
   F. B and D
10. **When using a REBOA catheter in obstetrics, typical timing to inflation of the occlusive balloon is as follows:**
    A. At the start of the operation
    B. Following delivery of the neonate
    C. Following removal of the uterus
    D. Once the uterus has been sewn closed
    E. Prior to incising the uterus
11. **Which of the below place a woman at highest risk for placenta accreta?**
    A. Prior C-section
    B. Placenta previa
    C. Multiparity
    D. A, B, and C
    E. C
12. **A 25-year-old female who was 36 weeks pregnant presented to the hospital with sudden vaginal bleeding and abdominal pain. She is found to have non-reassuring fetal heart tones. The patient was admitted for placental abruption and taken to the OR for urgent cesarean delivery. During the C-section, the patient was noted to have hematuria in her Foley bag and oozing from her IV sites. What are the expected laboratory findings?**
    A. Increased platelets, increased PT, increased PTT, increased fibrinogen, increased D-dimer
    B. Decreased platelets, decreased PT, increased PTT, decreased fibrinogen, decreased D-dimer
    C. Decreased platelets, decreased PT, decreased PTT, decreased fibrinogen, increased D-dimer
    D. Decreased platelets, increased PT, increased PTT, decreased fibrinogen, increased D-dimer

13. **A 28-year-old female at 39 weeks had a spontaneous vaginal delivery. She continues to have vaginal bleeding with greater than 500 mL of blood initially and ongoing blood loss. The patient's heart rate was 115 beats/min with blood pressure 86/56. In addition to starting resuscitation, which of the following is recommended for management in postpartum hemorrhage?**
    A. Give nitroglycerin
    B. Administer TXA
    C. Give calcium
    D. Give FFP and cryoprecipitate
14. **A patient experiences postpartum hemorrhage after delivery. Uterine atony is thought to be the cause of hemorrhage. Fundal massage was started, and oxytocin infusion was increased to 40 units/L. Despite these interventions, the patient continues to hemorrhage; what is the best next step?**
    A. Continue to increase oxytocin dosage
    B. Look for other sources of bleeding
    C. Place Bakri balloon for tamponade
    D. Place a central line for IV access
15. **A patient has ongoing postpartum hemorrhage, despite medical management and vacuum-induced suction device use. The patient is then brought to the OR for further intervention. Which of the following agents does not contribute to uterine atony?**
    A. Sevoflurane
    B. Desflurane
    C. Nitric oxide
    D. Halothane

Answers and Explanations

1. **C.** REBOA catheters in obstetrics are typically deployed in zone III, in the aorta just proximal to the aortic bifurcation [1]. Placement in this location allows for hemorrhage control without ischemia to the abdominal viscera, minimizing systemic insult to the patients while still achieving hemorrhage control.
2. **D**. Zone I is located between the left subclavian and celiac arteries. In zone I, the REBOA catheter functions as a "cross-clamp" on the aorta, concentrating perfusion to the heart and brain and excluding flow distal to the inflated balloon [2]. Placement in zone I is reserved for the management of severe hypotension and may have a role in ACLS [3, 4]. Because of the distal ischemia caused by aortic occlusion at this level, inflation times are limited.
3. **D**. This patient presented with hemorrhagic shock. She also has evidence of coagulopathy, which may be precipitated by her hemorrhage or could also be secondary to underlying hepatic insufficiency. Her INR is elevated, and she is anemic with evidence at presentation of ongoing hemorrhage. This patient needs goal-directed resuscitation and source control of her hemorrhage with operative intervention.

4. **B**. Pregnant patients are hypercoagulable and at increased risk for thrombotic events even in the setting of hemorrhage. REBOA catheters disrupt the flow of blood distal to the inflated balloon catheter and may precipitate clot formation. Heparin, either systemically administered or via the catheter sheath in an infusion, is recommended to reduce the risk of arterial thrombosis while the REBOA catheter is in use [1]. Initial management may include crystalloids to emergently address her hypotension, but this is only a temporizing measure. Blood products should be ordered and administered expeditiously, and hemodilution with crystalloids should be discontinued at the earliest opportunity [5]. Currently identified coagulopathy should be corrected with fresh frozen plasma. Additional laboratory assessments, including fibrinogen, a CBC, and thromboelastogram, if available, help to further determine the extent of coagulopathy and target discrete points of intervention. This patient's history of hepatitis C and preeclampsia should prompt concern for possible thrombocytopenia. She is also at risk for the development of DIC, and ongoing surveillance throughout the course of resuscitation should be performed to ensure optimal treatment of acute blood loss anemia. Fibrinogen and platelet levels may help to guide diagnosis and intervention. Additional agents, including tranexamic acid and prothrombin complex concentrate, may also serve as adjuncts to resuscitation and hemorrhage control [6].
5. **F**. Thromboelastograms (TEG) help to guide resuscitation in real time, expediting targeted intervention and optimizing transfusion with rapid correction of coagulopathy. Visual aids and calculated variables provide feedback to the user to identify specific deficits in the coagulation cascade that, when repleted, facilitate robust clot formation and cessation of bleeding.

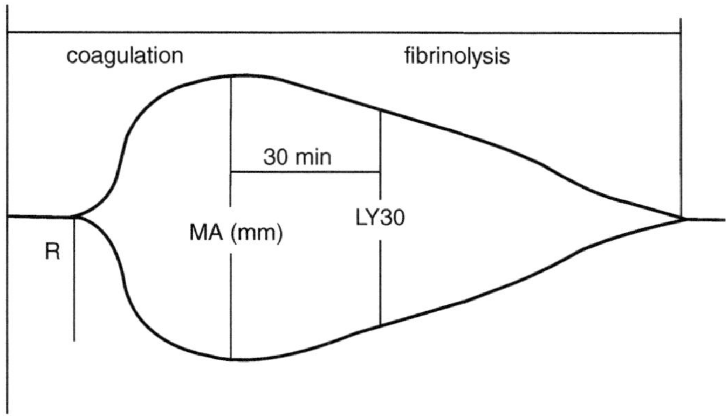

6. **B**. Uterine atony may occur after delivery. Globally, uterine atony is one of the top five causes of maternal death and accounts for nearly 70% of cases of postpartum hemorrhage [7]. Retained placenta may contribute to delayed uterine contraction and hemostasis. Strategies to facilitate appropriate uterine contraction include evacuation of the placenta and retained products of conception,

uterine massage with low-level traction on the umbilical cord, and the use of oxytocin infusion [8]. Additional treatments include the administration of methylergonovine, 15-methyl-PGF2-alpha (Hemabate), misoprostol, and dinoprostone [7, 8]. Uterine packing or the use of a Bakri balloon may provide tamponade by direct pressure. If hemostasis is unable to be achieved, surgery may be required for uterine curettage, uterine or hypogastric artery ligation, compression sutures, or hysterectomy. TEG reports display the progression of clot formation and dissolution, reporting on the viscoelasticity of the specimen. R-value or R-time marks the interval to initiate clot formation with fibrin formation. This event is facilitated by clotting factors II, VII, IX, and X, and coagulopathy in this phase may be treated with the administration of fresh frozen plasma. K-time corresponds to a period of clot strengthening that is influenced by the availability of coagulation factors and fibrinogen. The efficacy of coagulation factors, fibrinogen, and platelets to form effective fibrin cross-linking and the strength of the clot are marked by the α angle and mA (or amplitude). Low angle or amplitude marks a need for cryoprecipitate and/or platelets to correct coagulopathy. Subsequent degradation and fibrinolysis are depicted in the LY30 value, which speaks to the duration of the clot and the rate at which it dissolves. Weak clot formation and rapid breakdown require treatment for DIC, with a recommendation for tranexamic acid administration [5].

7. **E**. A systematic review and meta-analysis of the literature performed by Ende et al. in 2021 revealed 47 variables that may contribute to uterine atony [7]. Six were found to be definite risk factors and included Asian race, history of postpartum hemorrhage, gestational or preexisting diabetes mellitus, placenta disorders, prolonged labor, and genital tract trauma sustained during delivery. Morbid obesity, although reported in prior studies as a contributor, was not found to be associated with uterine atony in this review. Blakemore drains are used for the treatment of esophageal and GE junction hemorrhage, and crystalloids should be limited or avoided in the setting of hemorrhage. Octreotide is used in the management of mesenteric GI bleeding. Phenylephrine does not promote selective vasoconstriction of the uterine vessels.
8. **D**. Short, large-bore access provides the best conduit for volume resuscitation. This is based on the physics of resistance calculated by $R = (þL)/A$, where resistance (R) equals the length (L) of a cylinder times the resistivity (þ) of the material from which the cylinder is made, divided by the cross-sectional area of the cylinder. Consequently, the longer and smaller the diameter of the catheter is, the higher the resistance and the slower the delivery of fluids. Gauge measurements, originating with the British wire industry in the nineteenth century, correspond inversely to the thickness of a material. The higher the gauge, the smaller the diameter of the catheter. Consequently, a 16 g peripheral catheter is wider than a 18, 20, or 22 gauge [9].

In the absence of adequate peripheral access, an intraosseous or I/O catheter may be placed. The flow rates of intraosseous access vary based on location but approximate that of a 21 g peripheral IV with a range from 20 to over 3000 mL/h under pressure. Pharmacokinetics and dynamics have been found to be comparable to administration via IV [10].

9. **F**. Balanced transfusion and ongoing resuscitation directed by thromboelastogram and laboratory monitoring of coagulation factors help to achieve hemostasis with source control. However, other variables may contribute to ongoing hemodynamic derangements and hemorrhage. Ongoing acidosis, marked by a high base deficit (particularly >12.5), and hypocalcemia (ionized calcium <1 mmol/L) contribute to ongoing hypotension [11]. Resuscitative efforts should include treatment of acidosis. Hypocalcemia and hypothermia also contribute to ongoing coagulopathy and hemorrhage. Calcium (1–2 grams) should be administered for every 6 units of packed red blood cells administered, and levels should be monitored throughout resuscitation [11].
10. **B**. REBOA catheters may be used to facilitate prevention and control of hemorrhage in obstetric cases where percreta and accreta are anticipated to complicate delivery [12]. Bleeding typically occurs with the removal and delivery of the placenta. Blood flow to the fetus should be preserved. Therefore, the REBOA catheter should not be inflated until after the baby's delivery.
11. **D**. Placenta accreta is the abnormal attachment of the placenta to the uterus that can cause massive postpartum hemorrhage during an attempt to remove the placenta during delivery. Women are at highest risk for placenta accreta when they have a previous history of a cesarean section causing myometrial damage and now a pregnancy with placenta previa. The risk for placenta accreta increases with the number of previous C-sections. A patient with placenta previa with one previous C-section has an approximately 10% risk of placenta previa, whereas if they have had four C-sections, the risk is >60% [13].
12. **D**. This patient has disseminated intravascular coagulation. DIC occurs in response to an underlying disorder such as placental abruption, HELLP syndrome, preeclampsia, retained stillbirth, postpartum hemorrhage, acute fatty liver, or amniotic fluid embolism. In overt DIC, both coagulation and fibrinolysis are increased, leading to overt bleeding and thrombosis. Laboratory findings that suggest DIC are thrombocytopenia, prolonged PT/PTT, and decreased fibrinogen with increased D-dimer [14].
13. **B**. National guidelines recommend administration of TXA along with uterotonics in women with postpartum hemorrhage within 3 h of delivery. When the placenta separates from the uterine wall during delivery, there is a change in maternal physiology leading to increased fibrinolytic activity. Therefore, TXA is recommended to counteract this physiologic change when treating postpartum hemorrhage. The World Maternal Antifibrinolytic Trial (WOMAN Trial) was a randomized controlled, double-blinded study that demonstrated decreased death in postpartum patients who received TXA without an increase in adverse events [15].
14. **C**. The initial steps for the management of uterine atony are uterine massage and pharmacologic interventions. If these interventions are ineffective, the next step is to perform a uterine tamponade with a tamponade balloon (such as a Bakri balloon) or vacuum-induced suction device [16].

15. **C**. In a study performed by Yoo et al., volatile anesthetics were found to cause a decrease in uterine contractility, worsening atony, and hemorrhage [17]. The depression of uterine contractility is dose-dependent to volatile anesthetics.

References

1. Hall C, et al. Massive transfusions and severe hypocalcemia: an opportunity for monitoring and supplementation guidelines. Transfusion. 2021;61(Suppl 1):S188–94.
2. Brenner M, et al. Resuscitative endovascular balloon occlusion of the aorta (REBOA) may be superior to resuscitative thoracotomy (RT) in patients with traumatic brain injury (TBI). Trauma Surg Acute Care Open. 2022;7(1):e000715.
3. Levis A, et al. Resuscitative endovascular balloon occlusion of the aorta (REBOA) during cardiopulmonary resuscitation: a pilot study. Resuscitation. 2020;156:27–34.
4. Teeter W, et al. Resuscitative endovascular balloon occlusion of the aorta improves cardiac compression fraction versus resuscitative thoracotomy in patients in traumatic arrest. Ann Emerg Med. 2018;72(4):354–60.
5. ACS TQIP Massive Transfusion in Trauma Guidelines. Trauma quality improvement program 2014 April 30, 2023; https://www.facs.org/media/zcjdtrd1/transfusion_guildelines.pdf.
6. Higgins N, Patel SK, Toledo P. Postpartum hemorrhage revisited: new challenges and solutions. Curr Opin Anesthesiol. 2019;32(3):278–84.
7. Ende HB, et al. Risk factors for atonic postpartum hemorrhage: a systematic review and meta-analysis. Obstet Gynecol. 2021;137(2):305–23.
8. Dahlke JD, et al. Prevention and management of postpartum hemorrhage: a comparison of 4 national guidelines. Am J Obstet Gynecol. 2015;213(1):76 e1–76 e10.
9. Milne A, et al. Performance assessment of intravenous catheters for massive transfusion: a pragmatic in vitro study. Transfusion. 2021;61(6):1721–8.
10. Leidel BA, et al. Is the intraosseous access route fast and efficacious compared to conventional central venous catheterization in adult patients under resuscitation in the emergency department? A prospective observational pilot study. Patient Saf Surg. 2009;3(1):24.
11. Lier H, et al. Preconditions of hemostasis in trauma: a review. The influence of acidosis, hypocalcemia, anemia, and hypothermia on functional hemostasis in trauma. J Trauma. 2008;65(4):951–60.
12. Ioffe YJM, et al. When the balloon goes up, blood transfusion goes down: a pilot study of REBOA in placenta accreta spectrum disorders. Trauma Surg Acute Care Open. 2021;6(1):e000750.
13. Wortman AC, Alexander JM. Placenta accreta, increta, and percreta. Obstet Gynecol Clin N Am. 2013;40(1):137–54.
14. Erez O, et al. DIC in pregnancy - pathophysiology, clinical characteristics, diagnostic scores, and treatments. J Blood Med. 2022;13:21–44.
15. Shakur H, et al. The WOMAN Trial (World Maternal Antifibrinolytic Trial): tranexamic acid for the treatment of postpartum hemorrhage: an international randomized, double blind placebo controlled trial. Trials. 2010;11:40.
16. Kaya B, et al. Balloon tamponade for the management of postpartum uterine hemorrhage. J Perinat Med. 2014;42(6):745–53.
17. Yoo KY, et al. The effects of volatile anesthetics on spontaneous contractility of isolated human pregnant uterine muscle: a comparison among sevoflurane, desflurane, isoflurane, and halothane. Anesth Analg. 2006;103(2):443–7. table of contents

Accidental Dural Puncture

Antonio Gonzalez-Fiol and Christopher Dextras

Questions

1. **What is the incidence of accidental dural puncture in parturient patients?**
   A. 1–2%
   B. 3–6%
   C. 7–15%
   D. 16–21%
2. **Which of the following is a common symptom of accidental dural puncture?**
   A. Urinary incontinence
   B. Pain radiating down the lower extremities
   C. Vertigo
   D. Saddle anesthesia
3. **The incidence of headache following accidental dural puncture by an epidural needle is:**
   A. 2%
   B. 10%
   C. 40%
   D. 80%
4. **Which of the following consistently improves postdural puncture headache (PDPH) symptoms?**
   A. Prophylactic epidural blood patch
   B. Placement of an abdominal binder
   C. Supine patient position
   D. Oral sumatriptan administration

A. Gonzalez-Fiol (✉)
Division of Obstetric Anesthesia, Yale School of Medicine, New Haven, CT, USA
e-mail: antonio.gonzalez-fiol@yale.edu

C. Dextras
Yale School of Medicine, New Haven, CT, USA

A. C. Sinha, I. F. Pasca (eds.), *Peripartum Care of the Pregnant Patient*,
https://doi.org/10.1007/978-3-031-62756-9_33

5. **Which of the following is associated with an increased risk of PDPH?**
   A. High-volume CSF removal
   B. Advanced maternal age
   C. Cigarette smoking
   D. Elevated body mass index
6. **Which needle gauge size is associated with the greatest risk of PDPH?**
   A. 27
   B. 24
   C. 22
   D. 20
7. **Which type of spinal needle has the lowest incidence of postdural puncture headache?**
   A. Whitaker
   B. Quincke
   C. Tuohy
   D. Greene
8. **Which of the following risk factors *decrease* the incidence of PDPH?**
   A. Cesarean delivery
   B. Vaginal delivery
   C. Obesity
   D. Female gender
9. **Which of the following is *not* a known risk factor for PDPH?**
   A. Age between 20 and 29
   B. Bevel orientation to the dural fibers
   C. Cutting needles (e.g., Quincke)
   D. Previous history of PDPH
10. **Compared to patients without accidental dural puncture, those with dural puncture are more likely to be readmitted due to which one of the following complication(s):**
    A. Cerebral venous thrombosis
    B. Subdural hematoma
    C. Bacterial meningitis
    D. All the above
11. **Following an accidental dural puncture, what is the ideal time for performing an epidural blood patch?**
    A. 12 h
    B. 24 h
    C. 24–48 h
    D. > 48 h
12. **Based on current evidence, what is the optimal volume of blood to be utilized in an epidural blood patch?**
    A. 5–10 mL
    B. 15 mL
    C. 20 mL
    D. 30 mL

13. **Which of the following is true regarding the epidural blood patch procedure?**
    A. Following the procedure, the patient should remain in a seated position for 1–2 h
    B. EBP placement should be 1–2 spinal levels cephalad to the initial puncture level
    C. Patients should avoid anticoagulant medication for 24 h following the procedure
    D. Headache symptoms typically dissipate within 1 min of procedure completion
14. **Which one of the following cranial nerves is most likely to be affected secondary to accidental dural puncture?**
    A. III
    B. IV
    C. VI
    D. VIII
15. **Which of the following is consistently true when converting to spinal analgesia utilizing an intrathecal catheter rather than resiting after an accidental dural puncture?**
    A. Reduced incidence of headache
    B. Reduced incidence of blood patch
    C. Easier establishment of analgesia
    D. Increased complications to establish neuraxial analgesia
16. **What percentage of patients who undergo a single therapeutic blood patch experience full resolution of symptoms without any recurrence?**
    A. Up to 10%
    B. Up to 20%
    C. Up to 80%
    D. Up to 100%
17. **Which parasympathetic ganglion block has been postulated as an alternative to epidural blood patch?**
    A. Sphenopalatine or pterygopalatine ganglion block
    B. Ciliary ganglion block
    C. Otic ganglion block
    D. Submandibular ganglion block
18. **Which imaging finding would *not* be expected on MRI in a patient with PDPH?**
    A. Pituitary gland enlargement
    B. Downward displacement of the brain
    C. Small ventricles
    D. Compressed cerebral venous sinuses

Answers and Explanations

1. **A**. In the obstetric population, accidental dural puncture complicates approximately 1.5% of epidural procedures performed every year, with that number being slightly higher for inexperienced clinicians, making **B**, **C**, and **D** incorrect [1].
2. **C.** Vertigo is commonly reported after accidental dural puncture, along with headache worsening in the upright position, nausea, neck pain, changes in vision, or radicular symptoms in the arms. Urinary incontinence (**A**) can be observed following spinal anesthesia. Pain radiating down the lower extremities (**B**) is a common feature of sciatica. Saddle anesthesia (**D**) is caused by cauda equina syndrome, most commonly from disc herniation [2].
3. **D**. Approximately 60–80% of patients experience headache following accidental dural puncture with an epidural needle, whereas approximately 10% (**B**) of patients experience headache after dural puncture with a spinal needle. **A** and **C** are incorrect [1, 3].
4. **C**. A headache that improves in the supine position is the classic exam finding for patients with PDPH. Studies on caffeine, theophylline, gabapentin, and hydrocortisone have shown decreased pain scores in PDPH. Placement of an abdominal binder (**B**) and oral sumatriptan administration (**D**) are not widely recommended. Prophylactic epidural blood patch placement (**A**) has not been shown to significantly prevent PDPH [2, 4].
5. **A**. High-volume CSF removal (>20 mL) is associated with PDPH. Advanced maternal age (**B**) is associated with a lower risk of PDPH. Cigarette smoking (**C**) and elevated BMI (**D**) are associated with other obstetric complications but not PDPH [5].
6. **D**. In needle size nomenclature, a lower gauge corresponds to a larger needle diameter. Of the options listed, the 20-gauge needle has the largest diameter, making **A**, **B**, and **C** incorrect. Of note, smaller spinal needles may bend more easily and may require the use of an introducer. Clinicians' access to resources and ability should always play a role in selecting instrumentation [6, 7].
7. **A**. Spinal needles can be divided into two classes: cutting and pencil tip. Whitaker and Sprotte have a pencil tip design with the opening located on the side of the needle and are associated with a lower incidence of PDPH. Quincke (**B**), Tuohy (**C**), and Greene (**D**) are examples of cutting needles with a sharp needle opening located at the tip, creating greater trauma upon entry [6, 7].
8. **A**. Cesarean delivery and not vaginal delivery has been associated with a decreased risk of postdural puncture headache, making **B** a false statement. Studies suggest that the Valsalva movements needed for vaginal delivery increase cerebrospinal fluid leakage. The inverse relationship between obesity (**C**) and PDPH has been challenged, and its validity remains inconclusive. Female gender (**D**) is a known factor related to increased PDPH [8].
9. **B**. Although parallel insertion of the needle through the dura has often been cited as a factor that can decrease PDPH, the physiology of the dura would

argue against this statement. Dural fibers do not follow a specific pattern of distribution. In addition, the needle also penetrates the arachnoid layer, which is composed of cells attached by tight junctions. Hence, bevel orientation has no effect on the risk for PDPH. On the other hand, young age (**A**), female sex, type of needle (cutting needle > pencil point) (**C**), and history of PDPH (**D**) are known risk factors for PDPH [9].

10. **D**. The incidence of cerebral venous thrombosis and subdural hematoma was noted to be 0.312% (1 of 320 PDPH cases) in a recent study by Guglielminotti et al. The mechanism related to this increase in complications is related to the decrease in cerebrospinal fluid, which leads to an increase in stress and rupture of the meningeal veins, ultimately resulting in subdural hematoma (**B**). The increased risk for cerebral vein thrombosis (**A**) is hypothesized to be secondary to the increased venous dilation to compensate for the decreased intracranial pressure and the hypercoagulable state of pregnancy. Bacterial meningitis (**C**), although rare (<10 cases; 1/40,000), had an adjusted risk 40-fold higher than that of patients without an accidental dural puncture (1/69,000) [10].
11. **D**. Patients who received an epidural blood patch within 24 (**A** and **B**), 24–48 (**C**), and >48 h (**D**) after an accidental dural puncture had permanent relief (no need for a second epidural blood patch) of 50%, 65%, and 86%, respectively. It has been postulated that during the first 48 h, a large pressure gradient and/or the amount of cerebrospinal fluid within the epidural space may limit the ability for a clot to form or adhere to the dura. Despite this information, experts recommend that patients should be counseled regarding the increased risk for the possible need for a second blood patch [11].
12. **C**. In a randomized, blinded clinical trial by Paech et al., patients received 15 mL (**B**), 20 mL (**C**), or 30 mL (**D**) of autologous blood. The incidence permanent or partial relief of headache was 61%, 73%, and 67%, respectively [12].
13. **D**. There is an almost immediate dissipation of the headache following a successful epidural blood patch. Following the procedure, the patient should remain in a supine position, with the head of the bead at a maximum of 30 ° (**A**). MR imaging has demonstrated that injected blood spreads more cephalad than caudad, making **B** incorrect. There are no standard recommendations that a patient should remain off anticoagulant medication following an epidural blood patch (**C**) [11].
14. **C**. The anatomic course of CN VI is susceptible to traction stress in the setting of intracranial hypotension due to its 90 ° bend over the petrous bone. Injury to the abducens results in 92–95% of all cranial nerve palsies due to PDPH [13].
15. **C**. When faced with an accidental dural puncture, there are two options: insert the catheter and convert to spinal anesthesia or remove the needle and resite the epidural catheter at another space. Regardless of selection, a lack of evidence surrounds the benefits related to a decreased incidence of headache (**A**) and/or need for a blood patch (**B**). Studies have shown that the use of spinal analgesia can be beneficial by reducing (not increasing) (**D**) complications such as repeat dural puncture and provides a rapid onset of action [14, 15].

16. **C.** It has been estimated that after an epidural blood patch, 20–30% (**C**) of patients will need a second blood patch and do not experience complete resolution after the procedure. The literature suggests that the success rate can be lower than 50% (**A**), putting the efficacy of an epidural blood patch somewhere approximately 35–80%, making **A**, **B**, and **D** false [12, 16].
17. **A**. The sphenopalatine ganglion (SPG) block, also known as the pterygopalatine block, is the only ganglion block mentioned above that has been utilized for the treatment of PDPH. The use of SPG has been previously described for the management of cluster headaches, and its benefits for the treatment of postdural puncture headache are at best inconclusive. There are some case reports that suggest that its use can ameliorate and resolve pain related to postdural puncture, yet a randomized controlled trial failed to demonstrate the efficacy of the block over placebo. It is the author's opinion that the SPG may be offered to patients as an alternative when an epidural blood patch is contraindicated, as in the case of local or systemic infection. After all, if SPG is to work, it will do so by preventing symptoms, yet it will not rectify the cerebrospinal fluid leak [17–19].
18. **D**. PDPH is diagnosed based on symptom presentation and patient history; imaging is almost never needed. However, an MRI would likely demonstrate pituitary gland enlargement (**A**), downward displacement of the brain (**B**), and small ventricles (**C**). These findings stem from loss of CSF as cushioning for the brain, leading to drooping. Cerebral venous sinuses would be engorged as a compensatory mechanism, making **D** incorrect. These imaging findings are like those of patients with spontaneous intracranial hypotension [20, 21].

References

1. Choi PT, et al. PDPH is a common complication of neuraxial blockade in parturients: a meta-analysis of obstetrical studies. Can J Anesth. 2003;50(5):460–9. https://doi.org/10.1007/bf03021057.
2. Vilming ST, et al. The significance of age, sex, and cerebrospinal fluid pressure in post-lumbar-puncture headache. Cephalalgia. 1989;9(2):99–106. https://doi.org/10.1046/j.1468-2982.1989.902099.x.
3. Del Pizzo K, et al. Post-dural puncture headache is uncommon in young ambulatory surgery patients. HSS J. 2017;13(2):146–51. https://doi.org/10.1007/s11420-017-9541-0.
4. Ona XB, et al. Drug therapy for treating PostDural puncture headache. Cochrane Database Syst Rev. 2020;9:2015. https://doi.org/10.1002/14651858.cd007887.pub3.
5. Smith JH, et al. CSF pressure, volume, and post-dural puncture headache: a case-control study and systematic review. Headache. 2019;59(8):1324–38. https://doi.org/10.1111/head.13602.
6. Vallejo MC, et al. Postdural puncture headache: a randomized comparison of five spinal needles in obstetric patients. Anesth Analg. 2000;91(4):916–20. https://doi.org/10.1097/00000539-200010000-00027.
7. Zorrilla-Vaca A, et al. The impact of spinal needle selection on postdural puncture headache: a meta-analysis and Metaregression of randomized studies. Obstet Anesth Dig. 2019;39(2):82. https://doi.org/10.1097/01.aoa.0000557666.40775.e4.

8. Jagannathan DK, et al. Effect of Neuraxial technique after inadvertent dural puncture on obstetric outcomes and anesthetic complications. Int J Obstet Anesth. 2016;25:23–9. https://doi.org/10.1016/j.ijoa.2015.09.002.
9. Barad M, Carroll I, Reina MA, et al. Did she have an epidural? The long-term consequences of postdural puncture headache and the role of unintended dural puncture. Headache. 2021;61(9):1314–23.
10. Guglielminotti J, et al. Major neurologic complications associated with postdural puncture headache in obstetrics. Anesth Analg. 2019;129(5):1328–36. https://doi.org/10.1213/ane.0000000000004336.
11. Booth JL, et al. A retrospective review of an epidural blood patch database: the incidence of epidural blood patch associated with obstetric neuraxial anesthetic techniques and the effect of blood volume on efficacy. Int J Obstet Anesth. 2017;29:10–7. https://doi.org/10.1016/j.ijoa.2016.05.007.
12. Paech MJ, et al. The volume of blood for epidural blood patch in obstetrics. Anesth Analg. 2011;113(1):126–33. https://doi.org/10.1213/ane.0b013e318218204d.
13. Hofer JE, Scavone BM. Cranial nerve VI palsy after dural-arachnoid puncture. Anesth Analg. 2015;120(3):644–6.
14. Heesen M, et al. Insertion of an intrathecal catheter following accidental dural puncture: a meta-analysis. Int J Obstet Anesth. 2013;22(1):26–30. https://doi.org/10.1016/j.ijoa.2012.10.004.
15. Orbach-Zinger S, et al. Risk factors for unintended dural puncture in obstetric patients. Anesth Analg. 2016;123(4):972–6. https://doi.org/10.1213/ane.0000000000001510.
16. Gupta A, Van de Velde M, et al. European practices in the management of Accidental Dural Puncture in Obstetrics Investigators. Factors associated with failed epidural blood patch after accidental dural puncture in obstetrics: a prospective, multicenter, international cohort study. Br J Anesth. 2022;129(5):758–66.
17. Cohen S, et al. Topical sphenopalatine ganglion block compared with epidural blood patch for postdural puncture headache management in postpartum patients. Reg Anesth Pain Med. 2018;43(8):880–4. https://doi.org/10.1097/aap.0000000000000840.
18. Pacheco J, Ribeiro M. Transnasal sphenopalatine ganglion block for treatment of postdural puncture headache in obstetric patients. 2019. https://doi.org/10.26226/morressier.5d1.cc24d57558b317a173613.
19. Sviggum HP. Faculty opinions recommendation of sphenopalatine ganglion block for the treatment of postdural puncture headache: a randomized, blinded, clinical trial. Faculty Opinions—PostPublication Peer Review of the Biomedical Literature. 2020. https://doi.org/10.3410/f.737776512.793577109.
20. Michali-Stolarska M, et al. Diagnostic imaging and clinical features of intracranial hypotension—review of literature. Polish J Radiol. 2018;83:16–23. https://doi.org/10.5114/pjr.2018.72970.
21. Hannerz J, et al. MR imaging with gadolinium in patients with and without post lumbar puncture headache. Acta Radiol. 1999;40(2):135–41. https://doi.org/10.3109/02841859909177728.

Amniotic Fluid Embolism (AFE)

Ashley Beem and Christia Del Rosario

Questions

1. **Which of the following is/are diagnostic criteria for AFE?**
   A. Sudden onset cardiopulmonary arrest
   B. Disseminated intravascular coagulation (DIC)
   C. Clinical onset during labor/placental delivery
   D. All the above
2. **What is the incidence of AFE?**
   A. 6 per 100,000 deliveries
   B. 10 per 100,000 deliveries
   C. 60 per 100,000 deliveries
   D. 100 per 100,000 deliveries
3. **Which of the following is NOT associated with AFE?**
   A. Western US region
   B. Oligohydramnios
   C. Grand multiparity
   D. Black and Asian race
4. **Pregnancy factors that are associated with AFE include all of the following EXCEPT:**
   A. Placenta accreta spectrum
   B. Placental abruption
   C. Uterine rupture
   D. Macrosomia

A. Beem (✉)
Loma Linda OBGYN Residency Program, Linda School of Medicine, Loma Linda, CA, USA

Riverside University Health System, Moreno Valley, CA, USA
e-mail: a.beem@ruhealth.org

C. Del Rosario
Department of Gynecology and Obstetrics, Loma Linda University School of Medicine, Riverside University Health System—Medical Center, Moreno Valley, CA, USA

A. C. Sinha, I. F. Pasca (eds.), *Peripartum Care of the Pregnant Patient*,
https://doi.org/10.1007/978-3-031-62756-9_34

5. **Delivery factors that are associated with AFE include the following:**
   A. Late term
   B. Spontaneous labor
   C. Operative delivery
   D. Cesarean delivery
   E. Both C and D
6. **Which of the following risk factors has the highest association with AFE?**
   A. Placenta accreta spectrum
   B. Intra-amniotic infection
   C. Preeclampsia
   D. Fetal demise
7. **What is the mortality rate of AFE in recent literature?**
   A. 10%
   B. 17%
   C. 25%
   D. 40%
8. **Which of the following cofactors increase/increases the AFE mortality rate above 30%?**
   A. Cardiac arrest
   B. ARDS
   C. Placenta increta/percreta
   D. All of the above
9. **What medications have been shown in case reports to help prevent DIC in cases of AFE?**
   A. Atropine
   B. Ondansetron
   C. Ketorolac
   D. All of the above
10. **What is the most common heart rhythm noted in AFE?**
    A. Pulseless electrical activity (PEA)
    B. Asystole
    C. Ventricular tachycardia
    D. Bradycardia
11. **American Heart Association Guidelines recommend beginning perimortem cesarean delivery within how many minutes of cardiac arrest?**
    A. 4 min with delivery of fetus by 5 min
    B. 8 min with delivery of fetus by 10 min
    C. 10 min with delivery of fetus by 15 min
    D. 15 min with delivery of fetus by 20 min
12. **Other causes of cardiopulmonary compromise include the following:**
    A. Acute pulmonary embolism (PE)
    B. Anaphylactic shock
    C. Septic shock
    D. All of the above
13. **DIC is present in what percentage of AFE cases?**
    A. 63%

B. 73%
C. 83%
D. 93%

14. **The analysis of the national registry states that this percentage of cases of AFE occurs during labor:**
    A. 60%
    B. 70%
    C. 80%
    D. 90%
15. **Which age range has the highest association with AFE?**
    A. ≤29
    B. 30–34
    C. 35–39
    D. ≥ 40

Answers and Explanations

1. **D.** The triad of sudden onset cardiopulmonary arrest (**A**), disseminated intravascular coagulation (**B**), and clinical onset of labor/placental delivery (**C**) make up the typical presentation of AFE [1].

Uniform diagnostic criteria for research reporting of amniotic fluid embolism	
1	Sudden onset cardiopulmonary arrest, or both hypotension (SBP <90 mmHg) and respiratory compromise (dyspnea, cyanosis, or peripheral capillary oxygen sat [SpO_2] <90%)
2	Documentation of overt DIC following appearance of these initial signs or symptoms, using scoring system of scientific and standardization committee on DIC of the ISTH
3	Clinical onset during labor or within 30 min of delivery of placenta
4	No fever (≥38.0 °C) during labor

2. **A**. The incidence of AFE slightly increased from 2016 to 2019 from 5.2 to 6.5 per 100,000 deliveries. Choices **B**, **C**, and **D** are too high [2].
3. **B**. Advanced maternal age (**A**), grand multiparity (**C**), and Black and Asian race (**D**) are all associated with increased incidence of AFE. Polyhydramnios, not oligohydramnios, is also associated with AFE [2].
4. **D**. Placenta accreta spectrum (PAS) (**A**), placental abruption (**B**), and uterine rupture (**C**) are all pregnancy factors that are associated with AFE. Other pregnancy factors associated are intra-amniotic infection, polyhydramnios, fetal demise, and fetal growth restriction [2].
5. **E (both C and D)**. Delivery factors that are associated with AFE are both operative and cesarean deliveries. Early gestational age, induction of labor, manual removal of the placenta, and cervical ripening are other delivery factors that are associated with AFE [2].

6. **A**. Placenta accreta spectrum (PAS) disorder has the highest association with AFE, with the more severe forms of PAS (increta/percreta) having a greater association [2].
7. **B**. The mortality rate of AFE in recent literature is 17% [2].
8. **D**. Cardiac arrest, ARDS, and placenta increta/percreta all increase the mortality of AFE rate to above 30% [2].
9. **D**. Atropine, ondansetron, and ketorolac have all been shown to help in DIC (A-OK regimen). Atropine (**A**) at a dose of 1 mg blocks vagal stimulation and counteracts parasympathetic effects that contribute to bradycardia. Ondansetron (**B**) at a dose of 8 mg blocks serotonin receptors, which are found in vagal terminals of the heart and lungs and cause pulmonary vasoconstriction. Ketorolac (**C**) at a dose of 30 mg blocks thromboxane, which is a major platelet activator [3, 4].
10. **A**. PEA is the most common initial heart rhythm noted in AFE at 24%, undescribed/normal sinus rhythm (24%), bradycardia (22%) (**D**), ventricular tachycardia/fibrillation (17%) (**C**), and asystole (13%) (**B**) [3].
11. **A**. The American Heart Association recommendation is to begin perimortem cesarean delivery at 4 min to effect delivery at 5 min of the fetus after failed resuscitative efforts. The other choices are incorrect; however, the above goal may not be possible [5].
12. **D**. Acute PE, anaphylactic, and septic shock are all other cases of cardiopulmonary compromise.
13. **C**. Although DIC is not seen in all cases of AFE, it is present in 83% of AFE cases [6].
14. **B**. 70% of cases of AFE occur during labor, 19% during cesarean delivery, and 11% after a vaginal delivery [6].
15. **D.** Maternal ages over 30 years old are at increased risk; however, those aged 40 or greater are at the highest risk of AFE [2].

References

1. Clark SL, Romero R, Dildy GA, Callaghan WM, Smiley RM, Bracey AW, Hankins GD, D'Alton ME, Foley M, Pacheco LD, Vadhera RB, Herlihy JP, Berkowitz RL, Belfort MA. Proposed diagnostic criteria for the case definition of amniotic fluid embolism in research studies. Am J Obstet Gynecol. 2016;215(4):408–12. https://doi.org/10.1016/j.ajog.2016.06.037. Epub 2016 Jun 29. PMID: 27372270; PMCID: PMC5072279
2. Mazza GR, Youssefzadeh AC, Klar M, Kunze M, Matsuzaki S, Mandelbaum RS, Ouzounian JG, Matsuo K. Association of pregnancy characteristics and maternal mortality with amniotic fluid embolism. JAMA Netw Open. 2022;5(11):e2242842. https://doi.org/10.1001/jamanetworkopen.2022.42842. PMID: 36399343; PMCID: PMC9675004
3. Leighton BL Amniotic fluid embolism, March of Dimes. 2013. http://www.marchofdimes.org/pdf/missouri/AFE_11-21-13.pdf.
4. Long M, Martin J, Biggio J. Atropine, ondansetron, and ketorolac: supplemental management of amniotic fluid embolism. Ochsner J. 2022;22(3):253–7. https://doi.org/10.31486/toj.21.0107. PMID: 36189093; PMCID: PMC9477128

5. Jeejeebhoy FM, Zelop CM, Lipman S, Carvalho B, Joglar J, Mhyre JM, Katz VL, Lapinsky SE, Einav S, Warnes CA, Page RL, Griffin RE, Jain A, Dainty KN, Arafeh J, Windrim R, Koren G, Callaway CW, American Heart Association Emergency Cardiovascular Care Committee, Council on Cardiopulmonary, Critical Care, Perioperative and Resuscitation, Council on Cardiovascular Diseases in the Young, and Council on Clinical Cardiology. Cardiac arrest in pregnancy: a scientific statement from the American Heart Association. Circulation. 2015;132(18):1747–73. https://doi.org/10.1161/CIR.0000000000000300. Epub 2015 Oct 6
6. Society for Maternal-Fetal Medicine (SMFM). Electronic address: pubs@smfm.org, Pacheco LD, Saade G, Hankins GD, Clark SL. Amniotic fluid embolism: diagnosis and management. Am J Obstet Gynecol. 2016;215(2):B16–24. https://doi.org/10.1016/j.ajog.2016.03.012. Epub 2016 Mar 14

Perinatal Depression

Ashley Beem

Questions

1. **In the United States, the prevalence of postpartum depression quoted in the literature is approximately:**
   A. 5%
   B. 10%
   C. 15%
   D. 25%
2. **When is postpartum depression most likely to occur?**
   A. Within 1 month of delivery
   B. 2–4 months after delivery
   C. 6 months after delivery
   D. 9–12 months after delivery
3. **True or false: Perinatal depression is defined as depression that develops during pregnancy or within the first 12 months after delivery.**
   A. True
   B. False
4. **The most common risk factor for postpartum depression is:**
   A. Prior history of anxiety
   B. Pregnancy loss
   C. History of depression
   D. History of psychiatric disorder
5. **What is the timeframe for "baby blues" to resolve after delivery?**
   A. 1–3 days after delivery
   B. 1 week after delivery

A. Beem (✉)
Loma Linda OBGYN Residency Program, Linda School of Medicine, Loma Linda, CA, USA

Riverside University Health System, Moreno Valley, CA, USA
e-mail: a.beem@ruhealth.org

A. C. Sinha, I. F. Pasca (eds.), *Peripartum Care of the Pregnant Patient*,
https://doi.org/10.1007/978-3-031-62756-9_35

   C. 2 weeks after delivery
   D. 2 months after delivery
6. **"Baby blues" includes all the following except:**
   A. Crying for no clear reason
   B. Feeling hopeless
   C. Trouble sleeping or eating
   D. Feeling overwhelmed with caring for baby
7. **What factor/factors can increase the development of postpartum depression?**
   A. Changes in hormone levels
   B. Fatigue
   C. Genetic predisposition
   D. Social stressors
   E. All the above
8. **When should you screen for perinatal depression?**
   A. During the first prenatal visit
   B. Each trimester of pregnancy
   C. During hospitalization after delivery
   D. At postpartum visit
   E. All the above
9. **What screening modality is preferred for postpartum depression?**
   A. EPDS
   B. PHQ-9
   C. PHQ-2
   D. Both A and B are validated tools for postpartum depression
10. **What is the cutoff for a positive screen using EPDS?**
   A. 8
   B. 10
   C. 17
   D. 22
11. **What is/are the consequences of untreated depression during pregnancy?**
   A. Small for gestational age (SGA) or intrauterine growth restriction (IUGR)
   B. Preterm labor
   C. Placental abruption
   D. Preeclampsia
   E. A and B
12. **What depression treatments is/are safe in pregnancy?**
   A. Support groups
   B. Psychotherapy
   C. Antidepressants
   D. All the above
13. **Which of the following is the least likely to be a risk factor for antepartum depression?**
   A. Unintended pregnancy
   B. Smoking during pregnancy
   C. Domestic violence

   D. Lower education level
   E. Medicaid insurance
14. **Which of the following factors is/are most likely to be associated with antepartum depression?**
   A. Life stressors
   B. Lack of social support
   C. Domestic violence
   D. All the above
15. **What is the incidence of antenatal depression in the United States?**
   A. 2%
   B. 5%
   C. 9%
   D. 15%
16. **Of the following, which patient would be at most risk for postpartum depression?**
   A. 23-year-old G1P1001 with full-term, uncomplicated vaginal delivery
   B. 40-year-old G5P5005 s/p emergency repeat cesarean section at 36 weeks due to placental abruption
   C. 30-year-old G3P3003 with uncomplicated vaginal delivery of a full-term surrogate pregnancy
   D. 16-year-old G2P0111 living in foster care s/p emergency primary cesarean section under general anesthesia at 30 weeks due to PPROM and breech presentation.
17. **True or false? Having adequate pain control with epidural during delivery has a protective effect against postpartum depression.**
   A. True
   B. False
18. **True or false? Undergoing general anesthesia at the time of cesarean delivery increases the risk of severe postpartum depression.**
   A. True
   B. False
19. **All the following are signs and symptoms of postpartum psychosis except:**
   A. Hallucinations
   B. Delusions
   C. Appetite suppression
   D. Suicidal or homicidal ideation
   E. Disorganized thoughts
20. **What is the most common first indication of impending postpartum psychosis?**
   A. Severe insomnia
   B. Pressured speech
   C. Delusions of grandeur
   D. Extreme anxiety

Answers and Explanations

1. **B**. The incidence of postpartum depression in the United States is quoted as 10% in the literature [1].
2. **A.** Postpartum depression is most likely to occur within the first month of delivery. According to a retrospective study, the findings of the time of postpartum depression onset are as follows [2]:
   - Postpartum month 1–54%.
   - Postpartum months 2 to 4–40%.
   - Postpartum months 5 to 12–6%.
3. **A.** True. Peripartum depression is defined as depressive episodes during pregnancy or in the first 12 months after delivery. While it is common to have baby blues in the first 2 weeks after delivery associated with sadness that gradually diminishes, peripartum depression has symptoms that continue to worsen and persist after 1 month and can be associated with hopelessness, intense sadness, and even thoughts of self-harm [1].
4. **C.** Multiple studies have found that the most common risk factor for the development of postpartum depression is a history of depression. The other items listed are also risk factors for postpartum depression but are not as significant as a personal history of depression [3].
5. **C.** Baby blues is a very common phenomenon that approximately 80% of women experience after delivery. Symptoms usually start within 2–3 days of delivery and resolve after 2 weeks [4].
6. **B.** All the other symptoms listed, including crying, sleep disturbances, and feeling overwhelmed, are common for baby blues. Hopelessness is more indicative of postpartum depression [4].
7. **E.** The exact pathogenesis of postpartum depression is unknown. Conflicting literature exists on exactly how postpartum depression differs from depression outside of pregnancy. Factors thought to influence postpartum depression are genetic susceptibility, hormonal changes, extreme fatigue, and social stressors [5].
8. **E.** According to the ACOG, screening for antepartum depression should be performed at least each trimester and during hospitalization and continued through the postpartum visit [1].
9. **A.** EPDS (Edinburgh Postnatal Depression Scale) is the screening modality preferred for postpartum depression. While both the EPDS and PHQ-9 are validated depression screening tools, the EPDS is a better tool for antepartum and postpartum depression according to systematic reviews on postpartum depression screening [6].
10. **B.** The cutoff for a positive depression screen on the EPDS is a score of 10 on 10 questions which each receives a value of 0–3 focusing on joy, laughter, self-blame, anxiety, fear, ability to cope, insomnia, sadness, crying, and thoughts of self-harm [6].

11. **E.** SGA, IUGR, and preterm labor are all consequences of untreated depression during pregnancy. Many studies have examined the pregnancy outcomes of those complicated by antenatal depression. Consistently, in the literature, there is an association between depression, small for gestational age (SGA), low birth weight (LBW) infants, and preterm labor. Preeclampsia and placental abruption have not been found to be complications of untreated depression [7].
12. **E.** While antepartum depression and postpartum depression are a very common problem, treatment is often not initiated in a timely manner, and patients may be undertreated due to their pregnancy and breastfeeding status. The ACOG recommends that both psychotherapy and pharmacologic treatment modalities be offered to patients [8].
13. **B.** Smoking during pregnancy does not correlate strongly with antepartum depression unlike maternal anxiety and negative life events which are strongly correlated. Smoking only has a small association with the development of antepartum depression [1]. See table below:

Antepartum depression risk factors:	
Factor	Strength of association
Maternal anxiety	Medium–large
Negative life events	Medium–large
Unintended pregnancy	Medium
Medicaid (USA)	Medium
Poor relationship quality	Medium
History of depression	Medium
Domestic violence	Small–medium
Lack of social support	Small–medium
Smoking	Small
Lower income	Small
Lower education	Small

14. **D.** Life stressors, lack of social support, and domestic violence are all risk factors for the development of depression in pregnancy [1]. See table above.
15. **C.** The incidence of depression developing in pregnancy in the United States is quoted at approximately 9% in the literature [7].
16. **D.** The patient described has multiple risk factors for postpartum depression: younger age, lack of social support, life stressors, traumatic birth experience, and delivery under general anesthesia [1, 9].
17. **B.** Multiple studies have examined the association between epidural analgesia for labor pain control and a protective effect on the development of postpartum depression. Epidural analgesia does not have a protective effect on the development of depression after delivery based on current literature [10].
18. **A.** Undergoing general anesthesia for cesarean delivery is a risk factor for development in postpartum depression. Usually, general anesthesia is used in an emergency that is associated with traumatic birth experience and unmet expectations of labor and delivery—both of which are risk factors for postpartum depression [9].

19. **C.** Appetite suppression is not a symptom of postpartum psychosis. Postpartum psychosis is a very rare and serious psychiatric emergency that usually occurs in the first few weeks after giving birth. The symptoms are delusions, hallucinations, and disorganized thinking and behavior [11, 12].
20. **A.** Patients with a history of bipolar disorder, schizophrenia, and prior postpartum psychosis are most at risk for developing psychosis after delivery. The onset typically occurs 24 h to 3 weeks after delivery and is worsened by sleep deprivation [12].

References

1. OBG Project: Screening for Perinatal Depression. https://www.obgproject.com/2017/03/16/screening-perinatal-depression/.
2. Altemus M, Neeb CC, Davis A, Occhiogrosso M, Nguyen T, Bleiberg KL. Phenotypic differences between pregnancy-onset and postpartum-onset major depressive disorder. J Clin Psychiatry. 2012;73(12):e1485–91. https://doi.org/10.4088/JCP.12m07693.
3. Banti S, Mauri M, Oppo A, Borri C, Rambelli C, Ramacciotti D, Montagnani MS, Camilleri V, Cortopassi S, Rucci P, Cassano GB. From the third month of pregnancy to 1 year postpartum. Prevalence, incidence, recurrence, and new onset of depression. The results from the perinatal depression-research & screening unit study. Compr Psychiatry. 2011;52(4):343–51. https://doi.org/10.1016/j.comppsych.2010.08.003. Epub 2010 Sep 23
4. Mayo Clinic: Postpartum Depression. https://www.mayoclinic.org/diseases-conditions/postpartum-depression/symptoms-causes/syc-20376617.
5. Viguera A. Postpartum unipolar major depression: epidemiology, clinical features, assessment and diagnosis. UpToDate Article. 7 April 2023. https://www.uptodate.com/contents/postpartum-unipolar-major-depression-epidemiology-clinical-features-assessment-and-diagnosis?search=postpartum%20depression&source=search_result&selectedTitle=1~146&usage_type=default&display_rank=1.
6. Sultan P, Ando K, Elkhateb R, et al. Assessment of patient-reported outcome measures for maternal postpartum depression using the consensus-based standards for the selection of health measurement instruments guideline: a systematic review. JAMA Netw Open. 2022;5(6):e2214885. https://doi.org/10.1001/jamanetworkopen.2022.14885.
7. Grigoriadis S. Antenatal depression: pregnancy and neonatal outcomes. UpToDate Article 7 April 2023. https://www.uptodate.com/contents/antenatal-depression-pregnancy-and-neonatal-outcomes?topicRef=1718&source=see_link.
8. ACOG Clinical Practice Guideline #5. Treatment and management of mental health conditions during pregnancy and postpartum. https://www.acog.org/clinical/clinical-guidance/clinical-practice-guideline/articles/2023/06/treatment-and-management-of-mental-health-conditions-during-pregnancy-and-postpartum.
9. Guglielminotti J, Li G. Exposure to general anesthesia for cesarean delivery and odds of severe postpartum depression requiring hospitalization. Anesth Analg. 2020;131(5):1421–9. https://doi.org/10.1213/ANE.0000000000004663.
10. Almeida M, Kosman KA, Kendall MC, et al. The association between labor epidural analgesia and postpartum depression: a systematic review and meta-analysis. BMC Womens Health. 2020;20:99. https://doi.org/10.1186/s12905-020-00948-0.

11. Payne J. Postpartum psychosis: epidemiology, pathogenesis, clinical manifestations, course, assessment and diagnosis. UpToDate Article. 23 July 2021. https://www.uptodate.com/contents/postpartum-psychosis-epidemiology-pathogenesis-clinical-manifestations-course-assessment-and-diagnosis?search=postpartum%20psychosis&source=search_result&selectedTitle=1~12&usage_type=default&display_rank=1.
12. ACOG. Summary of Perinatal Mental Health Conditions. https://www.acog.org/programs/perinatal-mental-health/summary-of-perinatal-mental-health-conditions.

Postoperative Nausea and Vomiting

Anjeleena Kumar Gupta

Questions

1. **What is the incidence of PONV in obstetric and gynecologic populations?**
   A. 10–20%
   B. 20–40%
   C. 40–80%
   D. 80–100%
2. **The pathophysiology of PONV includes activation of the vomiting center by stimulation of all the following afferent pathways except:**
   A. Dopaminergic
   B. Histaminergic
   C. Serotonergic
   D. Nicotinergic
3. **Risk assessment for PONV in a patient scheduled for surgery is based on the following scoring system:**
   A. Glasgow score
   B. Apfel score
   C. Rockall score
   D. SAPS II score
4. **In females, all are independent risk factors for PONV except:**
   A. Age ≥ 50 years
   B. Previous chemotherapy
   C. Estrogen-positive breast tumor
   D. African ethnicity
5. **The increased incidence of PONV in pregnant compared to nonpregnant patients is due to the following:**

A. K. Gupta (✉)
Institute of Anaesthesiology, Pain and Perioperative Medicine, Sir Ganga Ram Hospital, New Delhi, India

A. C. Sinha, I. F. Pasca (eds.), *Peripartum Care of the Pregnant Patient*,
https://doi.org/10.1007/978-3-031-62756-9_36

A. Decrease in gastrin secretion
B. Reduction in esophageal sphincter pressure
C. Decreased gastrointestinal transit time
D. Decreased progesterone levels

6. **Which of the following risk factors demonstrates a positive association with PONV?**
   A. Female
   B. Obesity
   C. Nasogastric tube
   D. Supplemental oxygen
7. **In obstetric patients, all are risk factors for PONV except for the following:**
   A. Preoperative fasting
   B. Intraoperative hypotension
   C. Intraoperative hypoxia
   D. Uterine exteriorization
8. **All the following are the known complications of PONV observed in a parturient post-cesarean section *except*:**
   A. Dehydration
   B. Electrolyte imbalance
   C. Metabolic acidosis
   D. Incisional hernia
9. **Polymorphism of the following receptor gene is linked to increased incidence of PONV:**
   A. HTR3B
   B. TPH
   C. DRD3
   D. COMT
10. **All the following are the recommended strategies to reduce the risk of PONV *except*:**
    A. Use of propofol total intravenous anesthesia (TIVA)
    B. Use of epidural anesthesia
    C. Avoid using nitrous oxide if the surgical duration is above 1 h
    D. Use of neostigmine for reversal of neuromuscular junction blockade
11. **First-line rescue antiemetic treatment for PONV is as follows:**
    A. Metoclopramide
    B. Dexamethasone
    C. Ondansetron
    D. Diclectin
12. **Which of the following statement is *false*?**
    A. Aprepitant, an antagonist of the NK1 receptor, has a $t½$ of 40 h
    B. Oral gabapentin 600–800 mg given 1–2 h before surgery decreases PONV
    C. Prevention of PONV by midazolam 2 mg given 30 min before the end of surgery is recommended
    D. The rescue dose for the 5-HT3 receptor antagonist is 25% of the prophylactic dose

13. **Which of the following is the recommended intravenous drug to be administered at the time of induction?**
    A. Dexamethasone (4 mg)
    B. Ondansetron (4 mg)
    C. Droperidol (0.625 mg)
    D. Dolasetron (12.5 mg)
14. **Mark the incorrect statement.**
    A. Administration of ondansetron can result in elevated liver enzymes
    B. Extrapyramidal syndrome is a known adverse effect of aprepitant therapy
    C. IV dexamethasone can cause vaginal itching or anal irritation
    D. Sedation is a common side effect of phenothiazines
15. **"Unsafe" QT prolongation has been reported with the use of:**
    A. Droperidol
    B. Ondansetron
    C. Amisulpride
    D. Dolasetron
16. **The following strategies are advocated to minimize opioid use and to reduce the risk of PONV, *except*:**
    A. Intraoperative infusion of short-acting β-blockers
    B. Intraoperative ketamine
    C. Intraoperative betahistine
    D. IV acetaminophen, if administered before the onset of pain
17. **Researched pharmacological interventions for the treatment of PONV include:**
    A. Total intravenous anesthesia (TIVA)
    B. Gabapentin
    C. Naloxone
    D. All of the above
18. **The following nonpharmacological strategies reduce the incidence of PONV:**
    (i) Supplemental crystalloids
    (ii) Carbohydrate loading
    (iii) Ginger
    (iv) Aromatherapy
    (v) Acupoint stimulation
    A. i and ii
    B. i and iii
    C. i and iv
    D. i and v
19. **According to the guidelines for the management of PONV, which of the following statements is false:**
    A. Administer prophylactic antiemetic therapy to patients with a moderate to high risk of PONV
    B. Consider combination antiemetics in patients with a high risk of developing PONV

C. For patients in whom prophylaxis was not given or has failed, antiemetics should be given as soon as feasible
D. If prophylaxis with one drug fails, a repeat dose of the same drug should be given as rescue therapy

20. **Intraoperative or Postoperative nausea and vomiting after cesarean delivery is decreased by all the following measures except:**
A. Prophylactic vasopressor infusion
B. Limiting uterine exteriorization
C. Using saline for abdominal irrigation
D. Administering two prophylactic antiemetics with different mechanisms of action

Answers and Explanations

1. **C**. The reported incidence of PONV in obstetric and gynecological surgical patients, especially those undergoing laparoscopic surgery, is 40–80% [1, 2]. However, in the general surgical population, this incidence increases in the presence of risk factors from 20–30% to 70% [3].
2. **D**. The vomiting center is activated by stimulation of the chemoreceptor trigger zone (CTZ), pathways from cerebral cortex (C2, C3), gastrointestinal system (cholinergic–muscarinic receptors), vestibular system, and midbrain via dopaminergic, histaminergic, serotonergic, and muscarinic receptors [4].
3. **B**. The Apfel score is a simplified risk scoring system for PONV. The predictors are female sex, nonsmoker status, history of PONV or motion sickness, and use of opioids. The incidence of PONV is 10, 21, 39, 61, and 78%, depending on whether none, one, two, three, or four of these risk factors are present [5].
4. **D**. Black-African ethnicity has been associated with a lower incidence of PONV, which could be influenced by cultural and pharmacogenomic factors [6]. Postmenopausal women (age > 50 years) and those with estrogen-positive breast tumors have a higher incidence of PONV that is linked to elevated estrogen levels. Genetic predisposition can increase the risk of PONV in patients who experience chemotherapy-induced nausea and vomiting [6].
5. **B**. Increased incidence of PONV in pregnant patients is linked to increased levels of progesterone during pregnancy. Progesterone causes smooth muscle relaxation, resulting in a reduction in esophageal sphincter pressure. It also causes increased gastrin secretion and prolongs gastrointestinal transit time [7].
6. **A**. Risk factors for PONV are show in Table 1 [8]. Each 30 min increase in surgical duration increases the risk of PONV by 60% [9].
7. **A**. The correlation of preoperative fasting to the occurrence of PONV is uncertain [8]. Intraoperative hypotension is a known risk factor for PONV. Cerebral ischemia secondary to hypotension activates the vomiting center in the medulla oblongata [10]. Uterine exteriorization is known to activate vagal afferents to induce nausea and vomiting [10].

Table 1 Factors correlating with PONV

Positive correlation	Female gender, younger age, nonsmoker, history of PONV or motion sickness, volatile anesthetics, nitrous oxide, opioids, duration and type of surgery (gynecological, laparoscopic, bariatric)
Conflicting correlation	ASA physical status, anesthesiologist's experience, menstrual cycle
Limited correlation	Anxiety
Uncertain correlation	Preoperative fasting, neostigmine
No correlation	Obesity, nasogastric tube, supplemental oxygen

8. **C**. Vomiting causes loss of gastric secretions (rich in chloride ions), which can lead to an increase in bicarbonate ions in the extracellular fluid with resultant metabolic alkalosis in extreme cases [11].
9. **A**. HTR3B receptor gene polymorphism is linked to increased chances of PONV. In contrast, polymorphisms of the serotonin receptor genes HTR3A, TPH, DRD3, and COMT are associated with a decreased incidence of PONV [12].
10. **D**. Neostigmine increases the baseline risk of PONV. A new Cochrane review identified a reduced risk of PONV with the use of sugammadex compared to neostigmine [13]. Propofol TIVA along with other prophylactic agents also decreases this risk (evidence A2) [8]. Epidural anesthesia provides good pain relief, avoiding the need for opioids, thereby reducing PONV risk [8]. The risk of PONV with the use of nitrous oxide is dose dependent. The number needed to treat decreases from 128 to 9 if the nitrous oxide use increases from less than an hour to over 2 h [8].
11. **C**. Ondansetron is recommended as first-line rescue antiemetic treatment; if unavailable, metoclopramide 10 mg IV is used as second-line treatment [14]. Diclectin is an antiemetic medication containing 10 mg doxylamine succinate (antihistamine) and 10 mg pyridoxine hydrochloride. It is a commonly used antiemetic considered safe in pregnancy [3].
12. **C**. Midazolam administration at the end of surgery is associated with a significantly reduced incidence of PONV; however, there are sedation-related side effects. Therefore, it is not recommended at that time [8, 15]. Options **A**, **B**, and **D** are true [3, 8].
13. **A**. Data support dosing of dexamethasone (4 mg) at induction for prevention of PONV (A1 evidence) [8]. A higher dose of dexamethasone has not been associated with a further significant reduction in the occurrence of PONV [16]. Recommendations for the administration of ondansetron, droperidol (A1 evidence), and dolasetron (A2 evidence) are at the end of surgery [8].
14. **B**. Adverse effects of aprepitant are headache, fatigue, elevated liver enzymes, and dizziness. Extrapyramidal syndrome, sedation, and hypotension are commonly observed with phenothiazine therapy. Headache, elevated liver enzymes, and lightheadedness are side effects of ondansetron [3].

15. **D**. Studies suggest transient or no prolongation of QT with antiemetic doses of droperidol, ondansetron, and amisulpride and these are, therefore, considered safe. The risk of sudden cardiac death has been documented with doses of droperidol exceeding 25 mg [17]. Dolasetron is no longer marketed in the USA secondary to the risk of QT prolongation [8].
16. **C**. Betahistine is an H2-receptor antagonist used along with ondansetron for PONV prophylaxis but is not associated with a decrease in opioid consumption [8]. Intraoperative β-blockers reduce opioid requirements and PONV risk (evidence A3), similar to that with intraoperative ketamine [8]. Prophylactic IV acetaminophen reduces nausea when used as part of multimodal analgesia (evidence A1).
17. **D**. Options **A**, **B**, and **C** have been reported as treatment modalities for PONV [6].
18. **D**. A recent Cochrane review supports the infusion of crystalloids (10–30 mL/kg) to reduce the risk of PONV (early and late) and the need for rescue antiemetics [18].

    Acupoint stimulation before or after induction of anesthesia is effective in reducing PONV [19]. Inconsistent results have been reported following the administration of carbohydrate loading, but overall, there is no reduction in the incidence of PONV. Similar results have been documented with aromatherapy and the use of ginger [8].
19. **D**. Administer a different class of antiemetic drug if prophylaxis with one class of drug fails. However, if PONV occurs more than 6 h postsurgery, a repeat dose of the initial prophylactic drug (except in the case of dexamethasone or transdermal scopolamine) may be considered [3]. 5-HT3 receptor antagonists alone or along with dexamethasone form the cornerstone of antiemetic prophylaxis [8].
20. **C**. Prophylactic vasopressors decrease the incidence of hypotension-associated IONV. Communication with the surgeon to limit uterine exteriorization may decrease IONV and avoid delayed return of bowel function. Surgical saline irrigation of the abdominal cavity may worsen IONV/PONV. Combination therapy of at least two antiemetics from two different classes may improve IONV/PONV with metoclopramide decreasing IONV but not PONV and dexamethasone decreasing PONV but not IONV due to delayed onset [20].

References

1. Apfel CC, Heidrich FM, Jukar-Rao S, Jalota L, Hornuss C, Whelan RP, Zhang K, Cakmakkaya OS. Evidence-based analysis of risk factors for postoperative nausea and vomiting. Br J Anaesth. 2012;109:742–53.
2. Mraovic B, Simurina T, Sonicki Z, Skitarelic N, Gyan TJ. The dose response of nitrous oxide used in postoperative nausea in patients undergoing gynecologic laparoscogric surgery—a preliminary study. Anesth Analg. 2008;107:818–23.

3. McCracken G, Houston P, Lefebvre G. Guideline for the management of postoperative nausea and vomiting. J Obstet Gynecol Can. 2008;30:600–7.
4. Denholm L, Gallagher G. Physiology and pharmacology of nausea and vomiting. Anaesth Intensive Care Med. 2018;19:513–6.
5. Apfel CC, Läärä E, Koivuranta M, Greim CA, Roewer N. A simplified risk score for predicting postoperative nausea and vomiting: conclusions from cross-validations between two centers. Anesthesiology. 1999;91:693–700.
6. Echeverria-Villalobos M, Fiorda-Diaz J, Uribe A, Bergese SD. Postoperative nausea and vomiting in female patients undergoing breast and gynecological surgery: a narrative review of risk factors and prophylaxis. Front Med. 2022;9:909982.
7. Jabalameli M, Honarmand A, Safavi M, Chitsaz M. Treatment of postoperative nausea and vomiting after spinal anesthesia for cesarean delivery: a randomized, double-blinded comparison of midazolam, ondansetron, and a combination. Adv Biomed Res. 2012;1:2.
8. Gan TJ, Belani KG, Bergese S, Chung F, Diemunsch P, Habib AS, Jin Z, Kovac AL, Meyer TA, Urman RD, Apfel CC, Ayad S, Beagley L, Candiotti K, Englesakis M, Hedrick TL, Kranke P, Lee S, Lipman D, Minkowitz HS, Morton J, Philip BK. Fourth consensus guidelines for the management of postoperative nausea and vomiting. Anesth Analg. 2020;131:411–48.
9. Sinclair DR, Chung F, Mezei G. Can postoperative nausea and vomiting be predicted? Anesthesiology. 1999;91:109–18.
10. Jelting Y, Klein C, Harlander T, Eberhart L, Roewer N, Kranke P. Preventing nausea and vomiting in women undergoing regional anesthesia for cesarean section: challenges and solutions. Local Reg Anesth. 2017;10:83–90.
11. Hailu S, Mekonen S, Shiferaw A. Prevention and management of postoperative nausea and vomiting after cesarean section: a systematic literature review. Ann Med Surg (Lond). 2022;75:103433.
12. Wesmiller SW, Sereika SM, Bender CM, Bovbjerg D, Ahrendt G, Bonaventura M, Conley YP. Exploring the multifactorial nature of postoperative nausea and vomiting in women following surgery for breast cancer. Auton Neurosci. 2017;202:102–7.
13. Hristovska AM, Duch P, Allingstrup M, Afshari A. Efficacy and safety of sugammadex versus neostigmine in reversing neuromuscular blockade in adults. Cochrane Database Syst Rev. 2017;8:CD012763.
14. Teshome D, Fenta E, Hailu S. Preoperative prevention and postoperative management of nausea and vomiting in a resource-limited setting: a systematic review. Int J Surg Open. 2020;27:10–7.
15. Safavi MR, Honarmand A. Low dose intravenous midazolam for prevention of PONV, in lower abdominal surgery–preoperative vs intraoperative administration. Middle East J Anesthesiol. 2009;20:75–81.
16. D'souza N, Swami M, Bhagwat S. Comparative study of dexamethasone and ondansetron for prophylaxis of postoperative nausea and vomiting in laparoscopic gynecologic surgery. Int J Gynecol Obstet. 2011;113:124–7.
17. Habib AS, Gan TJ. Food and drug administration black box warning on the perioperative use of droperidol: a review of the cases. Anesth Analg. 2003;96:1377–9.
18. Jewer JK, Wong MJ, Bird SJ, Habib AS, Parker R, George RB. Supplemental perioperative intravenous crystalloids for postoperative nausea and vomiting. Cochrane Database Syst Rev. 2019;3:CD012212.
19. Frey UH, Scharmann P, Löhlein C, Peters J. P6 acustimulation effectively decreases postoperative nausea and vomiting in high-risk patients. Br J Anaesth. 2009;102:620–5.
20. Bollag L, Lim G, Sultan P, Habib AS, Landau R, Zakowski M, Tiouririne M, Bhambhani S, Carvalho B. Society for obstetric anesthesia and perinatology: consensus statement and recommendations for enhanced recovery after cesarean. Anesth Analg. 2021;132(5):1362–77.

Further Reading

Gan TJ, Belani KG, Bergese S, Chung F, Diemunsch P, Habib AS, Jin Z, Kovac AL, Meyer TA, Urman RD, Apfel CC, Ayad S, Beagley L, Candiotti K, Englesakis M, Hedrick TL, Kranke P, Lee S, Lipman D, Minkowitz HS, Morton J, Philip BK. Fourth consensus guidelines for the management of postoperative nausea and vomiting. Anesth Analg. 2020;131:411–48.

Obstetric Hyperthermia

Wyatt McGilvery and Ioana F. Pasca

Questions

1. **Identify the etiology driving intrapartum hyperthermia induced by epidural anesthesia.**
   A. Elevated levels of IL-6 and altered thermoregulation
   B. Peripheral vasodilation below the level of neuraxial blockade
   C. Reflexive parasympathetic nervous system activation
   D. Type I hypersensitivity to analgesic drug components
2. **During uncomplicated labor, maternal temperature can be expected to ______.**
   A. Increase by 2.5%
   B. Increase by 1–2 °C
   C. Decrease by 2.5%
   D. Decrease by 1–2 °C
   E. No change
3. **What percentage of laboring patients receiving neuraxial epidural anesthesia will develop an intrapartum fever?**
   A. 33%
   B. 20%

W. McGilvery
A.T. Still University Health Osteopathic Medicine in Arizona, Mesa, AZ, USA

I. F. Pasca (✉)
Riverside University Health System, Moreno Valley, CA, USA

Department of Anesthesiology, Critical Care, and Neurocritical Care, Loma Linda University at Riverside University Health System, Loma Linda, CA, USA

University of California San Diego, San Diego, CA, USA

University of California Riverside, Riverside, CA, USA
e-mail: i.pasca@ruhealth.org

A. C. Sinha, I. F. Pasca (eds.), *Peripartum Care of the Pregnant Patient*,
https://doi.org/10.1007/978-3-031-62756-9_37

C. 50%
D. 5%

4. **True or false: Anesthesia physicians wanting to avoid increasing the risk of epidural-associated intrapartum hyperthermia could use remifentanil patient-controlled analgesia (RPCA) as an alternative method of pain control.**
   A. True
   B. False
5. **Identify the prevalence of epidural hyperthermia among all intrapartum hyperthermia causes.**
   A. 20%
   B. 25%
   C. 33%
   D. 50%
   E. 75%
6. **Identify all the correct criteria for diagnosing intrapartum hyperthermia.**
   A. Core temperature during labor of ≥37 °C on one occasion
   B. A core temperature of ≥37 °C was maintained for at least 3 h
   C. One-time temperature of ≥37.5 °C
   D. Core temperature of ≥37.5 °C taken 2 h apart
7. **A 26-year-old G3P1101 is being evaluated in Labor and Delivery 4 h following successful placement of epidural anesthesia. The cervix was 7 cm dilated, 90% effaced, and anterior. She reports adequate pain control and is not in any acute distress, and she looks comfortable. Vital signs revealed a temperature of 38.3 °C, 112/82 BP, 87 HR, 12 RR, and 97% SpO_2 on room air. The patient denies any complaints aside from dull pelvic pressure occurring with each contraction. A physical exam is significant only for decreased sensation of the bilateral lower extremities. All the following are required *except*:**
   A. Begin broad-spectrum antibiotics (i.e., ampicillin and gentamicin regimen)
   B. Reassurance that the patient is asymptomatic and likely has intrapartum hyperthermia secondary to epidural analgesia
   C. Administer acetaminophen
   D. Draw blood cultures and perform complete blood count
8. **One day later, you are rounding on the same patient described in question number 7. Today, she feels well following an uncomplicated vaginal delivery, and her pain has been well controlled on scheduled acetaminophen and PRN morphine. Her vital signs were all within normal limits, including her temperature. All lab results are unremarkable. Her newborn baby is feeding well, voided twice, passed meconium, and remains afebrile. Based on the most likely diagnosis of her fever yesterday, what could have prevented her rise in body temperature?**
   A. Prophylactic acetaminophen
   B. Using dexmedetomidine as an epidural adjunct

C. Adequate prenatal care
D. Prophylactic methylprednisolone
E. Prophylactic ampicillin

9. **As defined by ACOG, all the following are involved in chorioamnionitis *except:***
   A. Endometrial decidua
   B. Fetal membranes
   C. Fetus
   D. Myometrium
   E. Placenta
10. **A 34-year-old G1P0 at 32 weeks pregnant was evaluated in the emergency department for progressing fever (38.5 °C), shortness of breath, dry cough, and myalgias. Symptoms began 72 h ago, which she originally attributed to shoveling the snow in her driveway Christmas morning. She received routine prenatal care; however, she declined to receive any vaccinations during this pregnancy.**
    CXR: Diffuse bilateral hazy infiltrates without consolidation.
    Labs: Hgb 10.5, WBC 12.5 K, PLT 412, K 4.2, Na 138, Cr 0.6, BUN 18.
    Vitals: Temp 38.5 °C, BP 121/88, HR 96, RR 21, SpO_2 94% on room air.
    Viral panel: Positive for H1N1.
    What is the next best step in management?
    A. Supportive care as the patient is 72 h outside of symptom onset
    B. Admit to the hospital for observation
    C. Discharge with 5 days of oseltamivir
    D. Discharge with 5 days of azithromycin
11. **Which of the following, if present, increases the parturient risk of developing intrapartum hyperthermia?**
    A. Epidural with reduced dosing of local anesthetics
    B. Epidural in place for greater than 5 h
    C. A patient who recently tested positive for *Streptococcus agalactiae*
    D. An epidural with a dexmedetomidine adjunct
12. **Bupivacaine has been shown to decrease the levels of this cytokine, ultimately leading to a proinflammatory state.**
    A. Interleukin-1
    B. Interleukin-6
    C. Interleukin-10
    D. Interleukin-17
13. **Select the most likely time of onset in which an intrapartum fever is likely to be attributed to an epidural.**
    A. Temperature increases begin within minutes of epidural placement
    B. A steady rise in temperature beginning 1 h after epidural placement
    C. Slow temperature rise beginning 5 h after epidural placement
    D. Sudden onset of fever (>38 °C) after 4 h of epidural placement

14. **True or false: Although epidural anesthesia-related hyperthermia poses an increased risk of morbidity to the parturient, there is little to no significant risk to the fetus.**
    A. True
    B. False
15. **Which of the following causes of intrapartum hyperthermia is the most prevalent (for a full-term pregnancy)?**
    A. Chorioamnionitis
    B. Preeclampsia
    C. Epidural anesthesia
    D. Urinary tract infections
16. **When performing a diagnostic evaluation on a routine patient with suspected intrapartum fever, what is the best location/method for obtaining an accurate temperature?**
    A. Tympanic
    B. Axillary
    C. Oral
    D. Rectal
    E. Pulmonary artery (Swan-Ganz catheter)
17. **Which patient population is at an increased risk for post-epidural hyperthermia?**
    A. Primigravid women
    B. Multiparous women
    C. A patient who has had multiple epidurals in the past
    D. A patient currently on 50 mg labetalol BID
18. **Pregnant women diagnosed with SARS-CoV-2 are less likely to present with which of the following when compared to the age-matched nonpregnant population?**
    A. Myalgias
    B. Cough
    C. Fever
    D. Dyspnea
    E. All the above
19. **Intrapartum hyperthermia carries an increased risk of all the following when compared to the normothermic parturient *except*:**
    A. Instrument-assisted deliveries
    B. Cesarean section
    C. Neonatal sepsis
    D. Uterine rupture
    E. Umbilical artery pH < 7.1
20. **The immunocompromised state of pregnancy is likely due to the large decrease in the quantity and function of _________.**
    A. Neutrophils
    B. Total white blood cell count
    C. T cells/B cells
    D. Monocytes/macrophages

Answers and Explanations

1. **A.** Although the precise mechanism of epidural hyperthermia remains unclear, the contemporary understanding of this phenomenon includes the release of IL-6 and loss of thermoregulation—a noninfectious, systemic inflammatory response to the epidural itself. Although peripheral vasodilation does occur due to neuraxial blockade, this has been shown to decrease temperature rather than lead to hyperthermia. Type I hypersensitivity reactions (IgE mediated) can rarely occur with epidural anesthesia. However, they would not have a presenting fever. Reflexive parasympathetic activation would not occur due to neuraxial blockade, nor would it result in increasing core body temperature [1].
2. **E.** Metabolic demand during uncomplicated labor can be expected to increase by 25%—deemed to be a physiologic response. However, this increase in metabolic demand is not large enough to cause a disturbance in the homeostatic temperature of the parturient. Thus, an intrapartum fever (one measurement of >38 °C or two measurements of >37.5 °C taken 2 h apart) requires extensive workup to rule out other pathologic causes, such as infection [2].
3. **B.** The literature has shown the incidence of epidural anesthesia intrapartum hyperthermia to be 20%. Compare this to the 5% incidence of intrapartum hyperthermia in those not receiving epidural anesthesia [2].
4. **B. False.** Multiple studies have shown that remifentanil patient-controlled analgesia (RPCA) does not lead to lower incidence of intrapartum hyperthermia when compared to epidural anesthesia. In addition, RPCA has demonstrated inferior efficacy and increased risk (hypoventilation) when compared to epidural anesthesia [3].
5. **D.** Of all intrapartum fevers, epidural causes account for approximately 50% of cases. In addition, 30% are due to a confirmed infection (chorioamnionitis), and the remaining 20% have multifactorial etiologies [2].
6. **D.** The diagnosis of intrapartum hyperthermia can be made when the patient's temperature meets any one of the two following criteria: hyperthermia with one temperature ≥38 °C or two temperatures of ≥37.5 °C taken at least 2 h apart. Other signs of maternal intrapartum infection include tachycardia (>100 bpm), tachypnea (>20 breaths per minute), hypoxia ($Pao_2/Fio_2 < 40$ kPa), hypotension (systolic blood pressure < 90 mmHg; mean arterial pressure < 70 mmHg or systolic blood pressure decrease > 40 mmHg), oliguria (urine output < 0.5 mL kg^{-1} h^{-1}), or impaired consciousness [2].
7. **B.** Although this patient may be experiencing epidural hyperthermia as indicated by a fever that came on quickly after epidural placement (within 4 h) and has a benign physical exam, this is not sufficient to adequately rule out infectious etiologies of this patient's fever. It is recommended that this patient undergo further diagnostic workup and be given a broad-spectrum antibiotic regimen before receiving a diagnosis of epidural hyperthermia [4].
8. **D.** This patient most likely experienced epidural hyperthermia. Current literature has shown that high-dose prophylactic methylprednisolone (100 mg every

4 h) reduces the risk of intrapartum hyperthermia. Although this is the correct answer, it is important to note that this prophylaxis cannot be recommended due to an increased rate of neonatal bacteremia. More research is needed before suggesting any prophylactic treatment [2].

9. **D.** ACOG defines chorioamnionitis as an infection with resultant inflammation of any combination of the amniotic fluid, placenta, fetus, fetal membranes, or decidua [5].
10. **C.** Given this patient's current symptoms/findings occurring in the winter months during pregnancy, her history of declining vaccinations, and positive H1N1, she has an influenza infection. Oseltamivir is the drug of choice for influenza in pregnancy. Although recommendations are to give oseltamivir within 48 h of symptom onset, it would still be appropriate to give this patient the medication due to her increased risk of morbidity due to pregnancy. Women are at an increased risk of severe disease that correlates directly with the duration of their pregnancy, with peak risk occurring during the second and third trimesters. This is suspected to be due to the physical characteristics of pregnancy (increased abdominal volume leading to altered respiratory physiology), as well as being relatively immunocompromised. According to the American College of Obstetricians and Gynecologists (ACOG), there is no time cutoff from symptom onset to treat pregnant women with antiviral medication. These recommendations are given for all pregnant women, regardless of gestational age, and include women who are up to 2 weeks postpartum [6, 7].
11. **B.** Recent prospective cohort studies have shown that there is a strong correlation between the length of time an epidural is in place and subsequent fever development. The length of time was deemed to be >5 h ($p < 0.001$). Those with an epidural in place for <5 h were not shown to be at an increased risk when compared to those who received no epidural at all. *Streptococcus agalactiae* (also known as GBS) is unlikely to lead to maternal fever—especially given that this patient previously tested positive for GBS, she would most likely be receiving intrapartum ampicillin prophylactically. Neither dexmedetomidine nor local anesthetics (i.e., lidocaine) have been shown to be correlated with hyperthermia [8].
12. **C.** Immunologic studies have shown that local anesthetics can modulate both the local and systemic immune systems via altered levels and functions of various cytokines. Of all the cytokines listed here, only interleukin-10 is an anti-inflammatory cytokine. Reduced levels of interleukin-10 would lead to higher levels of inflammation. Answers **A**, **B**, and **D** are all examples of proinflammatory cytokines. Reduced levels of these cytokines would lead to less inflammation [9].
13. **A.** Temperature rises associated with epidural anesthesia begin immediately after epidural placement, with an average rise of 0.18 °C/h (0.33 °F). Parturients with an epidural-associated fever (≥38 °C) reach this temperature within 4 h of exposure, and the temperature increases with the duration of epidural anesthesia [10].

14. **B. False.** Intrapartum hyperthermia, regardless of etiology, poses a threat to the morbidity and mortality of the parturient and the fetus. Fetal complications can be myriad but most commonly include bacteremia, neonatal sepsis, neonatal respiratory distress syndrome (NRDS), and a higher rate of more invasive medical intervention that carries its own risk of complications, such as cesarean and instrumental deliveries.
15. **C**. Epidural anesthesia accounts for 50% of intrapartum hyperthermia cases. Infectious causes of intrapartum hyperthermia account for 30%. Causes from UTI are shown to be rare, and preeclamptic cases are exceedingly rare, although they carry significant risks to the parturient and fetus. This is based on a population in which one-third of parturients have epidural analgesia, and the incidences of epidural hyperthermia and intrapartum infection are 20% and 5%, respectively [2].
16. **C.** Oral sublingual temperature recorded via an electric contact thermometer is accurate, and it is the most reasonable/convenient method for detecting intrapartum maternal fever. Axillary temperature has been shown to record a temperature that is 1.0–2.0 °C lower than oral temperature. Tympanic temperatures are highly inaccurate and vary greatly depending on the amount of cerumen impaction. Last, while the pulmonary artery temperature recorded via catheterization is the reference standard for true core body temperature, this would be a highly invasive and unnecessary procedure for a routine intrapartum patient. In addition, oral temperature has proven to be closely tied to intrauterine temperature [11].
17. **A.** Primigravidas have been shown to be at a higher risk of experiencing epidural hyperthermia. Although the exact cause of this correlation is unknown, it is believed to be because primigravidas are more likely to undergo a longer duration of labor than their multiparous counterparts. The longer an epidural is left in place throughout labor, the higher the likelihood of experiencing intrapartum hyperthermia. By this logic, multiparous women would be at a decreased risk of fever. There is no literature to support that women who have undergone multiple epidurals are at an increased risk of intrapartum hyperthermia. Last, beta-blockade (as seen with labetalol) is not shown to place a patient at increased risk of intrapartum hyperthermia. In fact, there are several studies demonstrating that beta-blockade may decrease the patient's ability to mount a stress fever [4, 12].
18. **E.** Compared to the general population, pregnant women have been shown to present with absent clinical manifestations of SARS-CoV-2 (COVID-19), including but not limited to cough, fever, dyspnea, and myalgias. This lack of symptomatology should not be mistaken for a decreased risk of morbidity and mortality of the parturient, as this population is at an increased risk of severe complications due to a COVID-19 infection [13].
19. **D.** Intrapartum hyperthermia has many known etiologies. However, the most common etiologies are due to epidural hyperthermia and intra-amniotic infections (chorioamnionitis). Retrospective cohort studies have found a strong correlation between intrapartum hyperthermia and the increased risk of instrumental

deliveries, cesarean section, neonatal sepsis, and an umbilical artery pH < 7.1 in the newborn. This is most likely to be correlated to the sequelae of underlying infection rather than the hyperthermia itself; however, this requires further research and investigation. Neither uterine rupture nor placenta accreta has been shown to be correlated with intrapartum hyperthermia [14].

20. **C.** The parturient is thought to exist in an immunocompromised state where they are particularly susceptible to viral infections. It is thought that the etiology of this is due to an overt decrease in lymphocyte (B and T cells) quantity and activity that progresses through pregnancy. White blood cell count is expected to *increase* during pregnancy (WBC of 9000–25,000 can be physiologic) primarily through the mechanism of increased neutrophils within the differential. (Neutrophil apoptosis is decreased during pregnancy.) Monocytes and macrophages play an important role in preventing fetal allograft rejection via decidual infiltration, thus leading to a potential reduction in serum levels of monocytes that carries no clinical sequelae [15].

References

1. Khanna P, Jain S, Thariani K, Sharma S, Singh AK. Epidural fever: hiding in the shadows. Turk J Anesthesiol Reanim. 2020;48(5):350–5. https://doi.org/10.5152/TJAR.2020.50. Epub 2020 Apr 27. PMID: 33103138; PMCID: PMC7556632
2. Mullington CJ, Malhotra S. Hyperthermia after epidural analgesia in obstetrics. BJA Edc. 2021;21(1):26–31. https://doi.org/10.1016/j.bjae.2020.08.004. Epub 2020 Oct 21
3. Lu G, Yao W, Chen X, et al. Remifentanil patient-controlled versus epidural analgesia on intrapartum maternal fever: a systematic review and meta-analysis. BMC Pregnancy Childbirth. 2020;20:151. https://doi.org/10.1186/s12884-020-2800-y.
4. Goetzl L. Epidural analgesia and maternal fever: a clinical and research update. Curr Opin Anesthesiol. 2012;25(3):292–9. https://doi.org/10.1097/ACO.0b013e3283530d7c.
5. Higgins RD, Saade G, Polin RA, Grobman WA, Buhimschi IA, Watterberg K, et al. Evaluation and management of women and newborns with a maternal diagnosis of chorioamnionitis: summary of a workshop. Obstet Gynecol. 2016;127:426–36.
6. Beigi RH, Venkataramanan R, Caritis SN. Oseltamivir for influenza in pregnancy. Semin Perinatol. 2014;38(8):503–7. https://doi.org/10.1053/j.semperi.2014.08.015. Epub 2014 Oct 1. PMID: 25281358; PMCID: PMC5745365
7. Oboho IK, Reed C, Gargiullo P, Leon M, Aragon D, Meek J, et al. Benefit of early initiation of influenza antiviral treatment to pregnant women hospitalized with laboratory-confirmed influenza. J Infect Dis. 2016;214:507–15.
8. Zhang Z, Deng C-M, et al. Effects of neuraxial labor analgesia on intrapartum maternal fever in full-term pregnancy and its influence on birth outcomes. Front Med. 2023;10:1208570. https://www.frontiersin.org/articles/10.3389/fmed.2023.1208570. https://doi.org/10.3389/fmed.2023.1208570.
9. Patel S, Ciechanowicz S, Blumenfeld Y, Sultan P. Epidural-related maternal fever: incidence, pathophysiology, outcomes, and management. Ajogorg. 2023. https://www.ajog.org/article/S0002-9378(22)00480-X/fulltext.
10. Lieberman E, Lang JM, Frigoletto F Jr, Richardson DK, Ringer SA, Cohen A. Epidural analgesia, intrapartum fever, and neonatal sepsis evaluation. Pediatrics. 1997;99(3):415–9. https://doi.org/10.1542/peds.99.3.415.

11. Banerjee S, Cashman P, Yentis SM, Steer PJ. Maternal temperature monitoring during labor: concordance and variability among monitoring sites. Obstet Gynecol. 2004;103(2):287–93. https://doi.org/10.1097/01.AOG.0000100155.85379.88.
12. Mayfield KP, Soszynski D, Kozak W, Kozak A, Rudolph K, Kluger MJ. Beta-adrenergic receptor subtype effects on stress fever and thermoregulation. Neuroimmunomodulation. 1999;6(4):305–17. https://doi.org/10.1159/000026389.
13. Allotey J, Fernandez S, Bonet M, Stallings E, Yap M, Kew T, Zhou D, Coomar D, Sheikh J, Lawson H, Ansari K, Attarde S, Littmoden M, Banjoko A, Barry K, Akande O, Sambamoorthi D, van Wely M, van Leeuwen E, et al. Clinical manifestations, risk factors, and maternal and perinatal outcomes of coronavirus disease 2019 in pregnancy: living systematic review and meta-analysis. BMJ. 2020;370:m3320. https://www.bmj.com/content/370/bmj.m3320?ijkey=a6b6a7604a45b236405e01c7f7fc1b18a8cf782d&keytype2=tf_ipsecsha
14. Ashwal E, Salman L, Tzur Y, Aviram A, Bashi TB-M, Yogev Y, Hiersch L. Intrapartum fever and the risk for perinatal complications—the effect of fever duration and positive cultures. J Matern Fetal Neonatal Med. 2018;31(11):1418–25. https://doi.org/10.1080/14767058.2017.1317740.
15. Chandra S, Tripathi AK, Mishra S, et al. Physiological changes in hematological parameters during pregnancy. Indian J Hematol Blood Transfus. 2012;28:144–6. https://doi.org/10.1007/s12288-012-0175-6.

Trauma and Critical Care

Mira Bishawi and John V. Agapian

Questions

1. **A 32-year-old G1P0 female at 34-week gestation was brought to the Emergency Department after an epigastric stabbing. ROS is negative except for some mild upper epigastric pain and nausea. She denies pain elsewhere. Vital signs were stable, and fetal heart monitoring was initiated. Which of the following is the next appropriate step for this patient?**
   A. Consult obstetrics to admit the patient
   B. CT abdomen/pelvis without contrast
   C. Observation of the patient in the ED for 6 h
   D. Speculum examination to evaluate for any occult bleeding
2. **At what volume of blood loss will a pregnant woman begin to exhibit clinical signs of hypovolemia?**
   A. 500 mL
   B. 1000 mL
   C. 1500 mL
   D. 750 mL
3. **Which of the following hemodynamic changes is *not* observed in pregnant patients?**
   A. Increased cardiac output
   B. Decreased systemic vascular resistance
   C. Increased ejection fraction
   D. Increased activation of the renin-angiotensin-aldosterone system (RAAS)

M. Bishawi
Riverside University Health System, Moreno Valley, CA, USA

J. V. Agapian (✉)
Riverside University Health System, Moreno Valley, CA, USA

Loma Linda University, Loma Linda, CA, USA
e-mail: john.agapian@gte.net

A. C. Sinha, I. F. Pasca (eds.), *Peripartum Care of the Pregnant Patient*,
https://doi.org/10.1007/978-3-031-62756-9_38

4. **Which of the following respiratory changes is observed during pregnancy?**
   A. $PaCO_2$ remains unchanged (expected ~40 mmHg)
   B. Tidal volume decreases
   C. Expiratory reserve volume (ERV) increases
   D. Functional residual capacity decreases
5. **Which of the following values may indicate early disseminated intravascular coagulation in a third trimester pregnant patient?**
   A. Fibrinogen 150 mg/dL
   B. Platelet count 140,000
   C. Decreased factor 12
   D. Normal PTT
6. **A 24-year-old G2P1 at 37-week gestation was brought to the ED by her husband for rhythmic "shaking" activity. The patient and her husband recently moved to the USA, and the patient had not received any prenatal care. The patient appears tired and is not at baseline mental status, per husband. Fetal heart tracings are initiated. Maternal vital signs were as follows: HR 95 bpm, BP 148/94 mmHg, RR 19, and SpO_2 97% on RA. Which of the following diagnostic tests should be prioritized?**
   A. CT head noncontrast
   B. Urinalysis
   C. STAT video EEG
   D. Pelvic US
7. **Upon the primary survey of a late pregnant trauma patient, which of the following measures should be immediately performed in the setting of hypotension?**
   A. Arterial line for a more accurate tracing
   B. Initiate vasopressors through the central line
   C. Manually displace the uterus to the left side
   D. Order 2 units of pRBCs
8. **A 28-year-old G1P0 female at 32-week gestation was brought into the ED after she was involved in an MVC. The patient was restrained with positive airbag deployment. The patient is complaining of abdominal pain diffusely across the lower abdomen. Her BP was 104/62 mmHg, and her HR was 94 bpm. She denied any vaginal bleeding or discharge. The fetal heart rate was 178 bpm. Uterine ultrasound does not reveal any signs of abruption. Which of the following is the most appropriate next step?**
   A. Admit for continuous fetal monitoring for 6 h
   B. Admit for continuous fetal monitoring for 24 h
   C. Discharge with close follow-up to OB-GYN
   D. Emergency cesarean section
9. **Which of the following is true regarding maternal fetal hemorrhage?**
   A. A single dose of anti-D IgG should immediately be administered to all Rh-pregnant trauma patients
   B. Rh alloimmunization is only of concern in major trauma cases
   C. Only anti-D IgG was administered after 12 weeks of gestation

D. The Kleihauer-Betke test should be used only in Rh-women if there is a high suspicion of maternal fetal hemorrhage

10. **Which of the following is false regarding CPR in a pregnant patient?**
    A. The uterus should be manually displaced to the left during compressions
    B. Chest compressions should be performed at a rate of 100/min
    C. Drugs of resuscitation should be administered according to standard ACLS guidelines
    D. Defibrillation should be avoided due to high fetal risk
11. **Which of the following is a diagnostic criterion for HELLP syndrome?**
    A. Platelets <100 K
    B. Total bilirubin >20
    C. LDH >100
    D. AST >20
12. **Which of the following hemodynamic parameters should be optimized for a pregnant patient with peripartum cardiomyopathy?**
    A. Reduce preload; reduce afterload; increase inotropy
    B. Increase preload; reduce afterload; increase inotropy
    C. Reduce preload; increase afterload; increase inotropy
    D. Reduce preload; reduce afterload; reduce inotropy
13. **A 40-year-old G1P0 undergoes spontaneous vaginal delivery of a healthy baby. Immediately after delivery of the placenta, the patient becomes dyspneic. Her BP was 75/40 mmHg, pulse was 123 bpm, and SpO_2 was 84% on RA. There is a small purpuric rash around her PIV on the left hand, which is oozing some blood. What is the most likely diagnosis?**
    A. Pulmonary embolus
    B. Amniotic fluid embolism
    C. Peripartum cardiomyopathy
    D. Sepsis
14. **Which of the following laboratory tests can be used to differentiate between acute fatty liver of pregnancy and HELLP syndrome?**
    A. Ammonia and proteinuria
    B. Creatinine and transaminases
    C. Creatinine and glucose
    D. Ammonia and glucose
15. **Which of the following reasons is *not* true regarding pulmonary edema in pregnancy?**
    A. Preeclampsia increases the risk of pulmonary edema
    B. Pulmonary vascular resistance increases in pregnancy, which increases susceptibility to pulmonary edema
    C. The colloid osmotic pressure to pulmonary capillary wedge pressure (PCWP) gradient is reduced, increasing the risk for pulmonary edema
    D. The increase in plasma volume during pregnancy places patients at a higher risk of pulmonary edema

Answers and Explanations

1. **B.** As the uterus enlarges in pregnancy, the intestines are pushed cephalad so they lie mostly in the upper abdomen. Any penetrating trauma to the upper abdomen during late gestation can result in complex intestinal injury. Furthermore, clinical signs of peritoneal irritation are less evident in pregnant women and must be further explored by imaging. The FAST exam is typically preferred and very sensitive in detecting intraperitoneal bleeding, but when it is not available, other imaging modalities should be considered. CT should not be delayed or deferred due to concerns of fetal radiation exposure. A, C, and D are all appropriate measures to eventually take in this patient, but it is essential to rule out any maternal intraperitoneal bleeding or injury first [1, 2].
2. **C.** Plasma volume increases steadily throughout pregnancy. Because of the increased intravascular volume, pregnant patients can lose a significant amount of blood before their vital signs can reflect this hemodynamic change (tachycardia, hypotension). Although maternal vital signs may appear stable, there can be a significant decrease in perfusion to the placenta and fetal distress. Thus, it is very important to recognize this and initiate early crystalloid resuscitation in pregnant patients when hypovolemia is suspected [3].
3. **C.** The ejection fraction remains unchanged in pregnancy. Although cardiac output is increased, contractility remains the same, which preserves left and right ventricular ejection fraction. (**A**) Cardiac output increases by approximately 1.0 to 1.5 L during pregnancy to compensate for the increase in plasma volume, systemic vasodilation, and increased perfusion requirements to the uterus and placenta, which require approximately 20% of the patient's cardiac output. (**B**) During pregnancy, there is a significant reduction in systemic vascular resistance (SVR) and afterload. It is believed that estrogen and relaxin stimulate the production of nitric oxide, which plays a major role in the systemic vasodilation observed during pregnancy. (**D**) In a normal pregnancy, there is a significant increase in the RAAS. As estrogen increases during pregnancy, as does renin, which eventually leads to an increase in angiotensin. This increase is important for blood pressure regulation in response to vasodilation [3, 4].
4. **D.** Functional residual capacity is the volume remaining in the lungs after a normal (tidal) expiration. It is a combination of the residual volume and expiratory reserve volume. Due to increased pressure from the gravid abdomen, the FRC substantially decreases. (**A**) Due to an increase in minute ventilation, it is expected that pregnant patients will demonstrate respiratory alkalosis. Normal $PaCO_2$ in pregnancy is approximately 28–32 mmHg. A $PaCO_2$ in the nonpregnant normal range (~40 mmHg) may indicate ventilatory failure and impending respiratory distress. (**B**) Tidal volume increases by approximately 30% in pregnancy. This is due to two main reasons. First, oxygen consumption and carbon dioxide production significantly increase during pregnancy. Second, progesterone directly acts on the central respiratory drive to increase minute ventilation. (**C**) Expiratory reserve volume is the additional volume of air that can be

expired after a normal expiration. Due to the compression of the diaphragm by the uterus, ERV will decrease in pregnancy [5].

5. **A.** Fibrinogen is significantly higher in pregnant patients than in the nonpregnant population. The pregnant patient is essentially in a hypercoagulable state to prevent postpartum hemorrhage. Fibrinogen levels almost double in late pregnancy, so a normal fibrinogen level is concerning for early disseminated intravascular coagulation (DIC).

   (**B**) Platelet counts typically drop by approximately 15% in pregnant patients. This is due to multiple factors but is mainly seen secondary to the dilutional effect (with increased plasma volume) and due to increased spleen size (spleen can increase up to 50% in pregnancy), where platelets can pool. A very low platelet count (<100,000 platelets) can be concerning for thrombocytopenic disorders and can be observed in DIC, but it is unlikely for a platelet count of 140,000 to raise immediate concern for DIC. (**C**) Most coagulation factors are increased in pregnancy due to the hypercoagulable state. (**D**) A normal PT is unlikely to be a cause of concern for DIC [2].
6. **B.** Eclampsia is a very serious condition in pregnancy. Although often a consequence of preeclampsia, some patients who have never had prenatal care are unaware of their condition. Preeclampsia was defined as hypertension (140/90 mmHg) in addition to proteinuria after 20 weeks of gestation. Some studies report that proteinuria is no longer a diagnostic marker for preeclampsia, as some patients have had advanced disease before the onset of proteinuria. However, it is essential to monitor and evaluate end organ dysfunction (renal dysfunction, liver dysfunction, CNS disturbances, pulmonary edema, or thrombocytopenia). Eclampsia is defined as the onset of new generalized tonic-clonic seizures in women with preeclampsia. Eclampsia can closely imitate head injury and thus must be carefully evaluated in any late pregnancy that presents with hypertension, proteinuria, and seizures. It is also important to also obtain a CT of the head to evaluate for any intracranial bleeding but remember not to mistake eclampsia for head injury [6].
7. **C.** Uterine compression of the IVC may reduce cardiac venous return, ultimately reducing preload and cardiac output. In any hypotensive pregnant woman, it is essential to manually displace the uterus to the left. IVF and blood products can be administered afterward. Vasopressors should be a last resort, as vasopressors can reduce uterine blood flow and result in fetal hypoxia [5].
8. **B.** Placental abruption is the second leading cause of fetal death, seen in 1–5% of minor trauma. Not all cases will present with the triad of vaginal bleeding, abdominal pain, and uterine irritability. Vaginal bleeding occurs in approximately 70% of cases. Ultrasound is not a sensitive test for placental abruption, and the diagnosis cannot be ruled out if it is negative. For patients with no risk factors for fetal risk, continuous fetal monitoring should occur for 6 h. For patients with one or more risk factors for fetal loss (FHR >160, maternal HR >110, mechanism of injury), continuous fetal monitoring should occur for at least 24 h [1, 7].

9. **A.** Rh immunoglobulin therapy should be administered to all injured Rh- mothers regardless of the severity of the trauma. The Kleihauer-Betke (KB) test measures the percentage of RBCs in the maternal circulation. Any result outside of 0 mL was considered positive. The KB test can also be used to predict the risk of preterm labor after maternal trauma and should not be limited to only Rh- mothers [1].
10. **D.** Cardiopulmonary resuscitation in a pregnant woman should not differ from that for a nonpregnant patient, and ACLS guidelines should be adhered to. The only difference seen in pregnant women is the manual displacement of the uterus to the left to allow for increased cardiac venous return to aid in resuscitation [5].
11. **A.** HELLP syndrome is a critical obstetric condition with a constellation of findings, including hemolysis, elevated liver enzymes, and low platelets. The syndrome is thought to be due to generalized endothelial injury from massive activation of the coagulation and complement cascades. This can lead to hepatic hemorrhage and necrosis, capsular tears, and intraperitoneal bleeding. Laboratory criteria were as follows: microangiopathic hemolysis with schistocytes, PLT count <100 K, bilirubin level of >1.2 mg/dL, serum LDH >500, and AST >70 [8].
12. **A.** Peripartum cardiomyopathy is a rare cause of heart failure observed in pregnant patients. To be characterized as peripartum cardiomyopathy, the following criteria must be met: (1) development of heart failure within the last 4 weeks of pregnancy or within 5 months of pregnancy, (2) no preexisting heart disease, (3) no other identifiable cases of heart failure, and (4) LV systolic dysfunction. Medical therapy should be aimed at the following: reduce preload, reduce afterload, and increase inotropy. Preload reduction is usually treated with nitrates. Diuretics can be used cautiously to avoid rapid changes in intravascular volume. Afterload reduction is achieved by vasodilators, such as hydralazine. ACE inhibitors are the preferred agent for pregnant women. Inotropy increase can be achieved by dobutamine, dopamine, or digoxin. Of note, it is important to avoid beta-blockers in patients with acute decompensated HF [8].
13. **B.** Amniotic fluid embolism (AFE) is a clinical diagnosis and must be immediately considered when a pregnant patient experiences dyspnea with signs of hypoxia, hypotension, or altered mental status during labor or immediately postpartum. AFE is believed to be caused by the introduction of amniotic fluid to the pulmonary vasculature, resulting in pulmonary vasospasm, pulmonary hypertension, right heart failure, DIC, and eventually cardiovascular collapse. Unfortunately, it is a catastrophic diagnosis with a very high mortality rate. The treatment is supportive and should be immediately implemented with a focus on cardiorespiratory resuscitation and correction of coagulopathy [8].
14. **D.** Acute fatty liver of pregnancy (AFLP) is a clinical diagnosis characterized by hepatic failure, usually during the third trimester of pregnancy. It is very common to confuse AFLP with HELLP syndrome due to the overlap of laboratory and clinical abnormalities. However, since AFLP is associated with liver failure, it is often associated with increased ammonia, hypoglycemia, abnormal

clotting (PT/PTT/INR), and more pronounced hyperbilirubinemia. The histological appearance of microvesicular fatty infiltration in hepatocytes can confirm the presence of AFLPs [8].

15. **B**. Pulmonary edema is a rare but life-threatening condition. The hemodynamic changes observed in pregnancy make a pregnant patient more susceptible to pulmonary edema. Pulmonary edema is commonly seen in conditions with increased cardiac preload, increased pulmonary capillary permeability (as seen in preeclampsia), or both. Due to the expansion of plasma volume by water and sodium retention, cardiac preload is increased. Pulmonary vascular resistance, such as systemic vascular resistance, is significantly *decreased* in pregnant patients. This increase in preload with a reduction in afterload makes pregnant patients hemodynamically more susceptible to pulmonary edema. Additionally, the colloid osmotic pressure to pulmonary capillary wedge pressure (PCWP) gradient is reduced. Although there is no increase seen in PCWP, serum osmotic pressure is decreased, which favors transudation of fluid into the lungs [9].

References

1. Maslovitz S, Aviv T, Dan Farine I, On T, Bujold E, Basso M, Bos H, Bc V. SOGC Clinical Practice Guidelines for the Management of a Pregnant Trauma Patient Maternal Fetal Medicine Committee. 2015. https://www.jogc.com/article/S1701-2163(15)30232-2/pdf.
2. Irving T, Menon R, Ciantar E. Trauma during pregnancy. *BJA*. Education. 2021;21(1):10–9. https://doi.org/10.1016/j.bjae.2020.08.005.
3. Sanghavi M, Rutherford JD. Cardiovascular physiology of pregnancy. Circulation. 2014;130(12):1003–8. https://doi.org/10.1161/circulationaha.114.009029.
4. Hall ME, George EM, Granger JP. The heart during pregnancy. Rev Esp Cardiol. 2011;64(11):1045–50. https://doi.org/10.1016/j.recesp.2011.07.009.
5. Madden A-M, Meng M-L. Cardiopulmonary resuscitation in the pregnant patient. BJA Educ. 2020;20(8):252–8. https://doi.org/10.1016/j.bjae.2020.03.007.
6. Magley M, Hinson MR. Eclampsia. PubMed; StatPearls Publishing. 2020. https://www.ncbi.nlm.nih.gov/books/NBK554392/.
7. American College of Surgeons, Committee on Trauma. ATLS: student course manual. American College of Surgeons; 2018.
8. Williams J, Mozurkewich E, Chilimigras J, Van De Ven C. Critical care in obstetrics: pregnancy-specific conditions. Best Pract Res Clin Obstet Gynecol. 2008;22(5):825–46. https://doi.org/10.1016/j.bpobgyn.2008.06.003.
9. Kaur H, Kolli M. Acute pulmonary edema in pregnancy—fluid overload or atypical preeclampsia. Cureus. 2021;13:e19305. https://doi.org/10.7759/cureus.19305.

Chronic Pain in Pregnancy

Ming J. Huang

Questions

1. **Which of the following is *incorrect* regarding musculoskeletal alterations during pregnancy that lead to development of low back pain?**
   A. Exaggerated lordosis of the lower back
   B. Increased forward flexion of the neck
   C. Increase in posterior tilt of the pelvis
   D. Increase in joint and ligament laxity
2. **What is the prevalence of pregnancy-related pelvic girdle pain in late pregnancy?**
   A. 10%
   B. 20%
   C. 25%
   D. 45%
3. **All the following risk factors are associated with pregnancy-related pelvic girdle pain *except*:**
   A. History of low back pain
   B. Lower educational level
   C. Older age
   D. Obesity
4. **Which of the following statements is *incorrect* regarding postpartum pelvic girdle pain?**
   A. The majority of the women recovered from pelvic girdle pain 6 months after delivery
   B. Emotional stress during pregnancy is associated with persistent pelvic girdle pain after delivery

M. J. Huang (✉)
Anesthesiology Loma Linda School of Medicine, Loma Linda, CA, USA

Riverside University Health System, Moreno Valley, CA, USA
e-mail: m.huang@ruhealth.org

A. C. Sinha, I. F. Pasca (eds.), *Peripartum Care of the Pregnant Patient*,
https://doi.org/10.1007/978-3-031-62756-9_39

   C. The recovery rate decreases with increasing levels of pain severity during pregnancy
   D. Women with cesarean birth are associated with lower rates of persistent pain postpartum
5. **Which of the following is most common peripheral neuropathy during pregnancy?**
   A. Cubital tunnel syndrome
   B. Carpal tunnel syndrome
   C. Femoral nerve neuropathy
   D. Fibular neuropathy
6. **Entrapment of which of the following nerves results in numbness and burning pain in the lateral aspect of the outer thigh?**
   A. Lateral femoral cutaneous nerve
   B. Obturator nerve
   C. Ilioinguinal nerve
   D. Genitofemoral nerve
7. **Which of the following statements is *incorrect* regarding the use of gabapentin during pregnancy in recent studies?**
   A. Strong association between early pregnancy exposure and major malformations
   B. Maternal use late in pregnancy is associated with an increased risk of preterm birth
   C. Increased risk in NICU admission of babies born to women exposed to gabapentin during pregnancy
   D. Gabapentin use during late pregnancy is associated with fetal lower birth weight
8. **In utero opioid exposure can result in neonatal abstinence syndrome (NAS). Which of following statements is *incorrect* regarding the treatment of NAS?**
   A. Avoidance of excessive environmental stimulation
   B. Frequent hypercaloric feeds
   C. Breastfeeding is generally not encouraged
   D. Morphine is the primary opioid used in the majority of centers
9. **Which of the following medications is considered an absolute contraindication for pain treatment of rheumatoid arthritis during pregnancy?**
   A. Sulfasalazine
   B. Glucocorticoids
   C. Hydroxychloroquine
   D. Methotrexate
10. **Which of the following statements is *incorrect* regarding opioid use during the breastfeeding period?**
   A. Breastfeeding should be encouraged for all mothers who are on a stable dose of opioids
   B. Methadone is generally safe to use in breastfeeding mothers
   C. Breastfeeding mothers should start feeding 1–2 h after taking the opioid

D. Breastfeeding may help decrease the duration of neonatal abstinence syndrome.

11. **Which of the statements is *false* about pregnancy and complex regional pain syndrome (CRPS)?**
    A. Pregnancy is the predisposed risk factor for developing CRPS
    B. Most CRPS involve the upper limbs
    C. Vitamin C helps prevent the development of CRPS after wrist fracture
    D. It is unclear whether preexisting CRPS is aggravated with subsequent pregnancy
12. **de Quervain tendinopathy can typically develop postpartum. Which of the following is *incorrect* regarding this condition?**
    A. The dominant hand is more likely to be affected
    B. It affects both the abductor pollicis longus and the extensor pollicis brevis
    C. Postpartum women tend to develop symptoms 4–6 weeks after delivery
    D. The etiology of de Quervain tendinopathy is not fully understood
13. **Pregnant women with headaches have been reported to have greater rates for all of the following *except*:**
    A. Preterm delivery
    B. Gestational HTN
    C. Preeclampsia
    D. Elective C-section
14. **Which of the following medications is *contraindicated* for treatment of migraine during pregnancy?**
    A. Opioids
    B. Ergotamine
    C. Metoclopramide
    D. Meclizine
15. **Which of the following statements is *incorrect* regarding the use of acetaminophen during pregnancy?**
    A. Acetaminophen is a first-line analgesic during pregnancy
    B. Acetaminophen is classified as a category A drug by the US Food and Drug Administration (FDA)
    C. Several studies have linked prenatal acetaminophen use with low birth weight
    D. Acetaminophen and its metabolites freely cross the placenta
16. **All of the following statements about treatment of low back pain during pregnancy are correct *except*:**
    A. Transcutaneous electrical nerve stimulation (TENS) has been safely used for pain relief during labor and delivery
    B. Benzodiazepine has teratogenic effects and should be avoided during pregnancy
    C. Physical therapy has demonstrated efficacy in treating low back pain
    D. Topic diclofenac gel is safe to use in the third trimester

Answers and Explanations

1. **C**. Many musculoskeletal changes in pregnancy are mediated by hormone relaxin. An increase in relaxin results in joint and ligament laxity (**D**). Other physical adaptations include increased lordosis of the lower back (**A**), forward flexion of the neck (**B**), and anterior tilt of the pelvis, not posterior tilt of the pelvis [1].
2. **D**. Pregnancy-related pelvic girdle pain is common among parturients, especially during late pregnancy. The average reported prevalence is 45.3% in 28 studies, making **D** the correct answer. The rates for **A**, **B**, and **C** are too low [2].
3. **C**. Risk factors including history of lower back pain (**A**) or pelvic girdle pain, being overweight/obese (**D**), younger age, and lower educational level (**B**) are associated with pregnancy-related pelvic girdle pain. Younger age is a risk factor not older age [3].
4. **D**. Cesarean birth does not lower the risk of postpartum pelvic girdle pain and is associated with higher rates of persistent postpartum pain. The other statements in **A**, **B**, and **C** are correct regarding postpartum pelvic girdle pain [4, 5].
5. **B**. Pregnancy can cause a variety of physiological changes related to the production of hormones that lead to weight gain and water retention. The most commonly occurring entrapment neuropathy is carpal tunnel syndrome. Cubital tunnel syndrome (**A**), femoral nerve neuropathy (**C**), and fibular neuropathy (**D**) are less common [6].
6. **A**. One of the most common peripheral neuropathies during pregnancy is meralgia paresthetica, which is characterized by numbness and burning pain in the lateral aspect of the outer thigh. A nerve block with local anesthetic and steroid can be both diagnostic and therapeutic for the condition. Neuropathies in other nerves, including the obturator nerve (**B**), ilioinguinal nerve (**C**), and genitofemoral nerve (**D**), have different clinical presentations [7].
7. **A**. In a recent large population-based cohort study, authors did not find an association between gabapentin exposure during early pregnancy and major malformations overall. Maternal use of gabapentin is associated with a higher risk of preterm birth (**B**), small for gestational age (**D**), and NICU admission (**C**) [8].
8. **C**. Both the American Congress of Obstetrics and Gynecology (ACOG) and the American Academy of Pediatrics (AAP) encourage breastfeeding, as it is associated with a lower incidence and severity of NAS. Quiet environment (**A**) and frequency feeds (**B**) to minimize hunger are nonpharmacologic strategies to manage NAS, while morphine (**C**) is the most common pharmacological treatment for NAS [9].
9. **D**. Methotrexate is considered a category X medication by the US FDA. It can lead to fetal defects in the heart, central nervous system, and skeleton. The other three medications **A**, **B**, and **C** are in category B, which suggests no evidence of risk in studies [10].

10. **C**. The lactating mother should avoid breastfeeding between 1 and 2 h after taking opioids. The other three statements in **A**, **B**, and **D** are correct regarding opioid use during the breastfeeding period [11].
11. **B**. Most CRPS cases in pregnancy involve the lower limbs. Pregnancy is a known predisposed risk factor for CRPS (**A**); however, there are limited data on whether preexisting CRPS is aggravated with subsequent pregnancy (**D**). The efficacy of vitamin C in preventing CRPS after wrist fracture or foot or ankle surgery is well established (**C**) [12].
12. **A**. The dominant hand is not more likely to be affected than the nondominant hand. It affects both the abductor pollicis longus and the extensor pollicis brevis (**B**). Postpartum women tend to develop symptoms 4 to 6 weeks after delivery (**C**). The etiology of de Quervain tendinopathy is not fully understood (**D**) [13].
13. **D**. The presence of headaches during pregnancy puts the patient at high risk for preterm delivery (**A**), gestational HTN (**B**), and preeclampsia (**C**). A prospective cohort study suggests that fewer women in the headache group had preterm elective cesarean section [14, 15].
14. **B**. Ergot and ergot alkaloids are contraindicated due to their known uterotonic and vasoconstrictive effects. Metoclopramide is commonly used during pregnancy without significant fetal side effects (**C**). Meclizine is an H1 antagonist preferred in pregnancy to relieve nausea associated with migraine (**D**). Opioids are a third-tier option for migraine treatment in pregnancy (**A**). All opioids pose risks for maternal addiction and neonatal withdrawal [16].
15. **B**. Acetaminophen is classified as a category B drug by the FDA (i.e., no risks observed in pregnant women). It is a first-line analgesic during pregnancy (**A**), with nearly two-thirds of pregnant women reporting taking the medication. Acetaminophen and metabolites have been shown to cross the placenta freely and have been found in fetal urine and liver (**C**). Several studies have linked prenatal acetaminophen use with preterm birth and low birth weight (**D**) [17].
16. **D**. Topical diclofenac gel is a medication in category C and should only be used in the first trimester per FDA recommendations. The TENS unit has been safely used for pain relief during labor and delivery when applied correctly (**A**). Benzodiazepine has teratogenic effects and should be avoided during pregnancy (**B**). Physical therapy has demonstrated efficacy in treating low back pain (**C**) [18].

References

1. Foti T, Davids JR, Bagley A. A biomechanical analysis of gait during pregnancy. J Bone Joint Surg Am. 2000;82:625.
2. Wu W-H, Meijer OG, Uegaki K, Mens J, Van Dieen J, Wuisman P, et al. Pregnancy-related pelvic girdle pain (PPP), I: terminology, clinical presentation, and prevalence. Eur Spine J. 2004;13(7):575–89.
3. Wuytack F, Begley C, Daly D. Risk factors for pregnancy-related pelvic girdle pain: a scoping review. BMC Pregnancy Childbirth. 2020;20:739.

4. Bjelland EK, Stuge B, Vangen S, Stray-Pedersen B, Eberhard-Gran M. Mode of delivery and persistence of pelvic girdle syndrome 6 months postpartum. Am J Obstet Gynecol. 2013;208(4):298.e1–7.
5. Bjelland EK, Stuge B, Engdahl B, Eberhard-Gran M. The effect of emotional distress on persistent pelvic girdle pain after delivery: a longitudinal population study. BJOG. 2013;120(1):32–40.
6. Ciafaloni E, et al. Entrapment neuropathy and pregnancy. In: Ciafaloni E, Thornburg LL, Bushnell CD, editors. Neurological diseases and pregnancy: a coordinated care model for best management. Online edition. New York, NY: Oxford Academic; 2018.
7. Mabie WC. Peripheral neuropathies during pregnancy. Clin Obstet Gynecol. 2005;48(1):57–66.
8. Patorno E, Hernandez-Diaz S, Huybrechts KF, Desai RJ, Cohen JM, Mogun H, Bateman BT. Gabapentin in pregnancy and the risk of adverse neonatal and maternal outcomes: a population-based cohort study nested in the US Medicaid analytic eXtract dataset. PLoS Med. 2020;17(9):e1003322.
9. Kraft WK, Stover MW, Davis JM. Neonatal abstinence syndrome: pharmacologic strategies for the mother and infant. Semin Perinatol. 2016;40(3):203–12.
10. Krause ML, Makol A. Management of rheumatoid arthritis during pregnancy: challenges and solutions. Open Access Rheumatol. 2016;8:23–36.
11. Committee on Obstetric Practice Breastfeeding Export Work Group. Acog Committee Opinion. Breastfeeding may help decrease the severity and d duration of neonatal abstinence syndrome. Obstet Gynecol. 2021;137(2):e3061.
12. Trikha A, Baidya DK, Singh PM. Complex regional pain syndrome and pregnancy. J Obstet Anaesth Crit Care. 2012;2:69–73.
13. Menendez ME, Thornton E, Kent S, Kalajian T, Ring D. A prospective randomized clinical trial of prescription of full-time versus as-desired splint wear for de Quervain tendinopathy. Int Orthop. 2015;39(8):1563–9.
14. Marozio L, Facchinetti F, Allais G, et al. Headache and adverse pregnancy outcomes: a prospective study. Eur J Obstet Gynecol Reprod Biol. 2012;161(2):140–3.
15. Facchinetti F, Allais G, Nappi RE, et al. Migraine is a risk factor for hypertensive disorders in pregnancy: a prospective cohort study. Cephalalgia. 2008;29:286–91.
16. Negro A, Delaruelle Z, Ivanova TA, et al. Headache and pregnancy: a systematic review. J Headache Pain. 2017;18:106.
17. Addo KA, Bulka C, Dhingra R, Santos HP Jr, Smeester L, O'Shea TM, Fry RC. Acetaminophen use during pregnancy and DNA methylation in the placenta of the extremely low gestational age newborn (ELGAN) cohort. Environ Epigenet. 2019;5(2):dvz010.
18. Bridwell R, Koyfman A, Long B. Pain in pregnancy. In: Cisewski D, editor. Pain management guide: evidence-based alternative analgesia. 1st ed; 2020.

Opioid and Substance Use Disorders

Antonio Gonzalez-Fiol and Kristen L. Fardelmann

Questions

1. **Which one of the following substances contributes most to teratogenicity in the United States?**
   A. Caffeine
   B. Cocaine
   C. Alcohol
   D. Marijuana
2. **Behavioral intervention for the management of nicotine use disorder is as follows:**
   A. Minimally associated with smoking cessation in late pregnancy
   B. Shown to produce no effect on birth weight
   C. Minimally associated with smoking cessation in late pregnancy and had no impact on birth weight
   D. Significantly associated with reduced smoking in the late term and reduced number of low-birth-weight infants
3. **When managing patients with medications (methadone, buprenorphine) for opioid use disorder (MOUD), current experts' opinion recommends ______.**
   A. Increasing MOUD dose
   B. Maintaining the current dose
   C. If on a partial agonist, switching to an agonist
   D. Tapering down during the last trimester

A. Gonzalez-Fiol (✉)
Division of Obstetric Anesthesia, Yale School of Medicine, New Haven, CT, USA
e-mail: antonio.gonzalez-fiol@yale.edu

K. L. Fardelmann
Yale School of Medicine, New Haven, CT, USA

A. C. Sinha, I. F. Pasca (eds.), *Peripartum Care of the Pregnant Patient*,
https://doi.org/10.1007/978-3-031-62756-9_40

4. **When compared to White parturients, Black and Hispanic individuals are likely to receive medications for opioid use disorder ______.**
   A. At a similar odds rate for receiving treatment and similar dosing
   B. At a higher odds rate for receiving treatment and higher dosing
   C. At a lower odds rate for receiving treatment and higher dosing
   D. At a lower odds rate for receiving treatment and lower dosing
5. **Which of the following is considered the most common modifiable risk factor to decrease adverse perinatal outcomes?**
   A. Cocaine
   B. Alcohol
   C. Tobacco
   D. Marijuana
6. **Patients presenting with acute cocaine intoxication may need blood pressure management. Which of the following is the most appropriate medication for blood pressure management of a patient with known or suspected acute cocaine intoxication?**
   A. Esmolol
   B. Nifedipine
   C. Propranolol
   D. Hydralazine
7. **Which of the following has become the most common illicit substance requiring medical treatment during pregnancy?**
   A. Methamphetamine (MDMA) and/or amphetamines
   B. Marijuana
   C. Cocaine
   D. Alcohol
8. **Which of the following illegal drugs can be clandestinely manufactured with the use of legally obtained products?**
   A. Marijuana
   B. Cocaine
   C. Methamphetamine
   D. Opioids
9. **Within the first 2 weeks postpartum, consumption of opioid tablets after cesarean delivery is as follows:**
   A. Linearly correlated with pain severity at the time of discharge
   B. Linearly correlated to pain severity the first week after discharge
   C. Inversely proportional to the number of pills prescribed
   D. Associated with the number of tablets prescribed and independent of pain severity at time of discharge
10. **A recent study showed that the median number of prescribed opioid tablets was 40 (interquartile range (IQR) 30–40) and the median number of leftover pills was 15 (IQR 3–26). What percentage of leftover pills were not properly disposed?**
    A. 5%
    B. 15%

C. 50%
D. 95%

11. **In a recent study that evaluated the effects of opioid use disorder on pain type and intensity, which one of the following had the highest correlation to pain intensity?**
A. Affective/evaluative
B. Nociceptive pain
C. Visceral
D. Neuropathic

12. **Based on postoperative opioid consumption patterns between patients receiving buprenorphine or methadone, which of the following is expected?**
A. Increased opioid consumption in patients prescribed buprenorphine
B. Decreased opioid consumption in patients prescribed buprenorphine
C. Increased opioid consumption in patients prescribed methadone
D. No significant difference in opioid consumption between patients prescribed buprenorphine and methadone

13. **Which of the following is/are recommended based on expert opinion for the postoperative management of patients with substance use disorder?**
A. Intrathecal morphine
B. Transverse abdominal plane block
C. Psychosocial services
D. All the above

14. **Which of the following biopsychosocial factors is associated with an increased risk of substance use disorder during pregnancy?**
A. Age > 25
B. Above poverty level income
C. High school or less education
D. Safe household environment

15. **As the legalization of marijuana has increased, so has its use by parturients who claim this drug may help with ______.**
A. Decreasing stress/anxiety
B. Nausea/vomiting
C. Decreasing chronic pain
D. All the above

16. **What percentage of parturients who smoke tobacco preconception quit during pregnancy?**
A. 15%
B. 33%
C. 50%
D. 90%

17. **In patients using cocaine (without concern for placental abruption), which of the following should be evaluated prior to administration of regional anesthesia?**
A. Complete blood count
B. Coagulation panel

C. Fibrinogen
D. Comprehensive metabolic panel

18. **The following diagnostic test should be performed during the preanesthesia evaluation for patients receiving methadone for opioid agonist treatment.**
    A. Electrocardiogram
    B. Complete blood count
    C. Comprehensive metabolic panel
    D. Coagulation panel
19. **During pregnancy and the first year postpartum, what percentage of maternal deaths are associated with illicit and prescription drug use?**
    A. 1–10%
    B. 11–20%
    C. 21–30%
    D. 31–40%
20. **All of the following risk factors for persistent opioid use following cesarean delivery were identified within the year prior to delivery and/or at the time of delivery *except*:**
    A. Cocaine abuse
    B. Migraine headaches
    C. Antidepressant use
    D. Repeat cesarean section
21. **Which of the following statements is most consistent with the American College of Obstetricians and Gynecologists recommendations for screening pregnant patients for substance use?**
    A. Universal screening at the first prenatal visit
    B. Selective screening for patients with poor adherence to prenatal care
    C. Selective screening for patients with prior adverse pregnancy outcomes
    D. Universal screening at every prenatal visit
22. **Acute effects of cannabinoids include all the following *except*:**
    A. Increased risk of respiratory events
    B. Altered mental status
    C. Increased risk of myocardial infarction
    D. Increased risk of hypotension
23. **Opioid agonist therapy is strongly recommended for pregnant patients with opioid use disorder. When compared to methadone use, use of buprenorphine is associated with all the following *except*:**
    A. Lower risk of neonatal abstinence syndrome
    B. Lower risk of preterm birth
    C. Lower risk of severe maternal complications
    D. Lower risk of small size for gestational age
24. **Exposure to cannabinoids in early pregnancy is associated with the following:**
    A. Normal gray matter volume in adolescence
    B. Decreased visual motor coordination in childhood

C. No difference in attention span
D. Normal sleep in adolescence

25. **All the following statements regarding cannabinoids are true *except*:**
A. Cannabinoid use increases the risk of preeclampsia
B. Cannabinoid use may be associated with postoperative hypothermia and shivering
C. Long-term use of cannabinoids may be associated with higher opioid analgesic requirements
D. Cannabinoids cross into breast milk

Answers and Explanations

1. **C**. Of the substance use disorders (SUDs) mentioned, alcohol is the greatest teratogen. Although other substances may be associated with birth defects, there is no specific syndrome associated with the use of the other substances in comparison to alcohol consumption and the potential for fetal alcohol syndrome disorders. Hence, although fetal anomalies may be related to the use of caffeine (**A**), cocaine (**B**), and marijuana (**D**), alcohol is the best-known SUD associated with the presence of neonatal facial features (e.g., small palpebral fissures, flat midface with a short, upturned nose, thin upper lip) and developmental and behavioral difficulties [1, 2].
2. **D**. The most effective modality of treatment for nicotine use disorder is behavioral therapy, more specifically cognitive behavioral therapy or contingency management. A Cochrane review study demonstrated that behavioral intervention significantly reduced smoking in late pregnancy, low birth weight, and preterm delivery, making **A**, **B**, and **C** false statements. Nicotine replacement therapy was minimally associated with smoking cessation in late pregnancy and did not produce improved perinatal outcomes (**A** and **B**) [3–5].
3. **B**. Despite the lack of robust evidence, expert opinion guidelines recommend continuing methadone and buprenorphine therapy throughout the peripartum and postpartum period. Guidelines discourage the increase (**A**), decrease, or discontinuation (**D**) of the patient's current medication, which should discourage substituting a partial (e.g., buprenorphine) for a full agonist (e.g., methadone), making **C** a false statement [6, 7]. The most effective modality of treatment for nicotine use disorder is behavioral therapy, more specifically cognitive behavioral therapy or contingency management. A Cochrane review study demonstrated that behavioral intervention significantly reduced smoking in late pregnancy, low birth weight, and preterm delivery, making **A**, **B**, and **C** false statements. Nicotine replacement therapy was minimally associated with smoking cessation in late pregnancy and did not produce improved perinatal outcomes (**A** and **B**) [3–5].
4. **D.** Treatment odds rates vary by substance and race, being higher for opioid use disorder (e.g., 34% for OUD versus 12% for alcohol use) and lower for Black and Hispanic individuals. Black and Hispanic patients have **lower** odds of

receiving treatment than White patients, making **A** and **B** false. When Black and Hispanic patients receive MOUD, they tend to receive lower doses than White individuals, making **C** false [3, 8].

5. **C.** The assessment of adverse neonatal outcomes is complicated secondary to cofounders, in this case polysubstance abuse. In a study that analyzed the adjusted population-attributable risk (PAR) proportions of polysubstance use (e.g., tobacco + alcohol, tobacco + alcohol + cocaine), tobacco (**C**) had the highest adjusted PAR for low birth weight (LBW), prematurity, and intrauterine growth restriction (IUGR) compared to any other substance of use studied. For LBW, the adjusted PAR % (confidence interval) was 5.57 (3.06–7.91) for tobacco and 1.72 (−0.73–4.06), 0.81 (−0.79–2.29), and 0.39 (−0.13–0.93) for alcohol, cocaine, and opiates, respectively. Similar trends were observed for prematurity and IUGR, for which tobacco had the highest adjusted PAR % [3.66 (0.87–6.53) and 13.79 (10.08–17.33), respectively], making options **A**, **B**, and **D** lower modifiable contributors [3, 9].
6. **D.** The use of beta-blockers for the blood pressure management of a patient with cocaine-induced hypertension is contraindicated, making options **A** and **C** false. Nifedipine is a calcium channel blocker, and the use of this drug family has been associated with potentiation of the toxic effects of cocaine, making **B** false. Hydralazine is the best choice from the options above, yet its use may cause further tachycardia, and caution is needed [10].
7. **A**. From 1994 to 2006, the number of admissions secondary to methamphetamines increased from 8% to 24%. Although the treatment admissions secondary to marijuana use increased during this period, they did not surpass those related to MDMA or amphetamine use (**B**). Alcohol (**D**) and cocaine (**C**) use throughout the studied period decreased [3, 11].
8. **C**. Methamphetamine can be synthesized using a clandestine laboratory utilizing pseudoephedrine and ephedrine, which are contained in over-the-counter medications for treating nasal congestion (e.g., SUDAFED). Although marijuana (**A**), cocaine (**B**), and opioids (**D**) can be prepared from *Cannabis sativa*, *Erythroxylum coca* leaves, and *Papaver somniferum*, the possession of these plants may be illegal. In some states, *cannabis* plants and *cannabis* are legalized [10, 12].
9. **D**. Bateman et al. showed that patients consumed opioid tablets in accordance with the number of tablets prescribed, and independently from the visual analog score pain, immediately after discharge or a week after, making **A**, **B**, and **C** false. Hence, the authors suggest that decreasing the number of opioid tablets may be a feasible alternative to lower opioid consumption without a subsequent increase in pain scores or affecting patient satisfaction [13].
10. **D**. A study looking into the patterns of opioid prescriptions showed that 95.3% of unused tablets are not disposed appropriately. This excess of prescription pills represents a risk for misuse of opioids by the patient or other household members [13].
11. **A**. Examples of pain type and descriptors are summarized in Table 1. For pain intensity and oxycodone use, patients with substance use disorder had

Table 1 Pain type and pain descriptor examples [6, 14]

Pain type	Descriptor examples
Nociceptive	"Sore"
Neuropathic	"Hot/burning," "electric shock"
Visceral	"Cramping"
Affective	"Sickening, "awful"

significant interactions with nociceptive (**B**), visceral (**C**), neuropathic (**D**), and affective (**A**) pain types, yet the highest coefficient relationship was affective/evaluative pain (**A**). This relationship suggests that it is possible that some patients with substance use disorder may benefit from psychosocial services rather than, or in addition to, opioids to cope with recovery after delivery; more research is needed to explore this relationship [6].

12. **D**. Although an increase in opioid consumption was noted in patients receiving buprenorphine (**A**), this did not result in a statistically significant increase when compared to patients receiving methadone, which makes **B** and **C** false statements. This finding highlights that buprenorphine does not need to be stopped or switched to another medication for opioid use disorder treatment peripartum [15].
13. **D**. There are scarce data related to the postoperative pain management of patients with opioid use disorder, as most randomized controlled trials exclude patients with such a past medical history. Although some anesthesiologists forego the use of intrathecal morphine due to the presumed availability of opioid mu-receptors, proponents recommend its use based on a lack of evidence to prove their inefficiency (**A**). Although no strong evidence supports the use of transverse abdominal plane (TAP) blocks for patients with substance use disorder, its use with liposomal bupivacaine (long-acting bupivacaine) has been proposed as part of a multimodal analgesic plan. As stated in question 12, the high correlation between pain intensity and affective pain highlights the need for psychosocial services as part of a multimodal and multidisciplinary pain management strategy [6, 16].
14. **C**. Some known biopsychosocial risk factors associated with substance use disorder include age < 25 years of age, income level at or below the poverty level, concurrent psychiatric disorders, trauma history (e.g., childhood or adult sexual abuse and domestic or interpersonal violence), polysubstance use (e.g., tobacco, marijuana, alcohol), and family history of substance use disorder [17].
15. **D.** As legalization and medical use of marijuana increases, so has the normalization of its use for relieving stress/anxiety (**A**), nausea and vomiting (**B**), and acute and chronic pain (**C**), among others [18].
16. **C.** It is estimated that 50% of patients who smoke tobacco will quit smoking during pregnancy. Approximately one-third (**B**) of these will resume smoking immediately postpartum and 90% (**D**) by 1 year postpartum [3, 19].
17. **A**. Cocaine-induced thrombocytopenia leading to prolonged bleeding has been reported; hence, a complete blood count is recommended before performing neuraxial anesthesia. On the other hand, prothrombotic effects (**B**) have also

been attributed to this drug, unless abruption is suspected. In cases where placental abruption is suspected, both a coagulation panel (**B**) and obtaining plasma fibrinogen levels (**C**) are recommended. Although unlikely to affect our ability to perform a neuraxial blockade, in pregnant ewes, the use of cocaine has been demonstrated to increase maternal and fetal plasma glucose (**D**) [20].

18. **A**. Methadone may lead to a prolonged QT interval, especially with increasing doses. Patients with a prolonged QT interval may be at risk for torsades de pointes and sudden cardiac death. An electrocardiogram would identify patients with a prolonged QT interval prior to administration of medications during labor and cesarean delivery. Common medications administered during anesthesia care may further prolong the QT interval and include ondansetron, volatile anesthetics, succinylcholine, nicardipine, glycopyrrolate, atropine, neostigmine, droperidol, albuterol, ephedrine, and phenylephrine. Medications commonly used in obstetric practice that may prolong the QT interval include azithromycin and terbutaline [21].
19. **B**. A recent study using death certificate records and ICD-10 codes from 33 states and the District of Columbia analyzed the prevalence of drug-related maternal deaths in the United States between 2010 and 2019. Drug-related (11.4%), suicide (5.4%), and homicide (5.4%) deaths accounted for approximately one in five deaths in pregnancy and the first year postpartum. Over the study period, the pregnancy-associated death ratio due to drug-related maternal deaths increased by 190% from 2.7 per 100,000 in 2010 to 7.8 per 100,000 in 2019. Non-Hispanic American Indians and Alaskan Natives are at highest risk for drug-related maternal death. Approximately one-third (34.3%) of drug-related maternal deaths occurred within pregnancy, with 19.2% within the first 42 days postpartum and 46.4% between postpartum days 43 and 365 [22].
20. **D**. It is estimated that 0.36–2.2% of opioid-naïve patients will become persistent opioid users following cesarean delivery. Risk factors associated with persistent opioid use include history of cocaine abuse (aOR 6.11), other illicit substance abuse (aOR 2.78), tobacco use (aOR 3.04), back pain (aOR 1.74), migraine headaches (aOR 2.14), antidepressant use (aOR 3.19), and benzodiazepine use (aOR 3.72) within the year prior to delivery. Nonelective cesarean section and repeat cesarean section were not identified as risk factors for persistent opioid use after cesarean delivery. Daily postoperative opioid consumption in all women with high inpatient opioid use postoperatively was similar for patients with scheduled versus unscheduled cesarean delivery [23–25].
21. **A**. The American College of Obstetricians and Gynecologists recommends universal screening of opioid use for all pregnant patients at the first prenatal visit. Selective screening based on specific factors such as poor adherence to prenatal care may lead to missed cases, stereotyping, and stigma. Obstetricians should also screen patients in the postpartum period, as it represents a vulnerable time for return to substance use. Screening tools for substance use in pregnancy include the 5A's for nicotine/tobacco, nonjudgmental screening for alcohol followed by AUDIT-C or T-ACE for positive results, and the 4P's Plus or 5P's and

NIDA Quick Screen followed by ASSIST, SURP-P, CRAFFT, and WIDUS for cannabis, opioids, amphetamines, cocaine, and benzodiazepines [3, 26, 27].

22. **D**. The 2021 SAMHSA National Survey on Drug Use and Health revealed that 7.2% of pregnant patients used marijuana within the past month. [SAMHSA] Cannabinoid receptors are present on maternal, placental, and fetal tissues and can impact maternal and fetal outcomes. Cannabinoid receptor 1 (CB1) agonism leads to sympathetic activation and parasympathetic inhibition, resulting in elevated norepinephrine plasma levels and systolic blood pressure, tachycardia, and increased cardiac output for 1–2 hours after use [28, 29].
23. **C**. Opioid agonist therapy is strongly recommended for pregnant patients with opioid use disorder. In a recent cohort study of more than 2.5 million pregnant patients with public insurance receiving either buprenorphine or methadone for opioid agonist therapy between 2000 and 2018, the risk of neonatal abstinence syndrome for patients who received buprenorphine within 30 days of delivery was lower than that for patients who received methadone (aRR 0.73) in the same time period. In patients with early exposure (0 through 19 weeks' gestation) and late exposure (20 weeks' gestation through delivery) to methadone or buprenorphine, neonatal outcomes in patients exposed to buprenorphine in both time periods included lower rates of preterm birth (aRR 0.58, 0.57), small size for gestational age (aRR 0.72, 0.75), and low birth weight (aRR 0.56, 0.56). There were no differences in the cesarean delivery rate or severe maternal complications between pregnant patients who received methadone and those who received buprenorphine in both early- and late-exposure populations [7].
24. **B**. Cannabinoids (Δ9-tetrahydrocannabinol (THC), cannabidiol (CBD), and other components of marijuana) readily cross the placenta and impact fetal neurodevelopment. Cannabinoid receptor 1 (CB1) is present in the fetal central nervous system at 14 weeks' gestation and increases with increasing gestational age. Exposure to cannabinoids in early pregnancy is associated with decreased problem-solving, visual-motor coordination, visual analysis, and attention span and behavior problems in early childhood. In adolescence and young adulthood, prenatal exposure to cannabis has been associated with psychopathology, sleep problems, lower cognition, and lower gray matter volume, leading to long-term concerns regarding neurodevelopment after prenatal cannabis exposure [28].
25. **A**. The use of synthetic cannabinoids may mimic preeclampsia, cerebral ischemia, and posterior reversible encephalopathy syndrome (PRES). There is no evidence that the use of cannabinoids increases the risk for preeclampsia. Cannabinoid use may be associated with postoperative hypothermia and shivering. Acute cannabinoid use may lower opioid analgesic requirements, while chronic cannabinoid use may increase opioid analgesic requirements. Cannabinoids cross into breast milk and may last for long periods of time in breast milk [28].

References

1. American Psychiatric Association. Chapter: substance related and addictive disorders, In: Diagnostic and statistical manual of mental disorders, 5th edition, Text Revision (DSM-5-TR). American Psychiatric Association Publishing; 2022.
2. Wright A, Walker J. Management of women who use drugs during pregnancy. Semin Fetal Neonatal Med. 2007;12(2):114–8.
3. Smid MC, Terplan M. What obstetrician–gynecologists should know about substance use disorders in the perinatal period. Obstet Gynecol. 2022;139(2):317–37.
4. Lumley J, Chamberlain C, Dowswell T, Oliver S, Oakley L, Watson L. Interventions for promoting smoking cessation during pregnancy. Cochrane Database Syst Rev. 2009;(3):CD001055.
5. Claire R, Chamberlain C, Davey M, Cooper SE, Berlin I, Leonardi-Bee J, et al. Pharmacological interventions for promoting smoking cessation during pregnancy. Cochrane Database Syst Rev. 2020;2020(3):CD010078.
6. Lim G, Soens M, Wanaselja A, Chyan A, Carvalho B, Landau R, et al. A systematic scoping review of peridelivery pain management for pregnant people with opioid use disorder: from the Society for Obstetric Anesthesia and Perinatology and Society for Maternal Fetal Medicine. Anesth Analg. 2022;135(5):912–25.
7. Suarez EA, Huybrechts KF, Straub L, Hernández-Díaz S, Jones HE, Connery HS, et al. Buprenorphine versus methadone for opioid use disorder in pregnancy. N Engl J Med. 2022;387(22):2033–44.
8. Gao YA, Drake C, Krans EE, Chen Q, Jarlenski MP. Explaining racial-ethnic disparities in the receipt of medication for opioid use disorder during pregnancy. J Addict Med. 2022;16(6):e356–65.
9. Bada HS, Das A, Bauer CR, Shankaran S, Lester BM, Gard CC, et al. Low birth weight and preterm births: etiologic fraction attributable to prenatal drug exposure. J Perinatol. 2005;25(10):631–7.
10. Kuczkowski KM. Anesthetic implications of drug abuse in pregnancy. J Clin Anesth. 2003;15(5):382–94.
11. Terplan M, Smith EJ, Kozloski MJ, Pollack HA. Methamphetamine use among pregnant women. Obstet Gynecol. 2009;113(6):1285–91.
12. Committee Opinion No. 479. Methamphetamine abuse in women of reproductive age. Obstet Gynecol. 2011;117(3):751–5.
13. Bateman BT, Cole NM, Maeda A, Burns SM, Houle TT, Huybrechts KF, et al. Patterns of opioid prescription and use after cesarean delivery. Obstet Gynecol. 2017;130(1):29–35.
14. Dworkin RH, Turk DC, Revicki DA, Harding G, Coyne KS, Peirce-Sandner S, et al. Development and initial validation of an expanded and revised version of the short-form McGill pain questionnaire (SF-MPQ-2). Pain. 2009;144(1–2):35–42.
15. Vilkins AL, Bagley SM, Hahn KA, Rojas-Miguez F, Wachman EM, Saia K, et al. Comparison of post-cesarean section opioid analgesic requirements in women with opioid use disorder treated with methadone or buprenorphine. J Addict Med. 2017;11(5):397–401.
16. Landau R. Post Cesarean Delivery Pain. Management of the opioid-dependent patient before, during and after cesarean delivery. Int J Obstet Anesth. 2019;39(Pediatrics 2017):105–16.
17. Cook JL, Green CR, de la Ronde S, Dell CA, Graves L, Ordean A, et al. Epidemiology and effects of substance use in pregnancy. J Obstet Gynecol Can. 2017;39(10):906–15.
18. Layoun V, Ohnona A, Tolosa JE. Pregnancy outcomes associated with use of tobacco and marijuana. Clin Obstet Gynecol. 2022;65(2):376–87.
19. Hawkins SS, Hacker MR. Trends in use of conventional cigarettes, E-cigarettes, and marijuana in pregnancy and impact of health policy. Clin Obstet Gynecol. 2022;65(2):305–18.
20. Kain ZN, Rimar S, Barash PG. Cocaine abuse in the parturient and effects on the fetus and neonate. Anesth Analg. 1993;77(4):835.
21. Kies SJ, Pabelick CM, Hurley HA, et al. Anesthesia for patients with congenital long QT syndrome. Anesthesiology. 2005;50(3):161–2.

22. Margerison CE, Roberts MH, Gemmill A, Goldman-Mellor S. Pregnancy-associated deaths due to drugs, suicide, and homicide in the United States, 2010–2019. Obstet Gynecol. 2022;139(2):172–80.
23. Peahl AF, Dalton VK, Montgomery JR, Lai YL, Hu HM, Waljee JF. Rates of new persistent opioid use after vaginal or cesarean birth among US women. JAMA Netw Open. 2019;2(7):e197863.
24. Prabhu M, Dolisca S, Wood R, James K, Bateman BT, Barth WH, et al. Postoperative opioid consumption after scheduled compared with unscheduled cesarean delivery. Obstet Gynecol. 2019;133(2):354–63.
25. Bateman BT, Franklin JM, Bykov K, Avorn J, Shrank WH, Brennan TA, et al. Persistent opioid use following cesarean delivery: patterns and predictors among opioid-naïve women. Am J Obstet Gynecol. 2016;215(3):353.e1–353.e18.
26. Committee Opinion No. 711. Obstet Gynecol. 2017;130(2):e81–94.
27. The American College of Obstetricians and Gynecologists. Statements of policy: opposition to criminalization of individuals during pregnancy and the postpartum period. Approved by the Board of Directors, December 2020. https://www.acog.org/clinical-information/policy-and-position-statements/statements-of-policy/2020/opposition-criminalization-of-individuals-pregnancy-and-postpartum-period.
28. Shah S, Schwenk ES, Sondekoppam RV, Clarke H, Zakowski M, Rzasa-Lynn RS, et al. ASRA pain medicine consensus guidelines on the management of the perioperative patient on cannabis and cannabinoids. Reg Anesth Pain Med. 2023;48(3):97–117.
29. SAMHSA. Center for Behavioral Health Statistics and Quality, National Survey on Drug Use and Health. 2021. https://www.samhsa.gov/data/report/2021-nsduh-detailed-tables. Accessed 20 Feb 2023.

Neonatal Physiology

Sumana Mahata, Joshua Vasquez, and Ioana F. Pasca

Questions

1. **What is one anatomic consideration to be aware of in neonates during airway management?**
   A. Obligate mouth breathers
   B. Decreased percentage of fat and muscles
   C. Relatively shorter epiglottis
   D. Proportionately smaller head
2. **Upon delivery, neonates have the greatest heat loss through which mechanism?**
   A. Conduction
   B. Radiation
   C. Brown fat metabolism
   D. Evaporation
3. **Which of the following is a characteristic of neonatal respiratory physiology that is important to consider during perioperative management?**
   A. Lower functional residual capacity (FRC)

S. Mahata
Riverside University Health System, Moreno Valley, CA, USA

J. Vasquez
Western University of Health Sciences College of Osteopathic Medicine of the Pacific, Pomona, CA, USA

I. F. Pasca (✉)
Riverside University Health System, Moreno Valley, CA, USA

Department of Anesthesiology, Critical Care, and Neurocritical Care, Loma Linda University at Riverside University Health System, Loma Linda, CA, USA

University of California San Diego, San Diego, CA, USA

University of California Riverside, Riverside, CA, USA
e-mail: i.pasca@ruhealth.org

A. C. Sinha, I. F. Pasca (eds.), *Peripartum Care of the Pregnant Patient*,
https://doi.org/10.1007/978-3-031-62756-9_41

B. Mature central control of ventilation
C. Lower rate of oxygen consumption
D. Slower induction and recovery from inhaled anesthetics

4. **In premature neonates, which of the following is true regarding their respiratory development?**
A. Surfactant production by type II pneumocytes begins at 30 weeks' gestation
B. Closing pressure of neonatal airways is low
C. Most alveoli are formed before birth
D. Anatomic dead space is 2 mL/kg

5. **Which would *not* be a concern with excess oxygenation in neonates?**
A. Bronchopulmonary dysplasia
B. Retinopathy of prematurity
C. Brain injury
D. Decreased DNA damage

6. **Another anatomical difference to consider with regard to neonatal respiratory function includes:**
A. Outward movement of rib cage during inspiration
B. Low cartilage content in the ribs
C. Ineffective accessory muscles due to horizontal rib angles
D. Decreased chest wall compliance

7. **A 5-day-old neonate, born at 39 weeks, under anesthesia has an increase in pulmonary vascular resistance and a re-opening of transitional circulation shunts, leading to persistent pulmonary hypertension of the neonate. Which of the following circumstances may have contributed to this patient's disease?**
A. Hypercarbia
B. Alkalosis
C. Hyperoxia
D. Hyperthermia

8. **The shape of the heart is complete by 6 weeks' gestation, but the myofibrillar density and maturation increase through the first year of postnatal life. This leads to the neonatal myocardium contracting less efficiently and increases the dependence on what factor to maintain cardiac output?**
A. Increased myocardial compliance
B. Vagal stimulation
C. Increase in heart rate
D. Hypoxia

9. **For what reason is it clinically relevant to be aware that the parasympathetic nervous system is predominant during the neonatal period?**
A. Postural changes can affect the heart rate
B. Marked bradycardia or asystole during laryngoscopy
C. Increased baroreceptor reflex
D. High cardiac stores of norepinephrine

10. **When considering resuscitation in neonatal hemorrhage, which of the following is appropriate in management of blood loss?**

A. Do not initiate treatment with colloid or crystalloid solution
B. Transfuse RBCs immediately after fluid initiation
C. Allowable blood loss = [estimated blood volume × (initial Hgb − lowest tolerated Hgb)]/initial Hgb
D. Disregard the surgical field when considering blood loss

11. **Which of the following characteristics of neonatal hemoglobin is different from that of adult hemoglobin?**
A. Lower hemoglobin values
B. Rightward shift of the oxyhemoglobin dissociation curve
C. Decreased concentration of 2,3-diphosphoglycerate (2,3-DPG)
D. The P50 of HgF is lower than adult Hgb

12. **Which of the following is true regarding the metabolism of pharmacologic drugs and protein binding of drugs in neonates?**
A. Lower concentration of serum protein
B. Hepatic metabolism of drugs approximates 30% of adult values at birth in a full-term neonate
C. Decreased concentration of free drugs
D. Higher serum albumin concentration

13. **A 15-day-old neonate, born at 39 weeks 3 days, is to undergo a procedure under anesthesia. When considering the neonate's immature liver development, which of the following would be appropriate for glucose management?**
A. 5–6 mg/kg/min glucose
B. Stopping TPN/PPN infusions
C. Running NS for maintenance
D. 3–5 mg/kg/min glucose

14. **When preparing a neonatal patient for induction, you prepare a larger initial dose of succinylcholine than you would for an adult patient. What characteristic of neonatal physiology is the reason for the higher initial dose?**
A. Lower percentage of total body water
B. Increased volume of distribution (Vd)
C. Higher serum blood level needed to achieve similar effects
D. Medications must be administered quickly to have an effect

15. **What is *not* a possible complication that neonates are susceptible to, given their renal physiology?**
A. Excessive sodium excretion
B. Hyperuricemia
C. Impaired response to acid-base changes
D. Aminoglycoside toxicity

16. **When conducting a neonatal preoperative evaluation, which of the following is *not* correct when gathering information and labs?**
A. Ask about cardiac congenital abnormalities
B. Check for micrognathia
C. Order BMP at a minimum
D. Ensuring fasting is >4 h for breast milk

17. **You are positioning a neonate before they are to undergo a procedure. What is important to consider when positioning this patient?**
    A. Neonates have soft and flexible skulls
    B. Using a gel headrest is critical
    C. Lines or tubing should not be padded
    D. The manner of draping is less important
18. **A 1.5 kg neonate comes in for a procedure. When considering airway management for this patient, which of the following is correct?**
    A. Intubation with a cuffed 2.5 ETT
    B. Ensuring there is no air leak when PPV is applied
    C. Intubation with a 3.0 uncuffed ETT
    D. Ensuring an air leak when 5–10 cm H_2O of pressure is applied
19. **You are determining your perioperative plan for a term neonate and are deciding what fluids to give the patient in the OR. What is correct in terms of selecting fluids?**
    A. Avoid glucose-containing fluids
    B. Give LR
    C. Give NS
    D. A fluid bolus cannot be delivered through saline flushes
20. **Which of the following is true regarding neonatal anesthesia induction with inhaled gases?**
    A. Smaller alveolar ventilation (VA) to FRC ratio
    B. Increased tissue/blood solubility and blood/gas solubility
    C. Prematurity increases MAC
    D. FA/FI increases more rapidly

Answers and Explanations

1. **B.** Compared to older children and adults, neonates have a lower percentage of fat and muscle [1]. In neonates, medications whose clinical effects are terminated by redistribution to these tissues may last longer [1]. For example, redistribution is necessary for waking following a single dose of propofol [1]. In addition, anatomical airway differences between adults/older children and neonates include proportionately larger head and tongue (**D**), narrower nasal passages, an anterior and cephalad larynx, a relatively longer, omega-shaped, epiglottis (**C**), and a shorter trachea and neck as shown in Fig. 1 [2, 3]. Nasal breathing is dominant in neonates because of these anatomical differences (**A**) [1]. Due to these differences, a neonate may be easier to intubate in a neutral or slightly flexed position as opposed to a sniffing position [3].
2. **D.** Because newborns have a greater surface area to weight ratio and a relatively thin layer of adipose tissue, they are more likely to experience thermal loss than adults when exposed to cold temperatures through radiation, evaporation, conduction, and convection. The greatest heat loss is from evaporation, necessitating rapid neonatal drying after delivery (**D**) [1, 2]. Neonates are not

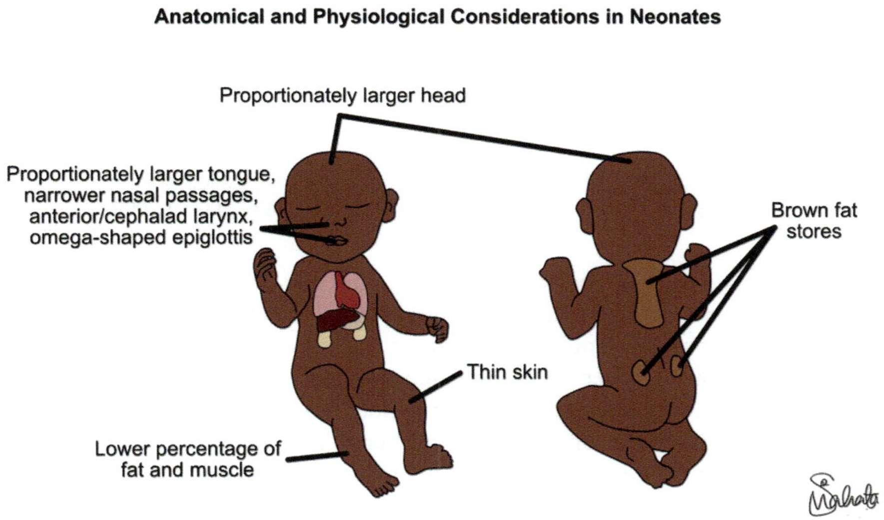

Fig. 1 Anatomic and physiologic differences between neonates and adults [2, 3]

able to shiver (**B**), and therefore rely on non-shivering thermogenesis to generate heat through the metabolism of brown fat [1]. Brown fat in neonates is located in the posterior neck along the interscapular and vertebral regions [2]. Thermoregulatory vasoconstriction can also limit heat loss (**A**) [1]. Techniques such as warming of the operating room and using radiant warmers to warm IV fluids, humidifying the airways, and forced air warming can also help keep newborns normothermic [1]. Underbody forced air warmers and warming lights are frequently used as well as hats if the head is not in the surgical field [1]. In addition, all fluids should be warmed. Hypothermia can lead to acidosis, myocardial depression, and delayed recovery from anesthesia [2]. Therefore, it should be ensured that no dramatic temperature changes occur in the neonate.

3. **A.** Neonates have an immature hypoxic response and lower FRC which limits oxygen reserves during the period of apnea and leads to rapid desaturation in a prolonged intubation attempt (**A**) [2]. The neonatal central control of ventilation is not completely developed (**B**) [2]. Peripheral feedback mechanisms are immature, and the neonatal oxygen consumption rate is 6 cc/kg per minute, which is twice the rate of a resting adult (**C**) [2]. A more rapid rise in FA/FI (fractional alveolar concentration/fractional inhaled concentrations) leads to a more rapid induction and recovery from inhaled anesthetics, and increased MAC (**D**) [2]. Several age-dependent respiratory variables, along with their normal values, are summarized in Table 1 [2].
4. **B.** Neonates have a high rate of desaturation and take a long time to recover after a desaturation episode, making them more prone to hypoxia during intubation [3]. Due to the very low closing pressure of the newborn's airways, alveolar closure occurs rapidly with a loss of ventilation which makes it difficult for the

Table 1 Range of age-dependent respiratory variables

Variable	Neonate	Adult
Respiratory rate (breaths/minute)	50 ± 10	12 ± 3
Tidal volume (mL)	16.5–26.4	400–500
Minute ventilation (mL/min)	66–99	5000–8000
Vital capacity (mL)	112–116	3000–5000
Functional residual capacity (L)	96–99	2000–4000
Total lung capacity (L)	203–210	4000–11,000

alveoli to reopen [3]. Therefore, video laryngoscopy may be an appropriate first choice. Anatomic dead space in neonates is >3 mL/kg (**D**) [4]. A lung-protective ventilation strategy should be used in neonates because newborns' lungs are structurally and biochemically immature and are thus prone to injury with positive pressure ventilation [4]. For these reasons, it is recommended to use PEEP to prevent atelectasis and to use a smaller tidal volume [4]. Neonates born before 34 weeks are at risk for apnea of prematurity, and if they are born before 28 weeks, the apnea can last past term [4]. Chronic apnea and intermittent hypoxemia can cause free radical formation, which can lead to long-term adverse health issues [4]. Although alveolar formation begins by the 36th post-conceptual week, most alveoli are formed postnatally (**C**) [1]. Around the 24th week gestation, type II pneumocytes start producing surfactant (**A**) [1]. This phospholipid-surfactant protein synthesis is essential for surface tension reduction and facilitating alveoli inflation [1]. However, alveolar maturation is incomplete in neonates and can take up to 8–10 years to mature [3].

5. **D.** Normally, fetal development takes place in a hypoxic environment in utero; therefore the transition to room air during birth poses a significant oxidative stress to the premature neonate [4]. Unfortunately, the shift from the womb's hypoxic environment to the extrauterine environment's relatively hyperoxic environment happens at a time when the extrauterine area is already sensitive to oxidative stressors [4]. Excess oxygen is harmful to neonates and can cause retinopathy of prematurity (**B**), bronchopulmonary dysplasia (**A**), brain injury (**C**), and DNA damage that can lead to cancer (**D**) [4]. One study showed no difference in mortality or BPD, ROP, or neurodevelopmental differences between a restrictive (spO_2 85–89%) and liberal (91–95%) oxygen group [4]. Therefore, there are currently no set guidelines of what the ideal oxygen saturation should be.
6. **C.** The ribs extend horizontally from the vertebral column in neonates, as opposed to caudally in adults [1]. Because of this, the accessory muscles for respiration are not effective in neonates [1]. Due to the high cartilage in the ribs of neonates (**B**), the rib cage tends to protrude inward during inspiration (**A**) [1]. Paradoxical chest wall movement is a common side effect of general anesthesia. This is caused by reduced intercostal muscle tone and upper airway obstruction [1]. Under general anesthesia, the diaphragm works harder to keep up with tidal volume, which can result in fatigue. During childhood and adolescence, the compliance of the chest wall decreases due to rib ossification and increases

in thoracic muscle mass (**D**) [1]. During this period, the elastic recoil pressure in the lung increases due to the growth of pulmonary elastic fibers [1].

7. **A.** The neonatal period is characterized by several changes to the cardiovascular system. Neonatal circulation is dynamic, transitioning into series circulation with spontaneous respiration and reduction of pulmonary vascular resistance as shown in Fig. 2 [2, 4]. This results in a rise in systemic vascular resistance and left atrial pressure. The dynamic circulation can revert to parallel fetal circulation at any point in time [4]. Neonatal pulmonary circulation is sensitive to hypoxia (**C**), hypercarbia, asphyxia, acidosis (**B**), hypothermia (**D**), hypo- or hyperglycemia, hypocalcemia, and sepsis after the first week of birth [4]. All these factors can lead to an elevation of pulmonary vascular resistance and a decrease in pulmonary blood flow, resulting in a reversal of fetal circulation [4]. Monitoring pre-ductal oxygen saturation on the right hand and post-ductal oxygen saturation on either leg may help detect a return to transitional circulation if pre-ductal oxygen saturation is higher than post-ductal oxygen saturation [4]. Pulmonary hypertension is one of the leading causes of neonatal anesthesia-related morbidity and mortality [4]. Adequate respiratory control and right ventricular dysfunction must be addressed to prevent long-term pulmonary hypertension in neonates [4].
8. **C.** At 6 weeks of gestation, the shape of the heart is fully developed [5]. During the first year of life, however, the density and maturation of myofibrils increase, resulting in an increase in the rate of protein synthesis and accelerated cell growth [5]. These processes necessitate an increase in intracellular concentrations of nuclei, mitochondria, and endoplasmic reticulum [5]. These changes lead to the neonatal myocardium being less compliant (**A**) and it contracts less efficiently than adult myocardium [2, 5]. Reduced ventricular compliance means that even small changes in final diastolic volumes result in large changes in total final diastolic pressures. The Frank-Starling mechanism to increase

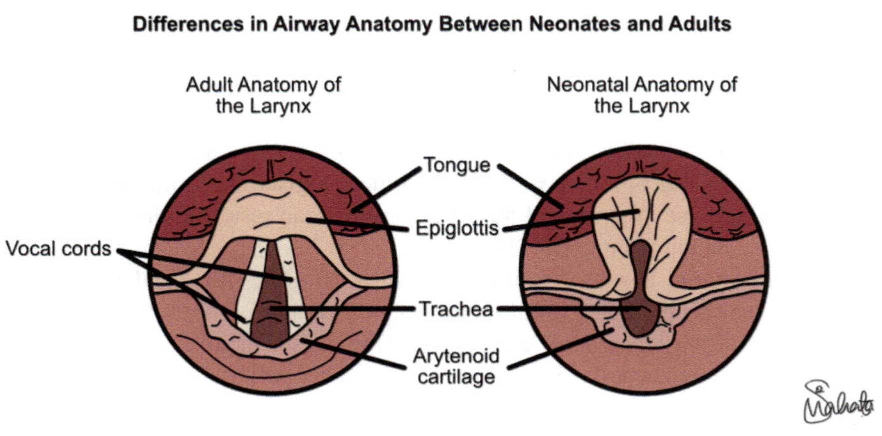

Fig. 2 Normal physiologic changes in neonatal circulation [4]

stroke volume is less efficient; therefore newborns are heart rate dependent for cardiac output [5]. Due to this decreased compliance, normal ranges for neonatal HR are 120–160 and SBP is 60–75 [1, 5]. The parasympathetic system is predominant in neonates; therefore vagal stimulus (**B**) by laryngoscopy and hypoxia (**D**) can cause bradycardia, so it needs to be treated aggressively when it occurs [1, 2].

9. **B.** In the early stages of life, the parasympathetic is the dominant nervous system, while the sympathetic is still developing. Adrenergic innervation of the human myocardium completes between 18 and 28 weeks' gestation [1, 5]. This imbalance is clinically significant and can be seen as marked bradycardia or even asystole during laryngoscopy, orogastric tube placement, or tracheal suctioning in the neonate [1]. Before airway instrumentation, many anesthesia providers will pretreat with anticholinergics such as atropine or glycopyrrolate [1]. As the fetal heart has low catecholamine stores (**D**) and is more sensitive to external norepinephrine, adrenergic reactions are present but reduced in neonates. In addition, the baroreceptor reflex is present but incompletely developed (**C**) [5]. Of note, postural changes do not change the heart rate in preterm infants (**A**) [5]. However, the chemoreceptor response is well-developed, and it is thought that the neonatal response to hypoxia is mediated through the chemoreceptor system [5].
10. **C.** Neonatal total blood volume ranges from 82 to 93 mL/kg for the term newborn to 90 to 105 mL/kg for the preterm newborn [1]. Blood volume then declines to approximately 70–80 mL/kg throughout the first year of life [1]. Crystalloid or colloid solutions are first choice treatment for blood loss to maintain adequate intravascular volume (**A**) [1]. Red blood cells should be transfused when the hematocrit (Hct) has reached the minimum acceptable Hct (**B**) [1]. The patient's age and coexisting conditions will determine the minimum acceptable Hct. For example, a higher Hct (30–45%) is desired in patients with congenital heart disease, significant pulmonary disease, and infants with apnea and bradycardia, or tachypnea and tachycardia [1]. Neonatal vasoconstriction is also less responsive to hemorrhage. A 10% decrease in blood volume can result in a 15% to 30% reduction in MAP, leading to less tolerance for blood loss and a decreased compensatory response to hemorrhage [1]. Neonatal blood volume is 90 mL/kg and preterm neonatal blood volume is 100 mL/kg [1]. For these patients, allowable blood loss = [estimated blood volume × (initial Hgb − lowest tolerated Hgb)]/initial Hgb [1]. Anesthesiologists watch the surgical field closely because even around 50–75 mL of loss can result in a loss of 20% of their circulating volume (**D**) [1].
11. **D.** The normal newborn hemoglobin is 14–20 g/dL (**A**). Fetal hemoglobin (HgF) makes up 70–80% of the hemoglobin at birth. HgF binds to oxygen with a higher affinity than adult hemoglobin. HgF causes the dissociation curve of oxyhemoglobin to shift to the left due to its higher affinity for oxygen [1]. HgF P50 is 18–20 mm Hg, and adult hemoglobin P50 is 27 mm Hg [1]. The difference in P50 between these two hemoglobin types facilitates the absorption of oxygen by the fetus at the placenta. The physiological nadir of hemoglobin is

9–12 weeks postpartum and is 10–11 g/dL in term infants where HgF is replaced by adult hemoglobin [1]. Once adult hemoglobin is generated, the decreased hemoglobin values do not affect oxygen delivery to tissues because the oxyhemoglobin dissociation curve begins shifting to the right (**B**) [1]. This rightward shift of the curve is due to an increase in 2,3-diphosphoglycerate (2,3-DPG) (**C**) and the replacement of HgF by adult hemoglobin (at approximately 2–3 months of age), which facilitates the unloading of oxygen in the tissues [1]. At approximately the age of 2, the hemoglobin concentration stabilizes at 11.5–12 g/dL. During puberty, the value gradually rises to adult values [1]. At birth, levels of the vitamin K-dependent coagulation factors II, VII, IX, and X range from 20% to 60% of adult levels [1]. A longer prothrombin time could be the outcome of this lower level. It may take many weeks for these components to return to normal levels because of the immature liver [1]. All newborns receive prophylactic intramuscular (IM) vitamin K. Additionally, a lack of vitamin K in the infant might be brought on by the mother taking certain medications, such as anticonvulsants and warfarin [1].

12. **A.** The metabolism of carbohydrates, proteins, and lipids and coagulation are all critically dependent on the liver [2]. However, the rates of hepatic oxidation, reduction, and hydrolysis function do not reach adult rates until 6 months. Due to the incomplete development of the degradation pathway, newborns may metabolize toxins and medications less efficiently [2]. This includes anesthetic medications. Protein binding is altered in newborns because they have lower levels of total serum protein, albumin, and alpha-1 acid glycoprotein (which reaches adult levels at about 1 year old) (**D**) [1, 2]. Substances that are lipid-soluble and pharmacologically active are converted by hepatic metabolism into typically inactive, nonlipid-soluble substances for excretion [1]. In neonates, blood flow to the liver is decreased, as is the activity of the majority of hepatic enzymes [1]. The hepatic metabolism of medications in a full-term neonate is around 50% of adult values (**B**) and increases quickly during the first month of life to close to adult values, with full development by 1–2 years of age [1]. Protein binding of drugs is also different between infants and adults. A part of this variation can be attributed to younger children's lower blood protein/albumin levels [1]. Additionally, compared to adults, neonates have a decreased affinity for protein-bound medicines in serum proteins [1]. Reduced protein binding causes an increase in the concentration of free drug (**C**), which increases the drug effect [1]. When it comes to highly protein-bound medications like phenytoin, bupivacaine, barbiturates, and diazepam, the impact of reduced protein binding is most apparent [1].
13. **D.** Glycogenolysis and gluconeogenesis may be impaired in newborns and preterm infants. Neonates are vulnerable to hypoglycemia even after brief periods of fasting because of their low glycogen stores [3]. Preterm neonates have an even greater risk for hypoglycemia. To sustain euglycemia, term newborns need 3–5 mg/kg/min of glucose, while preterm neonates need 5–6 mg/kg/min (**A**) of glucose [3]. D10 water and D10 0.2% NaCl are common choices for IV fluids in neonates (**C**) [3]. If administered during the preoperative period, TPN and

PPN, both glucose-containing solutions, should be continued intraoperatively [3]. Acute hypoglycemia can occur if TPN/PPN infusions are stopped (**B**) [3]. During anesthesia for all infants younger than 6 months old, D5 LR at maintenance rates can be run since isotonic fluids are preferred intraoperatively [3].

14. **B.** Neonates have a different distribution of total body fluid components than adults. The intracellular and extracellular fluid compartments in neonates account for roughly 45 and 33% of the total body weight, respectively [2]. Pharmacokinetics are also impacted by differences in body composition. Compared to older children and adults, preterm and term neonates have a higher percentage of total body water (**A**) [1, 2]. The volume of distribution is increased as a result. When the Vd is increased, a larger initial dose of medication is required to achieve the same therapeutic serum level and pharmacologic effect [1]. Digoxin, succinylcholine, and antibiotics all need higher starting doses in neonates [1]. Fentanyl is another important example of an anesthetic medication for neonates that requires higher first dosages [1]. Additionally, infants and neonates may be more susceptible to the side effects of some medications and require lower serum blood levels to have the same effects (**C**) [1]. The dosage of medications should be given gradually and titrated to achieve the desired effects (**D**) [1].
15. **B.** Acid-base homeostasis and fluid electrolyte balance are maintained by the kidneys. Age-dependent increases in GFR and reabsorption require 6–12 months to reach adult values [2]. After birth, the placenta is replaced by the kidneys in the maintenance of metabolic homeostasis [1]. At birth, the glomerular filtration rate (GFR) ranges from 15% to 30% of adult values and rises to 50% between days 5 and 10. At 1 year of age, adult values are reached [1]. The neonate's ability to excrete salt, water loads, and several medicines is impacted by the low GFR (**A**) [1]. After 34 weeks of pregnancy, the tubular system begins to function. The kidney's ability to fully reabsorb bicarbonate has a lower threshold since the tubules are still developing. This is associated with the young infants' incapacity to respond to an acid load and the slightly decreased values of plasma bicarbonate (22 mEq/L) and pH (7.37) (**C**) [1]. Additionally, infants' concentration ability is decreased, and their urea synthesis and excretion are low. Because less urea is being produced, blood urea nitrogen (BUN) stays within normal range (**B**) [1]. If renal function is normal, creatinine soon after birth equals the maternal value and drops to levels of 0.5 mEq/L or less within the first 48 h [1]. The kidneys of neonates become more efficient with time. Drugs that need the kidney for excretion, such as aminoglycosides, have delayed elimination half-times in newborns due to underdeveloped glomerular and tubular activity [1]. At 20 weeks, glomerular and tubular function is almost entirely developed, and at 2 years, it is completely developed [1].
16. **C.** Labs to order for a neonatal preoperative evaluation include the following: Hgb at minimum, BMP to check for electrolytes, CBC, and clotting factors [2]. It is also prudent to ask about perinatal history (prematurity, apnea, hypoxic episode history, how long they needed oxygen, neurological damage), congenital anomalies, and any lung disease or cardiac pathology (**A**) [2]. Anatomically,

factors like micrognathia, restricted neck movement, and macroglossia might cause a difficult airway (**B**) [2]. During the cardiorespiratory exam, the focus should be on breathing sounds, any new murmurs, and cardiac congenital defects. Necrotizing enterocolitis, hyaline membrane syndrome, cardiac pathologies, sepsis, and neuromuscular conditions are examples of concurrent disorders that can increase anesthetic risk [2]. To evaluate physical status, height, weight, and head circumference can be assessed. Some genetic abnormalities that have consequences for anesthesia are linked to microcephaly [2]. Acceptable NPO time is 2 h for clear liquids, 4 h for breast milk, and 6 h for formula/non-human milk (**D**) [2]. Fasting increases the risk of hypoglycemia and dehydration in neonates, especially since they feed more often. Thus dextrose-containing maintenance fluids can be started perioperatively [2].

17. **A.** Neonates can conform to the shape of whatever surface they are on because they have soft, flexible heads, thin skin, and relatively little fat storage [3]. Gel headrests may result in hair loss and pressure necrosis (**B**) [3]. Neonates are prone to red marks and pressure injuries, so all lines, monitors, and tubing should be appropriately padded (**C**) [3]. Once draped, any adjustment may interrupt surgical colleagues (**D**); therefore communication is critical [3]. It is important to know where all lines and monitors are placed just in case management intraoperatively requires access.
18. **C.** With respect to intubation, generally neonates who weigh more than 1 kg should receive a 3.0 uncuffed ETT, and neonates who weigh less than 1 kg should receive a 2.5 uncuffed ETT (**A**) [5]. The correct size ETT should have a slight air leak when a positive pressure of 20–30 cm H_2O is applied (**B, D**) [5]. Using excessively large ETTs has the potential to cause serious, lifelong laryngeal and subglottic damage, especially in children with inflammatory lesions of the upper airway such as laryngotracheobronchitis [5]. Uncuffed ETTs typically create a sufficient seal in children under the age of 5 due to the more malleable tracheal cartilage and relative subglottic constriction [5]. However, a cuffed tube is preferable if the patient has lung illness that necessitates higher ventilation pressure. Younger patients are typically fitted with small cuffed ETTs in the ICU; however it is important to make sure that there is a small air leak at 25–30 cm H_2O [5]. Cuffed tubes will typically stop the air leak surrounding an ETT, but overinflating the cuff could obstruct venous flow and injure the airway [5].
19. **B.** In order to prevent hyponatremia and anomalies in serum potassium values, the preferred fluid in the OR should be isotonic [1]. The two most popular isotonic solutions for pediatric patients are lactated Ringer's solution and Plasma-Lyte A (**C**) [1]. The most frequent colloid given to pediatric patients is 5% albumin, but there are disagreements on its effectiveness in comparison to isotonic crystalloid administration [1]. Neonatal patients should be given D10W or D10 0.2% NaCl on the ward, followed by D5 LR in the operating room [1]. They require 3–5 mg/kg/min glucose if they are term and 5–6 mg/kg/min glucose if they are preterm (**A**) [1]. Normal saline (NS) or lactated Ringer's (LR) solution (without glucose) can be used to administer fluid boluses [1]. An

approach that is frequently employed is to administer a fluid bolus to a neonate through 10 mL normal saline flushes multiplied by their weight in kilograms [1]. For example, by administering four 10 mL NS flushes, you can give a 3.8 kg baby 40 mL of normal saline (10 mL/kg fluid bolus) (**D**) [1].

20. **D.** The ratio of alveolar (FA) to inspired (FI) anesthetic concentration is known as FA/FI. FA is zero and FI is large at the start of an inhaled induction of anesthesia [1]. Anesthesia is induced as the FA/FI moves closer to 1. Anesthesia can be induced more quickly in neonates because the FA/FI ratio rises more quickly compared to adults [1]. In comparison to adults, newborns have a higher alveolar ventilation to FRC ratio (VA/FRC), which causes FA/FI to rise more quickly [1]. In neonates, the ratio is 5:1, whereas in adults, it is 1.5:1 [1]. Additionally, neonates have less blood/gas solubility and less blood/tissue solubility (**B**) [1]. Neonates have an 18% lower blood solubility of highly soluble inhaled anesthetics (isoflurane). As a result, there is less absorption from the alveoli, and FA/FI increases more quickly [1]. Neonates and adults have the same blood solubility for the less soluble inhaled anesthetics, such as sevoflurane and desflurane, and FA/FI does not rise as quickly in infants [1]. Right-to-left shunts also delay the induction of anesthesia and slow the increase in FA/FI [1]. This is more pronounced with less soluble anesthetics like sevoflurane and desflurane [1]. Minimum alveolar concentration (MAC) varies with age. Infants aged 1–6 months have the highest MAC for inhaled anesthetics [1]. For isoflurane and desflurane, the MAC is 30% lower in full-term neonates. Sevoflurane MAC at term is equivalent to that at 1 month of age. The presence and severity of prematurity result in a decrease in MAC (**C**) [1]. The central nervous system's immaturity or neurohumoral variables may be to blame for this. Developmental delay and cerebral palsy both reduce the MAC by 25% [1].

References

1. Pardo M, Miller RD. Chapter 34: pediatrics. Basics of Anesthesia E-Book: Elsevier; 2017.
2. Barría RM. Neonatal Care for Anesthesiologists. In: Selected topics in neonatal care. London: IntechOpen; 2018.
3. Boyer TJ, Kritzmire SM. Neonatal anesthesia—StatPearls—NCBI Bookshelf. www.ncbi.nlm.nih.gov/books/NBK541030/. Accessed 30 Aug 2023.
4. Bang SR. Neonatal anesthesia: how we manage our most vulnerable patients. Korean J Anesthesiol. 2015;68(5):434. https://doi.org/10.4097/kjae.2015.68.5.434.
5. Miller RD, et al. Chapter 79—Pediatric and neonatal critical care. In: Anesthesia: 2-volume set. London: Elsevier Health Sciences; 2013.

Neonatal Resuscitation

Nidhi Bhatia

Questions

1. **The following is not true with regard to umbilical cord management in a newborn:**
   A. For preterm infants not requiring resuscitation at birth, it is reasonable to delay cord clamping for longer than 30 s.
   B. For term infants not requiring resuscitation at birth, it may be reasonable to delay cord clamping for longer than 30 s.
   C. For infants born at <28 weeks of gestation, cord milking is recommended.
   D. For term and preterm infants requiring resuscitation at birth, there is insufficient evidence to recommend delayed vs early cord clamping.
2. **At what temperature should newborn babies be maintained?**
   A. 350–360 °C
   B. 36.5–37.5 °C
   C. 37.5–38.5 °C
   D. 38–39 °C
3. **Which is the best modality for assessing a newborn's heart rate during resuscitation?**
   A. Electrocardiography (ECG)
   B. Auscultation
   C. Palpation
   D. Pulse oximetry
4. **Which of the following is not true regarding positive pressure ventilation (PPV) during neonatal resuscitation?**
   A. Should be provided in neonates who are persistently bradycardic, with heart rate <100/min.
   B. Needs to be provided with excessive peak inflation pressures.

N. Bhatia (✉)
Department of Anesthesia & Intensive Care, PGIMER, Chandigarh, India

A. C. Sinha, I. F. Pasca (eds.), *Peripartum Care of the Pregnant Patient*,
https://doi.org/10.1007/978-3-031-62756-9_42

   C. PEEP should be provided in neonates receiving PPV.
   D. A peak inflation pressure of 20–25 cm of water should be used.

5. **In neonates requiring resuscitation, positive pressure ventilation (PPV) should be provided at the following rates:**
   A. 20–30/min
   B. 30–40/min
   C. 40–60/min
   D. 60–80/min
6. **During neonatal resuscitation, what are the recommendations for oxygen administration in newborn infants requiring respiratory support**?
   A. 100% oxygen is required in term and late preterm neonates requiring respiratory support.
   B. 100% oxygen is required in preterm neonates <35 weeks of gestation requiring respiratory support.
   C. All neonates requiring respiratory support should be administered 50% oxygen.
   D. Inspired oxygen concentration should be increased to 100% if there is no response to PPV with lower oxygen concentrations during chest compressions.
7. **What measures should be taken in a neonate who is breathing spontaneously, with a heart rate of >100/min, but has labored breathing?**
   A. No intervention is required.
   B. Give continuous positive airway pressure.
   C. Administer positive pressure ventilation.
   D. Intubate the baby.
8. **The need for intervention in a newborn is based on the initial assessment of the following:**
   A. Observing tone and color
   B. Assessing adequacy of breathing
   C. Assessing heart rate
   D. Assessing tone, color, breathing, and heart rate
9. **Acceptable preductal oxygen saturation at 5 min of birth is:**
   A. 65–70%
   B. 70–75%
   C. 75–80%
   D. 80–85%
10. **Positive pressure ventilation (PPV) with chest compressions in a neonate should be initiated if:**
   A. Heart rate <100/min
   B. Heart rate <60/min despite adequate ventilation for at least 30 s
   C. Heart rate <30/min despite adequate ventilation for at least 60 s
   D. Only if the neonate is pulseless
11. **Immediately following birth, the initial intervention that can stimulate breathing in a neonate with ineffective breathing effort is as follows:**
   A. Positive pressure ventilation (PPV)

   B. Vigorous suctioning
   C. Tactile stimulation
   D. Endotracheal intubation
12. **What is the compression-ventilation ratio in a neonate undergoing resuscitation?**
   A. 30:2
   B. 15:2
   C. 5:1
   D. 3:1
13. **The best technique for giving chest compressions in a neonate is as follows:**
   A. Two-thumb encircling hands technique
   B. Two-finger technique
   C. Two-hand technique
   D. One-hand technique
14. **The recommended route of achieving vascular access in a newborn requiring resuscitation is as follows:**
   A. Intravenous access to the forearm
   B. Femoral vein cannulation
   C. Central venous cannulation
   D. Umbilical venous catheterization
15. **Which of the following is true with regard to administration of medications during resuscitation of a newborn?**
   A. Medications are frequently needed.
   B. Medications are rarely needed.
   C. Medications should be administered early in resuscitation.
   D. There is no role of any medication in neonatal resuscitation.
16. **During neonatal resuscitation, which is the first drug that is administered?**
   A. Atropine
   B. Glucose
   C. Epinephrine
   D. Sodium bicarbonate
17. **The following are true of intravenous epinephrine during neonatal resuscitation <u>except</u>:**
   A. It is indicated if heart rate continues to remain <60/min despite adequate ventilation and chest compressions
   B. Following the first dose, intravenous epinephrine is repeated every 3–5 min
   C. The dose of endotracheal epinephrine is the same as that of intravenous epinephrine
   D. Intravenous epinephrine is given at a dose of 0.01–0.03 mg/kg
18. **The fluid of choice for volume replacement in a neonate undergoing resuscitation is:**
   A. 0.9% sodium chloride
   B. Ringer lactate
   C. Colloids
   D. 0.9% sodium chloride or blood

19. **The next preferred route of emergency access for administering drugs/fluids in neonates with difficult umbilical venous access is as follows:**
    A. Peripheral venous access
    B. Intraosseous access
    C. Central venous access
    D. Endotracheal route
20. **The best parameter for assessing the adequacy of ventilations is:**
    A. Increase in heart rate
    B. Increase in oxygen saturation
    C. Change in the baby's color
    D. Change in ton

Answers and Explanations

1. **C**. Early cord clamping, within 30 s, is known to interfere with healthy transition as, rather than filling the newborn's circulating volume, it leaves fetal blood in the placenta. Delayed cord clamping is known to be associated with higher hematocrit at birth, better iron levels in infancy, and improved survival. Hence, options **A** and **B** are correct statements. There are currently insufficient studies in newborns requiring resuscitation before cord clamping to make a recommendation. Hence, option **D** is a correct statement. Cord milking is being studied as an alternative to delayed cord clamping but should be avoided in babies less than 28 weeks' gestational age, as it is associated with brain injury. Thus, for infants born at <28 weeks of gestation, cord milking is not recommended. Therefore, option **C** is not true [1].
2. **B**. The temperature of newly born babies should be maintained between 36.5 °C and 37.5 °C after birth during stabilization. Hypothermia (temperature <36 °C) and hyperthermia (temperature >38 °C) are associated with an increased risk of adverse outcomes and hence should be avoided. Thus, options **A**, **C**, and **D** are incorrect [2, 3].
3. **A**. Because ECG provides the most reliable and accurate measurement of the newborn's heart rate during resuscitation. Identifying a rapid and reliable method to measure the newborn's heart rate is critically important during neonatal resuscitation, as the newborn's heart rate is used to assess the effectiveness of spontaneous respiratory effort, the need for interventions, and the response to interventions, including chest compressions. Clinical assessment of heart rate by palpation or auscultation may be unreliable and inaccurate. Furthermore, pulse oximetry is slower in detecting heart rate changes and tends to be inaccurate during the first few minutes after birth. Hence, options **B**, **C**, and **D** are incorrect [1].
4. **B**. In newborn infants who are gasping, apneic, or bradycardic (heart rate <100/min), PPV should be initiated without delay. Peak inflation pressures of 20–25 cm of water are required to inflate the lungs and increase the heart rate, with administration of PEEP aiding in lung aeration and preventing airway

collapse. Hence, options **A**, **C**, and **D** are true statements. However, excessive peak inflation pressures can be potentially detrimental and should be avoided [1, 4, 5].

5. **C**. Providing PPV at a rate of 40–60/min is based on expert opinion and corresponds to the natural breathing pattern of both term and preterm neonates [1].
6. **D**. In neonates requiring respiratory support at birth, term and late preterm neonates should initially be given 21% oxygen, and preterm neonates should be administered 21–30% oxygen initially. Subsequent oxygen titration should be based on pulse oximetry. The literature has shown no difference in the neurodevelopmental outcome of neonates who received 21% versus those who received 100% oxygen during resuscitation. Excess oxygen concentrations can, on the contrary, be harmful. However, it is reasonable to use high oxygen concentrations during chest compressions [6–8].
7. **B**. Some newborn infants experience respiratory distress or labored breathing. This is more common in preterm neonates. Providing respiratory support in the form of CPAP helps keep their lungs open. Hence, option B is correct. Since the baby has labored breathing, some intervention is needed. However, as the neonate is breathing spontaneously and has a heart rate of >100/min, PPV or intubation is not needed [1, 9].
8. **D**. Immediately after birth, the initial assessment of the neonate is based on assessing all three, i.e., tone (and color), adequacy of breathing, and heart rate. Based on these three factors, the neonate can be placed in one of the three groups: (a) satisfactory transition, good tone, vigorous breathing/crying, and heart rate ≥100/min; (b) incomplete transition, reduced tone, inadequate breathing/apnea, and heart rate < 100/min; and (c) poor transition, floppy and/or pale, inadequate breathing/apnea, and heart rate <60/min [9].
9. **D**. Following birth, the acceptable preductal oxygen saturation at different time intervals is 60–65% at 1 min; 65–70% at 2 min; 70–75% at 3 min; 75–80% at 4 min; 80–85% at 5 min; and >85% at 10 min [1, 9].
10. **B**. Neonates who are apneic or gasping or have a heart rate of <100/min need PPV. Therefore, **A** is incorrect, as a neonate with a heart rate <100/min requires PPV. However, if, despite adequate PPV, the heart rate is <60/min, chest compressions should be immediately initiated along with PPV (**B**). **C** and **D** are incorrect, as it is not recommended to wait until the heart rate drops to less than 60 beats/min or the baby becomes pulseless before starting chest compressions [1].
11. **C**. Tactile stimulation, such as drying the neonate and rubbing the back/soles of the baby, is known to stimulate breathing. Hence, **C** is correct. PPV is indicated after the initial steps, including tactile stimulation, drying and suctioning (when indicated) fail, and the baby continues to have ineffective breathing/apnea/heart rate <100/min. Therefore, **A** is incorrect. Suctioning is indicated if there are secretions causing airway obstruction. Endotracheal intubation is not an initial intervention and is indicated if all initial measures, including PPV, fail. Therefore, options **B** and **D** are not correct [5, 10].

12. **D**. A compression-ventilation ratio of 30:2 is indicated in adult (single-rescuer/two-rescuer) resuscitation as well as in single-rescuer pediatric (including infants and children) resuscitation, whereas a ratio of 15:2 is indicated in two-rescuer pediatric (including infants and children) resuscitation. Hence, **A** and **B** are incorrect. A compression-ventilation ratio of 5:1 is not recommended in any age group. In neonatal resuscitation, it is recommended to use a compression-ventilation ratio of 3:1 [1].
13. **A**. Chest compressions in a neonate can be administered by using either the two-thumb encircling hands technique or the two-finger technique. However, the two-thumb encircling hands technique is known to be associated with better blood pressure generation and less rescuer fatigue. The one-hand technique is used in small children, and the two-hand technique is used in both children and adults [1, 9].
14. **D**. The recommended route for securing vascular access in a newborn is umbilical vein catheterization. In a compromised neonate, peripheral venous access is likely to be difficult to achieve and suboptimal for vasopressor administration. The umbilical vein, on the other hand, offers rapid vascular access. Central venous cannulation in a newborn is technically extremely challenging, time-consuming, and associated with significant complications. Furthermore, central venous cannulation is not recommended during resuscitation, as it requires interruption of chest compressions. Hence, **A**, **B**, and **C** are incorrect [9].
15. **B**. A low heart rate in a newborn is usually due to low oxygen levels. Therefore, establishing adequate ventilation most often corrects the low heart rate. Hence, medications are rarely needed. Thus, **B** is the correct answer, and **A**, **C**, and **D** are incorrect. Medications have a role but are mostly required late during resuscitation of a newborn [1].
16. **C**. Intravenous epinephrine is the first-line drug that is administered during neonatal resuscitation, if needed. Glucose is indicated in prolonged resuscitation to reduce the likelihood of hypoglycemia, and sodium bicarbonate is indicated in established metabolic acidosis. There is no role of atropine in cardiac arrest. It is indicated in bradyarrhythmia [9].
17. **C**. Intravenous epinephrine, at a dose of 0.01–0.03 mg/kg, is indicated during neonatal resuscitation if the heart rate continues to remain below 60/min despite optimal ventilation with 100% oxygen, preferably through an endotracheal tube and adequate chest compressions. Intravenous epinephrine is repeated every 3–5 min. Thus, **A**, **B**, and **D** are correct statements. In cases where intravenous access has not been established, epinephrine can be administered endotracheally, but the dose is greater (0.05–0.1 mg/kg) than the intravenous dose [1, 11, 12].
18. **D**. In neonates who respond poorly to resuscitation and in whom blood loss is suspected, initial volume expansion is performed with normal saline. In cases of suspected substantial blood loss, 10–20 mL/kg of blood is transfused [1].
19. **B**. The next best route, after umbilical vein catheterization, is intraosseous access. Securing peripheral venous access is difficult, and placing a central venous cannula is not recommended in neonates undergoing resuscitation.

Endotracheal tubes can be used as an emergency route for administering certain drugs in cases where venous/intraosseous access is difficult/not possible [1, 9].

20. **A**. In neonates undergoing resuscitation, the adequacy of ventilation is best assessed by the increase in heart rate. Measuring oxygen saturation or seeing the changes in tone/color may be unreliable and at times inaccurate [1, 9].

References

1. Aziz K, Lee HC, Escobedo MB, Hoover AV, Kamath-Rayne BD, Kapadia VS, et al. Part 5: neonatal resuscitation: 2020 American Heart Association guidelines for cardiopulmonary resuscitation and emergency cardiovascular care. Circulation. 2020;142:S524–50.
2. Laptook AR, Bell EF, Shankaran S, Boghossian NS, Wyckoff MH, Kandefer S, et al. Generic and moderate preterm subcommittees of the NICHD neonatal research network. Admission temperature and associated mortality and morbidity among moderately and extremely preterm infants. J Pediatr. 2018;192:53–9.
3. Lyu Y, Shah PS, Ye XY, Warre R, Piedboeuf B, Deshpandey A, et al. Canadian Neonatal Network. Association between admission temperature and mortality and major morbidity in preterm infants born at fewer than 33 weeks' gestation. JAMA Pediatr. 2015;169:e150277.
4. Mian Q, Cheung PY, O'Reilly M, Barton SK, Polglase GR, Schmölzer GM. Impact of delivered tidal volume on the occurrence of intraventricular hemorrhage in preterm infants during positive pressure ventilation in the delivery room. Arch Dis Child Fetal Neonatal Ed. 2019;104:F57–62.
5. Ersdal HL, Mduma E, Svensen E, Perlman JM. Early initiation of basic resuscitation interventions including face mask ventilation may reduce birth asphyxia related mortality in low-income countries: a prospective descriptive observational study. Resuscitation. 2012;83:869–73.
6. Welsford M, Nishiyama C, Shortt C, Isayama T, Dawson JA, Weiner G, et al. International liaison committee on resuscitation neonatal life support task force. Room air for initiating term newborn resuscitation: a systematic review with meta-analysis. Pediatrics. 2019;143(1):e20181825. https://doi.org/10.1542/peds.2018-1825.
7. Welsford M, Nishiyama C, Shortt C, Weiner G, Roehr CC, Isayama T, et al. International liaison committee on resuscitation neonatal life support task force. Initial oxygen use for preterm newborn resuscitation: a systematic review with meta-analysis. Pediatrics. 2019;143(1):e20181828. https://doi.org/10.1542/peds.2018-1828.
8. Escobedo MB, Aziz K, Kapadia VS, Lee HC, Niermeyer S, Schmölzer GM, et al. 2019 American Heart Association focused update on neonatal resuscitation: an update to the American Heart Association guidelines for cardiopulmonary resuscitation and emergency cardiovascular care. Circulation. 2019;140:e922–30.
9. Madar J, Roehr CC, Ainsworth S, Ersdal H, Morley C, Rüdiger M, et al. European resuscitation council guidelines 2021: newborn resuscitation and support of transition of infants at birth. Resuscitation. 2021;161:291–326.
10. Lee AC, Cousens S, Wall SN, Niermeyer S, Darmstadt GL, Carlo WA, et al. Neonatal resuscitation and immediate newborn assessment and stimulation for the prevention of neonatal deaths: a systematic review, meta-analysis and Delphi estimation of mortality effect. BMC Public Health. 2011;11(suppl 3):S12. https://doi.org/10.1186/1471-2458-11-S3-S12.
11. Halling C, Sparks JE, Christie L, Wyckoff MH. Efficacy of intravenous and endotracheal epinephrine during neonatal cardiopulmonary resuscitation in the delivery room. J Pediatr. 2017;185:232–6.
12. Vali P, Chandrasekharan P, Rawat M, Gugino S, Koenigsknecht C, Helman J, et al. Evaluation of timing and route of epinephrine in a neonatal model of asphyxial arrest. J Am Heart Assoc. 2017;6:e004402. https://doi.org/10.1161/JAHA.116.004402.

Fetal Surgery and the EXIT Procedure

Aditi Jain and Kajal Jain

Questions

1. **Which of the following does <u>not</u> lead to compromised uteroplacental blood flow?**
   A. Hypotension
   B. High uterine tone
   C. Left lateral displacement of the uterus
   D. Kinking of the umbilical cord
2. **Which factor is <u>not</u> responsible for drug transport to the fetus?**
   A. Fetal blood pH
   B. Lipid solubility
   C. Molecular size of blood
   D. Maternal hypotension
3. **Which of the following drugs has the lowest fetal to maternal ratio?**
   A. Isoflurane
   B. Vecuronium
   C. Propofol
   D. Fentanyl
4. **Which blood group is transfused to the fetus in case of loss during midgestational open procedures?**
   A. O-negative blood crossmatched with sibling blood
   B. O-negative blood crossmatched with fetal blood
   C. O-negative blood crossmatched with paternal blood

A. Jain
Department of Anaesthesia and Intensive Care, Government Medical College and Hospital, Chandigarh, India

K. Jain (✉)
Department of Anesthesia and Intensive Care, Postgraduate Institute of Medical Education and Research, Chandigarh, India

A. C. Sinha, I. F. Pasca (eds.), *Peripartum Care of the Pregnant Patient*,
https://doi.org/10.1007/978-3-031-62756-9_43

   D. O-negative blood crossmatched with maternal blood
5. **Which of the following is true regarding fetal cardiac physiology?**
   A. The majority of cardiac output comes from the right ventricle.
   B. The left and right circulations are in series.
   C. The myocardium is more compliant than in adults.
   D. The PVR is much lower than the SVR.
6. **Which of the following is true regarding the EXIT procedure when compared to open midgestation surgery?**
   A. There is an equal risk of postoperative pulmonary edema.
   B. Postoperative tocolysis is not needed.
   C. MAC is kept at <1.
   D. Fetal analgesia is not warranted in open midgestational procedures.
7. **The following is true of fetal cardiovascular physiology:**
   A. A leftward shift of the oxygen dissociation curve.
   B. There is relative anemia compared to maternal blood.
   C. Cardiac output is dependent on afterload.
   D. Pulmonary shunting is less than after delivery.
8. **The following can lead to flip-flop circulation after birth <u>except</u>:**
   A. Hypercapnia
   B. Hyponatremia
   C. Hypothermia
   D. Hypoxia
9. **Which of the following is <u>not</u> a prerequisite for fetal surgery?**
   A. The fetal abnormality would lead to fetal demise if left untreated before birth, and intervening before birth would benefit the neonatal outcome.
   B. The maternal risk is acceptably low.
   C. Absence of severe genetic defects.
   D. Availability of MRI facility for fetal MRI.
10. **Which of the following is <u>not</u> a complication following fetal surgery?**
    A. Preterm labor
    B. Pulmonary edema
    C. Cholestasis
    D. Chorioamnionitis
11. **The following is true regarding intrauterine transfusion:**
    A. Can be performed at any period of gestation.
    B. The umbilical vein is the preferred site for sampling.
    C. Generally, performed under GA.
    D. Target hematocrit is 30–35%.
12. **Which of the following is <u>not</u> a useful device for fetal monitoring?**
    A. Fetal Doppler
    B. Pulse oximeter
    C. Fetal ECHO
    D. Fetal capnometry
13. **In utero fetal temperature is most dependent on:**
    A. Ambient temperature

   B. Maternal temperature
   C. Fetal shivering and movement
   D. Amount of brown fat

14. **All the following are accepted routes for atropine administration to the fetus <u>except</u>:**
   A. Intracardiac
   B. Intramuscular
   C. Intravenous
   D. Intratracheal

15. **Which of the following is <u>not</u> a result of high concentrations of volatile anesthetic?**
   A. Maternal hypotension
   B. Fetal cardiac dysfunction
   C. Increased uterine tone
   D. Abnormal umbilical artery flow

16. **What is a contraindication to fetal surgery?**
   A. ASA 2 maternal status
   B. Mirror syndrome
   C. Hypoplastic left heart syndrome
   D. GDM

17. **What is the normal range of oxygen saturation (%) for a fetus?**
   A. 10–30
   B. 30–70
   C. 70–80
   D. >85

Answers and Explanations

1. **C**. Uteroplacental flows can be decreased due to preplacental, placental, and postplacental causes. Preplacental issues are most often associated with maternal conditions such as maternal hypotension or high uterine tone (**A**, **B**) [1]. Kinking of the umbilical cord (**D**) and fetal manipulation are the postplacental reasons for decreased uteroplacental flow. In cases of fetal distress, left lateral displacement of the uterus can relieve aortocaval compression and help increase uteroplacental flow [1].
2. **D**. Maternal-fetal exchange across the placenta occurs by one of four mechanisms: passive diffusion, facilitated diffusion, transporter-mediated mechanisms, and vesicular transport. Most drugs have molecular weights of less than 1000 daltons and cross the placenta by diffusion if the drug is not ionized. The rate of diffusion and peak levels in the fetus depend on maternal-fetal concentration gradients, maternal protein binding, molecular weight, lipid solubility, and the degree of drug ionization. Drug ionization in turn depends on the pKa of the drug and fetal blood pH. The maternal blood concentration of a drug is

typically the primary determinant of how much drug will ultimately reach the fetus [2].

3. **B**. Drug fetal to maternal ratios are given below [1]:

Drug administered	Fetal to maternal ratio
Halothane	0.7–0.9
Isoflurane	0.7
Nitrous oxide	0.83
Thiopental	0.1–1.1
Propofol	0.5–0.85
Diazepam	1–2
Midazolam	0.76
Morphine	0.61
Fentanyl	0.16–1.2
Remifentanil	0.29–0.88
Vecuronium	*0.06–0.11*
Glycopyrrolate	0.22
Ephedrine	0.7

4. **D**. Blood transfusion may be required for open fetal procedures as even loss in milliliters can lead to a decrease in perfusion and fetal distress. For this O-negative blood crossmatched with the maternal blood is transfused to the fetus. The antibodies from maternal circulation are passed to the fetus, so the blood is crossmatched with the mother to minimize the possibility of a hemolytic transfusion reaction in the fetus [3].
5. **A**. The fetal circulation is notable for being a parallel system before transitioning to serial circulation at birth (**B**) [1]. A normal human fetus has a CCO of 425–550 mL/kg/min, with the right ventricle contributing 60–70% of the total output (**A**) [4]. The fetal myocardium has a greater proportion of noncontractile elements and is also stiffer with impaired relaxation compared with the adult myocardium (**C**) [4]. Since the lungs are compressed and fluid-filled, the PVR is high, resulting in the diversion of blood through the ductus arteriosus.
6. **B**. The ex-utero intrapartum procedure is carried out just before the delivery of the fetus or as a bridge to ECMO [3]. As the baby is delivered after the procedure, tocolysis is not required (**B**). Midgestational open procedures have an increased risk of pulmonary edema compared to EXIT procedures and may warrant careful fluid therapy (**A**). For adequate uterine relaxation, the MAC of inhalational agents can be kept as high as two to three when they are used as a sole agent and 1.5 when supplemented with intravenous agents (**C**). Pain perception during fetal life is controversial, although analgesia during fetal surgeries has been seen to lead to a decrease in stress hormones in fetal blood and is now practiced (**D**) [1].
7. **A**. Fetal hemoglobin has a greater affinity than maternal adult hemoglobin for oxygen to facilitate transplacental transfer of oxygen (**A**). Fetal blood has higher hematocrit to maintain oxygen delivery (**B**). Fetal cardiac output is largely heart rate dependent (**C**). Most fetal blood is diverted from the lungs to decrease the shunt fraction (**D**) [5].

8. **B**. The cardiac shunts in fetal life undergo physiological closure on transition to neonatal life. However, certain conditions can lead to a reopening of these shunts and reversal of blood flow from neonatal to fetal circulation. These include prematurity, hypercarbia, hypoxia, and hypothermia (**A**, **C**, **D**) [5].
9. **D**. The prerequisites for fetal surgery include the following: (1) the fetal lesion is accurately diagnosed; (2) the progression and severity of the anomaly are predictable and well understood; (3) other severe associated anomalies that would contraindicate fetal intervention are excluded; (4) the fetal abnormality would lead to fetal death, irreversible organ damage, or severe postnatal morbidity if left untreated before birth, and intervening before birth would benefit the neonatal outcome; (5) the maternal risk is acceptably low; (6) animal models have demonstrated the feasibility of the surgical technique; (7) fetal interventions are performed at specialized multidisciplinary institutions using protocols approved by the center's ethics committees with maternal informed consent; and (8) the patient has access to highly specialized multidisciplinary care, including bioethical and psychological counseling [6–8].
10. **C**. Pulmonary edema, acute respiratory distress syndrome, chorioamnionitis, abruptio placentae, and preterm labor have all been reported after intrauterine fetal procedures, with maternal complications occurring mostly postoperatively rather than intraoperatively. Cholestasis of pregnancy has not been reported after the EXIT procedure (**A**, **B**, **D**). Potential fetal morbidities include infection, heart failure, intracranial hemorrhage, oligohydramnios, and fetal demise [3].
11. **B**. Fetal blood sampling from the umbilical vein just before starting the intrauterine transfusion (IUT) is the gold standard for determining the degree of fetal anemia (**B**). IUT is not used before 18 weeks' GA because umbilical vein access is not reliable (**A**). IUTs are typically performed using local anesthesia and require minimal maternal sedation and analgesia (**C**). The rate of transfusion is typically 5–10 mL/min with a target hematocrit of 45–55%. Steady intravascular location of the needle tip can be assessed with Doppler imaging throughout the transfusion injection (**D**) [9].
12. **D**. Fetal heart rate monitoring is performed during fetal procedures to ensure well-being. During fetal procedures, echocardiography, pulse oximetry, and ultrasound imaging of umbilical artery flow are the primary methods for fetal assessment. During EXIT procedures, pulse oximetry and fetal scalp electrodes help monitor fetal heart rate. Intraoperative ultrasonography allows imaging of FHR, cardiac contractility, and cardiac filling, as well as Doppler assessment of flow in the ductus arteriosus and umbilical artery flow. During fetal surgeries, since the fetus is on placental support, the lungs are not ventilated, and capnometry is redundant [10].
13. **B**. In utero, the fetus is unable to thermoregulate and depends on maternal body temperature secondary to placental circulation and surrounding amniotic fluid (**B**). Thermogenesis ex-utero in neonates is dependent on brown fat, and shivering develops even later (**C**, **D**) [1].

14. **C**. Drugs are most commonly administered intramuscularly in the fetus (**B**). During EXIT procedures, they can also be administered intravenously after securing an intravenous line (**C**). During fetal resuscitation, emergency medication, such as atropine and adrenaline, was also given intracardially (**A**) [1]. The intratracheal route of administration is not effective during fetal life, as the lungs are filled with water and the alveoli are not well perfused (**D**).
15. **C**. Inhalational agents are kept at a high MAC during the fetal procedure to keep the uterine tone low and provide tocolysis (**C**). Their side effects include cardiac dysfunction and maternal hypotension that can lead to decreased utero-placental perfusion and abnormal umbilical artery flow (**A**, **B**, **D**) [11].
16. **B**. Controlled medical conditions are not a contraindication for fetal surgeries if the risk to maternal health is reasonably low (**A**, **D**). Hypoplastic left heart syndrome is one of the indications for fetal surgeries (**C**). Since mirror syndrome is potentially life-threatening for both the mother and fetus due to edema in the mother and fetus, it forms a contraindication for fetal surgery [1, 12].
17. **B**. The normal oxygen saturation in a fetus is 30–70% and quickly rises to 90–95% in the first few minutes after delivery. Adult pulse oximeters have limited accuracy for fetal measurements due to calibration ranges, light interference, and decreased fetal pulse pressures [1].

References

1. Hoagland MA, Dean KA, Chatterjee D. Anesthesia for fetal surgery. In: Davis PJ, editor. Smith's anesthesia for infants and children. 10th ed. Elsevier; 2022. p. 709–31.
2. Myllynen P, Pasanen M, Pelkonen O. Human placenta: a human organ for developmental toxicology research and biomonitoring. Placenta. 2005;26(5):361–71.
3. Ferschl MB, Rollins MD. Anesthesia for fetal surgery and other fetal therapies. In: Gropper MA, et al., editors. Miller's anesthesia, 2-volume set. 9th ed. Elsevier; 2019. p. 2042–70.
4. Rychik J. Fetal cardiovascular physiology. Pediatr Cardiol. 2004b;25(3):1–9.
5. Waberski A, Unegbu C, Deutsch N. Cardiovascular physiology. In: Davis PJ, editor. Smith's anesthesia for infants and children. 10th ed. Elsevier; 2022.
6. Partridge EA, Flake AW. Maternal-fetal surgery for structural malformations. Best Pract Res Clin Obstet Gynecol. 2012;26:669–82.
7. Harrison MR, Filly RA, Golbus MS, et al. Fetal treatment 1982. N Engl J Med. 1982;307:1651–2.
8. Sudhakaran N, Sothinathan U, Patel S. Best practice guidelines: fetal surgery. Early Hum Dev. 2012;88:15–9.
9. Papantoniou N, Sifaki S, Antsaklis A. Therapeutic management of fetal anemia: review of standard practice and alternative treatment options. J Perinat Med. 2013;41:71–82.
10. Subramanian R, Mishra P, Subramaniam R, Bansal S. Role of anesthesiologist in ex utero intrapartum treatment procedure: a case and review of anesthetic management. J Anesthesiol Clin Pharmacol. 2018;34(2):148.
11. Garcia PJ, Olutoye OO, Ivey RT, Olutoye OA, Riou B. Case scenario: anesthesia for maternal-fetal surgery: the ex utero intrapartum therapy (EXIT) procedure. Anesthesiology. 2011;114:1446–52.
12. Duci M, Pulvirenti R, Fascetti Leon F, Capolupo I, Veronese P, Gamba P, Tognon C. Anesthesia for fetal operative procedures: a systematic review. Front Pain Res (Lausanne). 2022;3:935427. https://doi.org/10.3389/fpain.2022.935427.

Suggested Reading

Ferschl MB, Rollins MD. Anesthesia for fetal surgery and other fetal therapies. In: Gropper MA, et al., editors. Miller's anesthesia, 2-volume set. 9th ed. Elsevier; 2019. p. 2042–70.

Hoagland MA, Dean KA, Chatterjee D. Anesthesia for fetal surgery. In: Davis PJ, editor. Smith's anesthesia for infants and children. 10th ed. Elsevier; 2022. p. 709–31.

Informed Consent in Obstetric Anesthesia

Shilpa Kasodekar and Aparajita Nathroy

Questions

1. **Regarding informed consent for labor analgesia, which of the following is true?**
   A. Informed consent should be obtained before the procedure.
   B. Women want to know rare but minor side effects.
   C. Women want to know rare but devastating complications.
   D. No neonatal risks should be mentioned.
2. **Which of the following is true about when obtaining consent for epidural analgesia in labor?**
   A. Only verbally discussing the procedure and the side effects to the patient
   B. Only giving written materials explaining the procedure and side effects
   C. Not only verbally discussing but also giving written materials to the patient for better understanding
   D. Explaining the procedure in short to the patient and enumerating the side effects to only the relatives
3. **The main elements of consent include the following:**
   A. Procedural description
   B. Potential risks and complications

S. Kasodekar (✉)
P D Hinduja Hospital and Medical Research Centre, Khar, Mumbai, Maharashtra, India

A. Nathroy
Hinduja Hospital Khar, Mumbai, Maharashtra, India

P D Hinduja Hospital and Medical Research Centre, Khar, Mumbai, Maharashtra, India

A. C. Sinha, I. F. Pasca (eds.), *Peripartum Care of the Pregnant Patient*,
https://doi.org/10.1007/978-3-031-62756-9_44

C. Benefits and alternate therapeutic options
D. All of the above

4. **The informed consent form for labor analgesia should include the following:**
A. Minor side effects only
B. Major side effects only
C. Both major and minor side effects
D. No side effects

5. **Informed consent for neuraxial analgesia for labor of a term pregnant patient should include the following concept:**
A. Neuraxial analgesia could increase the duration of labor, increase the need for forceps delivery, and eventually increase the incidence of cesarean section.
B. Neuraxial analgesia could increase the duration of labor and increase the need for forceps delivery but will not modify the incidence of cesarean section.
C. Neuraxial analgesia does not increase the duration of labor, although it does increase the need for forceps delivery and the incidence of cesarean section.
D. Neuraxial analgesia does not affect the duration of labor, the need for forceps delivery, or the incidence of cesarean section.

6. **Which of the following statements is false?**
A. Despite the stress of labor, women believe they are capable of consenting and accurately recalling information as readily as other patient populations.
B. Recall is not hindered by pain level or opioid premedication.
C. Information provided during the consent process was able to be recalled months after the process.
D. Level of education, age, and previous epidural analgesia experience improved recall.

7. **The disadvantage of written forms during informed consent have the following:**
A. No requirement of verbally interacting with the patient and relatives
B. Convenient method of enumerating all the risks and benefits
C. Makes disclosure more convenient
D. Beneficial from a medicolegal point of view

8. **Informed consent should be explained and written in the language best understood by:**
A. The patient
B. The relatives
C. The local dialect
D. The doctors and the nursing staff

9. **How can the information in the consent form of labor analgesia be conveyed to the patient?**
A. Positive, factual, and thorough explanations
B. By enumerating the actual consequence of every side effect
C. By using harsh words and making sure that the patient does not deviate from the decision of labor analgesia
D. By using the nocebo method of communication

10. **In which year was the concept of informed consent introduced?**
    A. 1998
    B. 1957
    C. 1963
    D. 1977
11. **In what percentage of cases will an epidural catheter need to be readjusted or replaced when inserted by experienced providers?**
    A. 5%
    B. 15%
    C. 10%
    D. 12%
12. **What is the incidence of inadvertent dural puncture during epidural anesthesia in obstetrics?**
    A. More than 2%
    B. 1.5%
    C. 0.5%
    D. Less than 0.2%
13. **Consent for sterilization should <u>not</u> occur ______.**
    A. More than 30 days before the anticipated due date
    B. While the patient is in labor
    C. In those aged >21 years
    D. If patient is deemed mentally competent
14. **During the active phase of labor, information regarding epidural analgesia is to be given to ______.**
    A. The patient at any time
    B. The relatives only
    C. Should not be given any information
    D. The patient between the contractions
15. **If a woman lacks a mental capacity to consent, which of the following should be done?**
    A. The doctor should consult only the family members.
    B. The doctor should consult an experienced colleague.
    C. An experienced colleague and where appropriate, seek ethics and legal advice on appropriate management, including applications to the court.
    D. The patient should be allowed to make her own decisions.

Answers and Explanations

1. **A**. Informed consent should be obtained immediately before surgery. Anesthetists are morally and legally obliged to obtain consent from women before performing regional analgesia in labor [1]. It is also part of good clinical practice. All women requesting epidural analgesia should be fully informed of the benefits, side effects, and risks involved before consenting to the procedure.

2. **C**. When obtaining consent for epidural analgesia in labor, written information, in addition to a verbal discussion, improves recall of the information given [1–3]. It may also act as written medicolegal evidence of the information women receive.
3. **D**. The main elements of consent include procedural description, potential risks, benefits, complications, and alternate therapeutic options [4]. Additionally, the clinician's recommendation in a noncoercive manner provides the patient with expert advice and reassurance.
4. **C**. Minor side effects include hypotension, nausea/vomiting, pruritus, and transient respiratory depression; shivering and an increase in body temperature may also occur. Headache could occur due to inadvertent dural puncture in experienced hands in <1% of cases. In cases of severe headaches, a combination of conservative management and an epidural blood patch could be used to treat discomfort.

   Rare major side effects are as follows: inadvertent high spinal block and IV injection of local anesthetic agents, which could result in arrhythmias, convulsions, or cardiorespiratory arrest. While enumerating these complications, the anesthetist must ensure that the patient is aware that an anesthetist is well versed to deal with such complications if any occur [5].
5. **B**. Epidural analgesia (EA) per se does not increase the likelihood of cesarean section. However, EA could slightly prolong the duration of the second stage of labor and increase the chances of assisted deliveries. Compared with other systemic analgesia methods, epidural analgesia has better neonatal blood gas values [5]. Currently, pregnant patients demand information, so it is important to recognize aspects that may affect their outcome. Neuraxial obstetric analgesia could interfere at multiple levels with relevant outcomes such as duration of labor, forceps delivery, and cesarean section rates.
6. **D**. Medical capacity, determined by the clinician, is the patient's ability to assimilate information, debate the risks/benefits, and communicate a decision. This stands in contrast to court-affirmed legal competence, which gives a person legal decision-making power. Some anesthesia providers argue that the pain and distraction of labor may limit a parturient's capacity [6]. Although recall of facts during consent may not equate to comprehension, information is at the heart of understanding. Despite the stress of labor, women believe they are capable of consenting [7] and accurately recalling information as readily as other patient populations [8]. Research shows that recall is not hindered by pain level or opioid premedication. Additionally, level of education, age, and previous epidural analgesia experience did not improve recall [8, 9]. Information provided during the consent process was able to be recalled months after the process [10].
7. **A**. Written forms give a scope of enumerating all the risks and benefits, thus making disclosure more convenient. However, the anesthetist must ensure that other than the printed forms, there is good verbal communication of the enumerated issues, which would also be beneficial from a medicolegal

documentation point of view. Using written forms, antenatal education can improve consent for obstetric anesthesia and analgesia [11].

8. **A**. There are many official languages in different parts of the world. However, countries such as India and South Africa, with the number of official languages in double digits and an even higher number of regional dialects and variations, are an exception. Likewise, there are more than 20 languages spoken in India, with Hindi being spoken by most Indians. The other widely spoken languages are Bengali, Marathi, Telugu, Tamil, Gujarati, Urdu, and Kannada. Per the constitution, there are 22 official languages in the country [12].

   Countries such as the United States of America, United Kingdom, and other European countries with a predominantly English-speaking population are also facing difficulties since migration has made communication and information sharing truly challenging [13]. According to the US Census Bureau, nearly 25 million people in the United States have limited English proficiency (LEP). Effective communication is such an important part of the treatment process as communication errors have been found to be the cause of 59% of serious adverse events reported to The Joint Commission [14].
9. **A**. Patients must be given every opportunity to have concerns addressed and questions responded to. However, it might be helpful to remain positive regarding outcomes on the day of surgery unless the patient asks specifically for clarification regarding risks. This is particularly relevant when suggesting symptoms such as pain, nausea, and itching, given that patients are particularly vulnerable to the effects of nocebo communications when anxious and anxiety tends to escalate as the time to anesthesia induction approaches [15]. Information should be provided to the patients in a way that is more reassuring rather than anxiety provoking. Positive affirmations have a great impact on the patient's mindset, which also aids in early recovery. Similarly, instead of telling the patients they should expect postoperative nausea and vomiting, we could just state to them that nausea and vomiting is common postoperatively but appropriate medications will be given to significantly lower that risk.
10. **B**. The concept of informed consent was introduced by the courts during a famous legal case in the United Kingdom in 1957. A patient had suffered paraplegia following translumbar aortography and maintained that he had not been informed of the dangers of the procedure. Following this case, it became the responsibility of the physician to explain the risks and benefits of the intended procedure and the alternatives. From 1957 to 1998, the so-called Bolam principle was applied, which stated that a doctor is not guilty of negligence if acting in accordance with a practice accepted as proper by a reasonable body of medical men skilled in that art. In 1998, following Pearce versus the United Bristol Healthcare NHS Trust, the premise was adopted for the first time that it was the opinion of a reasonable patient, and not that of the court or the medical profession, that was crucial [16].
11. **C**. In terms of pain relief, the patient can expect that, in experienced hands, 90% of epidural catheters will provide excellent pain relief in the very first attempt, and this mode of analgesia is better than any other method employed in labor.

In the remaining 10% of cases, it can either be a patchy block or poor analgesia, which may require further intervention. This could be in the form of withdrawal of the catheter (1–2 cm) or top up with local analgesics with the patient lying on the affected side, or there could be a requirement of reinserting the epidural catheter [5].

12. **B**. The incidence of inadvertent dural puncture during epidural catheter placement for parturients is 1.5%. Of those patients, approximately half will develop postdural puncture headaches. Postdural puncture headache can occur as early as day 1 and as late as day 7 post-procedure [17].
13. **B**. Care must be taken when obtaining consent for sterilization so that the consent is obtained at least 30 days before the due date. Where possible, women should be informed of their contraceptive options in the prenatal period. Consent to be sterilized should not be obtained while a woman is in labor. In the United States, the patient must be 21 years old and deemed mentally competent, and 30 days must pass between sterilization consent and elective sterilization [18].
14. **D**. When consent must be obtained from a woman during painful labor, such as to perform a vaginal examination, episiotomy, and operative delivery or to place an epidural, information should be given between contractions. If appropriate, upon admission for induction of labor, consideration should be given concerning possible procedures and interventions. Women should be encouraged to express their views and questions about such procedures [19].
15. **C**. Where the woman lacks mental capacity to consent, where there has been appropriate dialog with family, carers, and multidisciplinary teams, and where differences of opinion about her best interests cannot be resolved satisfactorily, the doctor should consult experienced colleagues and, where appropriate, seek legal advice on appropriate management, including applications to the court. Management of the patient using the Mental Capacity Act 2005 allows the appointment of an independent mental capacity advocate to speak for a person who lacks capacity and who does not have a family member or friend to assist the patient in consideration of their treatment choices if time allows [20, 21]. In the case of a woman losing mental capacity after refusing consent to a treatment following previous discussion during pregnancy, even if this is at the expense of the fetus, her wishes should be respected in the same way as if she were competent [19, 20]. Where there is substantial doubt as to whether the woman foresaw the present circumstances when making her wishes known, the hospital ethics team should be consulted.

References

1. Black JD, Cyna AM. Issues of consent for regional analgesia in labor: a survey of obstetric anesthetists. Anesth Intensive Care. 2006;34:254–60.
2. Gerancher JC, Grice SC, Dewan DM, Eisenach J. An evaluation of informed consent prior to epidural analgesia for labor and delivery. Int J Obstet Anesth. 2000;9:168–73.

3. Hoyt MR, Wissler RN. Do we need written consent for labor analgesia? SOAP Newsletter, Spring; 1998. http://www.soap.org/media/newsletter_spring1998.pdf. Accessed 27 June 2008.
4. Hoehner PJ. Ethical aspects of informed consent in obstetric anesthesia: new challenges and solutions. J Clin Anesth. 2003;15:587–600.
5. Dyer RA, Hodges O. Informed consent for epidural analgesia in labor. Southern Afr J Anesth Analg. 2007;13(1):27–34. https://doi.org/10.1080/22201173.2007.10872462.
6. Black JD, Cyna AM. Issues of consent for regional analgesia in labor: a survey of obstetric anesthetists. Anaesth Intensive Care. 2006;34:254–60.
7. Brooks H, Sullivan WJ. The importance of patient autonomy at birth. Int J Obstet Anesth. 2002;11:196–203.
8. Affleck PJ, Waisel DB, Cusick JM, Van Decar T. Recall of risks following labor analgesia. J Clin Anesth. 1998;10:141–4.
9. Cheng WYC, Cyna AM, Osborn KD. Risks of regional anesthesia for cesarean section: women's recall and information sources. Anaesth Intensive Care. 2007;35:68–73.
10. Grice SC, Eisenach JC, Dewan DM, Robinson ML. Evaluation of informed consent for anesthesia for labor and delivery. Anesthesiology. 1988;69:A664.
11. Saunders TA, Stein DJ, Dilger JP. Informed consent for labor epidurals: a survey of Society for Obstetric Anesthesia and Perinatology anesthesiologists from the United States. Int J Obstet Anesth. 2006;15:98–103.
12. Constitutional Provisions Relating to Eighth Schedule. https://Mha.gov.in/Sites/Default/Files/Eighth_Schedule.Pdf.
13. Jaeger F, Pellaud N, Laville B, Klauser P. The migration-related language barrier and professional interpreter use in primary health care in Switzerland. BMC Health Serv Res. 2019;19:429.
14. Wasserman M, Renfrew M, Green A, Lopez L, Tan-McGrory A, Brach C, et al. Identifying and preventing medical errors in patients with limited English proficiency: key findings and tools for the field. J Healthc Qual. 2014;36:5–16.
15. Lang EV, Hatsiopoulou O, Koch T, et al. Can words hurt? Patient–provider interactions during invasive procedures. Pain. 2005;114:303–9.
16. Plaat F, McGlennan A. Women in the 21st century deserve more information: disclosure of material risk in obstetric anaesthesia. Int J Obstet Anesth. 2004;13(2):69–70.
17. Choi PT, Galinski SE, Takeuchi L, Lucas S, Tamayo C, Jadad AR. PDPH is a common complication of neuraxial blockade in parturients: a meta-analysis of obstetrical studies. Can J Anaesth. 2003;50(5):460–9. https://doi.org/10.1007/BF03021057.
18. Raine SP. Federal sterilization policy: unintended consequences. Virtual Mentor. 2012;14(2):152–7. https://doi.org/10.1001/virtualmentor.2012.14.2.mhst1-1202.
19. Association of Anesthetists of Great Britain and Ireland. Consent for anesthesia. London: AAGBI; 2006.
20. Department for Constitutional Affairs. The mental capacity act 2005. Code of practice. London: The Stationery Office; 2007.
21. Royal College of Obstetricians and Gynecologists Law and Ethics in Relation to Court-Authorized Obstetric Intervention. Ethics Committee Guideline No. 1. London: RCOG; 2006.

Diversity, Equity, and Inclusion in Obstetric Care

Katharine Stolz, Gabrielle Pina, and Leonard J. Soloniuk

Questions

1. **Which of the following groups has the lowest maternal** mortality **rate in the United States?**
   A. Non-Hispanic White women
   B. Non-Hispanic Black women
   C. Hispanic women
   D. Non-Hispanic Asian women
   E. Non-Hispanic Native American or Alaska Native
2. **The general fertility rate is a measure of the number of live births among women 15–44 years of age. Which of the following statements is true regarding women incarcerated in the United States?**
   A. Preterm births are less likely in incarcerated women.
   B. The general fertility rate of incarcerated women is the same as that of the general population.
   C. Cesarean deliveries are more common in incarcerated women than in the general population.
   D. The prevalence of pregnancy on incarceration is higher than that in the general population.

K. Stolz
Riverside University Health System, Moreno Valley, CA, USA
e-mail: K.Stolz@ruhealth.org

G. Pina · L. J. Soloniuk (✉)
Loma Linda University, Loma Linda, CA, USA

Riverside University Health System, Moreno Valley, CA, USA
e-mail: g.pina@ruhealth.org; l.soloniuk@ruhealth.org

A. C. Sinha, I. F. Pasca (eds.), *Peripartum Care of the Pregnant Patient*,
https://doi.org/10.1007/978-3-031-62756-9_45

E. The rate of ectopic pregnancies in incarcerated women is higher than that in the general population.

3. **The ICE score measures the extent to which an area's population is concentrated into extremes of deprivation versus privilege. The ICE score ranges from −1 (everyone in the least privileged group) to 1 (everyone in the most privileged group). In California, USA, after adjustment for confounding variables (such as age, education, nativity, prenatal care visits, pregnancy BMI, cigarette use, alcohol and drug use, infection, diabetes, hypertension, depression, parity, and previous preterm births), women from the lowest quintile ICE score neighborhoods had an adjusted odds ratio for preterm births of:**
   A. 1
   B. 1.05
   C. 1.25
   D. 1.8
   E. 2.5
4. **An increase of $10,000 in the median income in a county in the United States is associated with which of the following?**
   A. No change in Black-White income disparity
   B. A decrease in low birth weight (LBW; <2500 g) births
   C. An increase in very low birth weight (VLBW; <1500 g) births
   D. The lowest effect on birth outcomes at the lowest income levels
   E. Increased maternal smoking
5. **Among the indigenous people of Canada (Inuit, First Nations, and Métis), which of the following adverse birth outcomes has lower rates compared to non-indigenous individuals?**
   A. Preterm birth
   B. Small-for-gestational-age birth
   C. Large-for-gestational-age birth
   D. Stillbirth
   E. Infant mortality
6. **Which of the following factors has been historically considered to have the largest impact on the risk for small-for-gestational-age (SGA) births in nulliparous women?**
   A. Low pregnancy weight gain
   B. Age
   C. Education
   D. Race-ethnicity
   E. Percent of neighborhoods with income below the poverty line
7. **Observational studies of the effect of racism on health outcomes do NOT include measurement of which of the following?**
   A. Self-reported racism experienced directly in interpersonal contact
   B. Racism directed toward a group (e.g., based on ethnicity/race/nationality) of which the person is a member

   C. Vicarious experiences of racism (e.g., witnessing racism experienced by family members or friends)
   D. Internalized racism (i.e., the incorporation of racist attitudes and/or beliefs within an individual's worldview)
   E. Exposures to race-related stress or discrimination distress (e.g., the extent to which racial discrimination was stressful/upsetting)

8. **The effect of racism on health is moderated the most by the following:**
   A. Age
   B. Sex
   C. Education level
   D. Birthplace
   E. Ethnicity
9. **Which region of the world has the highest percentage of HIV-related maternal deaths as a subset of all maternal deaths?**
   A. Australia and New Zealand
   B. Europe
   C. Eastern and Southeastern Asia
   D. North America
   E. Sub-Saharan Africa
10. **In office visits with physicians, race-concordant visits (White patients meeting White physicians and Black patients meeting Black physicians) are compared to race-discordant visits; which of the following is true?**
    A. Patient satisfaction is lower.
    B. Ratings of patient-centered communication are higher.
    C. Visits are longer.
    D. Had faster speech in the dialogue of both physician and patient.
    E. Physician verbal dominance was lower.
11. **In the United States and other countries, racial and ethnic disparities in severe maternal morbidity have been explained by the "healthy immigrant effect" (HIE) and the "salmon" effect. Which of the following statements about these terms is correct?**
    A. The "healthy immigrant" effect refers to healthier immigrants being able to return to their home of origin.
    B. The "salmon" effect refers to healthier migrants being able to move more readily between their home of origin and their immigrant home.
    C. The "healthy immigrant" effect refers to immigrants improving their health status after moving to their migrant home and attaining an improved socio-economic status.
    D. The "salmon" effect refers to less healthy immigrants being more likely to die in their destination country.
    E. The "healthy immigrant" effect refers to healthier people being more likely to become immigrants.
12. **Globally, the lifetime risk for a 15-year-old girl dying of a <u>maternal</u> cause is:**
    A. 1 in 10
    B. 1 in 37

C. 1 in 105
D. 1 in 190
E. 1 in 400

13. **The use of labor neuraxial analgesia for vaginal delivery is associated with a lower rate of severe maternal morbidity (SMM). Which of the following statements is correct about the use of labor neuraxial analgesia?**
    A. Black and Hispanic women have the same reduction in risk of SMM as White women.
    B. The reduction in risk of SMM occurred only for women with a high risk of SMM.
    C. Fetal heart rhythm abnormalities were associated with a lower rate of use of labor neuraxial analgesia.
    D. Induced labor was associated with a lower rate of use of labor neuraxial analgesia.
    E. Over 75% of the reduction in risk was associated with a reduction in postpartum hemorrhage.
14. **In the United States, which of the following groups has the highest prevalence of smoking at any time during pregnancy?**
    A. Non-Hispanic White
    B. Non-Hispanic Black
    C. Hispanic
    D. Non-Hispanic Native Hawaiian or Other Pacific Islander
    E. Non-Hispanic American Indian or Alaska Native
15. **Compared to heterosexual cisgender women, which of the following statements is true about LGBTQ women?**
    A. They have a decreased risk for cardiovascular disease.
    B. They have a decreased risk for diabetes mellitus.
    C. They have increased allostatic load.
    D. They have a decreased risk of venous thromboembolism.
    E. They have a decreased likelihood of requesting an elective cesarean section because of gender dysphoria.
16. **Medical comorbidities increase the risk of severe maternal morbidity. Which of the following groups of women has the largest number of comorbid conditions per patient?**
    A. Asian
    B. Black
    C. Hispanic
    D. White
    E. Others
17. **For women serving in the US military, which of the following statements is correct?**
    A. They have a higher rate of unintended pregnancy than civilian women.
    B. They have the same financial access to abortion as the civilian population with commercial health insurance.

C. When on active deployment, they have a lower rate of unintended pregnancy than when non-deployed.
D. Hispanic servicewomen are more likely to have unintended pregnancies than non-Hispanic White servicewomen.
E. Women serving in the Air Force are more likely to have unintended pregnancies than servicewomen serving in the Navy, Army, or Marine Corps.

18. **Low-risk cesarean rate is defined as the number of singleton, term (37 or more weeks of gestation), cephalic, cesarean deliveries to women having a first birth per 100 women delivering singleton, term, cephalic, first births. Which of the following groups has the lowest rate of cesarean births for low-risk teenage pregnancies?**
    A. Hispanic
    B. Non-Hispanic Black
    C. Non-Hispanic American Indian or Alaska Native
    D. Non-Hispanic Native Hawaiian/Pacific Islander
    E. Non-Hispanic Asian
    F. Non-Hispanic White
19. **For non-Hispanic Black women in the United States, what is the leading cause of maternal mortality?**
    A. Hypertensive disorders
    B. Hemorrhage
    C. Infection
    D. Accident
    E. Homicide
20. **Published studies of implicit racial/ethnic bias in healthcare providers have shown which of the following?**
    A. Education in implicit bias has been shown to improve provider behavior, patient care delivery, and patient outcomes.
    B. Black healthcare providers are more likely to demonstrate no implicit bias compared to Whites and other minorities.
    C. Higher implicit bias does not lead to poorer patient-provider interactions.
    D. Interventions to reduce implicit bias demonstrate post-intervention reduction in implicit bias.
21. **Of the following, which are the top three leading causes of pregnancy-related deaths? (Choose three.)**
    A. Pulmonary conditions
    B. Cardiac/coronary conditions
    C. Embolism-thrombotic
    D. Hemorrhage
    E. Hypertensive disorders of pregnancy
    F. Mental health conditions
    G. Infection
22. **Of the following, which are the two strongest indicators for pregnancy-related mortality? (Choose two.)**
    A. Level of education

B. Household income
C. Food insecurity
D. Unemployment
E. Low birth weight

23. **A maternal death is defined by the World Health Organization as "the death of a woman while pregnant or within 42 days of termination of pregnancy, irrespective of the duration and the site of the pregnancy, from any cause related to or aggravated by the pregnancy or its management, but not from accidental or incidental causes." Maternal mortality rate (MMR) is the number of maternal deaths per 100,000 live births. How did the maternal mortality rate (MMR) change in the United States between 2018 and 2020 compared to other first-world countries?**
    A. The MMR trended downward by 24.8%, following the global trend of decreasing MMR.
    B. The MMR trended upward by 24.8%, not following the global trend of decreasing MMR.
    C. The MMR stayed stable in both the United States and the world.
    D. Not possible to determine.
24. **How do implicit biases and assumptions based on negative and false stereotypes contribute to the peripartum experience of patients of color? (Choose one or more.)**
    A. Higher likelihood of undergoing general anesthesia for cesarean delivery
    B. Assumption of lower adherence to management leading to lower rates of prescribing progesterone in Black parturients at risk of preterm birth
    C. Assumption of biological differences between White patients and patients of color such as thicker skin and underestimation of pain
    D. Undertreatment of pain
    E. All of the above
25. **According to the National Center for Health Statistics, what is the maternal mortality rate for non-Hispanic Black women in 2020?**
    A. 5 deaths per 100,000 live births
    B. 10 deaths per 100,000 live births
    C. 22 deaths per 100,000 live births
    D. 41 deaths per 100,000 live births
26. **What percentage of pregnancy-related deaths are preventable?**
    A. 20%
    B. 40%
    C. 60%
    D. 80%
27. **Which of the following is the leading cause of pregnancy-related death in Hispanic women following pregnancy?**
    A. Mental health conditions
    B. Cardiomyopathy
    C. Hemorrhage
    D. Respiratory complications

28. **Maternal death is defined by the World Health Organization as "the death of a woman while pregnant or within ___ days of termination of pregnancy, irrespective of the duration and the site of the pregnancy, from any cause related to or aggravated by the pregnancy or its management, but not from accidental or incidental causes."**
    A. 30
    B. 42
    C. 55
    D. 67

Answers and Explanations

1. **C**. The Hispanic paradox is sometimes used to describe the findings that Hispanic women in the United States have both a lower maternal mortality rate and a lower severe maternal morbidity (SMM) prevalence than Black and White women. Despite having socioeconomic profiles that are comparable to Black women, Hispanic women in the United States have either a comparable or better proportion of maternal morbidity, proportion of mortality, and birth outcomes than White women. The maternal mortality rate (deaths per 100,000 live births) is 14.9 for non-Hispanic White women, 37.3 for non-Hispanic Black women, and 11.8 for Hispanic women [1].
2. **A**. The US national average of preterm births is nearly 10% of live births. For incarcerated women, 6% of live births are preterm. The general fertility rate was 62 per 1000 women in the United States in 2016. A rough estimate of the general fertility rate for incarcerated women is 18 per 1000 women (**B**). The rate of cesarean deliveries is the same in the incarcerated population as in the general population (**C**). The prevalence of pregnancy on incarceration, 3%, is the same as that in the general population (**D**). The rate of ectopic pregnancies in incarcerated women is the same as that in the general population (**E**) [2, 3].
3. **C**. Even after adjusting for other confounding variables, neighborhoods experiencing racial and economic segregation have a 25% increase in preterm births [4].
4. **B**. An increase in the median income in a county in the United States is associated with decreased Black-White income disparity, decreased LBW births, and decreased VLBW births. Gains in income are associated with reduced LBW incidence, partly by increasing prenatal care and decreasing maternal smoking. Infants born LBW, particularly below 1500 g, are at increased risk of impaired cognitive functioning, low academic achievement, and cardiovascular disease. Disparities in LBW (e.g., by economic factors, race/ethnicity, and geography) have implications for lifelong disparities in health and well-being. A large increase in county median income of $10,000 is associated with 0.34 and 0.10 fewer LBW and VLBW incidents per 100 live births, respectively, and a smaller Black-White disparity in LBW and VLBW of 0.58 and 0.17 cases per 100, respectively. Cash transfers to low-income households and minimum wage

increases have been shown to reduce the incidence of LBW. Policies leading to median income growth may improve birth outcomes for the population and reduce Black-White disparities [5].

5. **B**. Except for small-for-gestational-age birth, adverse birth outcomes occurred more frequently among First Nations, Inuit, and Métis women than among non-indigenous women. Analyses of the disparities in birth outcomes in indigenous women (studied primarily in Australia, Canada, and the United States) have shown higher risks for adverse birth outcomes compared to non-indigenous women. Associated factors include: (1) reduced access to prenatal care, (2) accurate estimation of gestational age, (3) preexisting medical conditions, (4) high rates of multiparity, (5) young maternal age, (6) marital status, and (7) low educational attainment. Other factors include the legacy of policies and resultant intergenerational trauma that has affected the physical and mental health of individuals, families, and communities [6, 7].
6. **A**. Studies of risk factors may adjust for standard confounding variables and detailed confounding variables. Standard confounders are participant's age, education, race-ethnicity, marital status, prepregnancy smoking, medical insurance, gravidity, preexisting diabetes, chronic hypertension, and use of assisted reproductive technologies. Detailed confounders are diet quality, nausea and vomiting, health literacy, depressive symptoms, perceived stress, anxiety, resilience, neighborhood walkability, neighborhood deprivation, proximity to grocery stores, and percent of neighborhoods with income below the poverty line. There, however, has been contestation of the idea that low pregnancy weight gain would have minimal impact on adverse pregnancy outcomes based on a large-scale prospective cohort study in 2023 observing several confounding variables such as peripartum weight gain [8].
7. **E**. Studies of racism distinguish between reported racism and other measures, such as general measures of discrimination, discrimination due to other reasons (e.g., gender, socioeconomic status), and exposures to race-related stress or discrimination distress (which measure the response to racism) [9].
8. **E**. Moderation of the effect of racism on health by age, sex, education level, and birthplace of study participants has been inconclusive in systematic reviews and meta-analyses. Ethnicity, however, significantly moderates the association between racism and depression, negative mental health, and negative physical health. There is evidence that the association between racism and negative mental health is stronger for Asian Americans and Latin Americans than for African Americans and that the association between racism and physical health is stronger for Latin Americans than for African Americans [9].
9. **B**. Most HIV-related maternal deaths occur in sub-Saharan Africa, but Europe has the highest percentage of HIV-related maternal deaths as a subset of all maternal deaths. In 2017 (the most recent year with available statistics), sub-Saharan Africa accounted for the largest proportion (89%) of global HIV-related indirect maternal deaths: 3200 out of 3600. Europe, however, had by far the highest proportion of HIV-related maternal deaths as a subset of all maternal deaths at 8.9%. The next highest region was sub-Saharan Africa (1.6%),

compared with Western Asia (0.13%), and there were no HIV-related maternal deaths in Australia and New Zealand. The HIV-related maternal mortality ratio (MMR; maternal deaths per 100,000 live births) for sub-Saharan Africa in 2017 is high, estimated at nine maternal deaths per 100,000 live births, compared with one in Southeastern Asia, Latin America, and the Caribbean, Oceania (excluding Australia and New Zealand), and Europe, and 0 (zero) in all other subregions [10].

10. **C**. Compared with race-discordant visits, race-concordant visits are longer by approximately 2.2 min and have slower speech speed in the dialogue of both the patient and physician. Race-concordant visits also have higher positive patient affect than race-discordant visits. There is no significant difference in physician positive affect in the type of visit. There is no relationship between race concordance and patient-centered interviewing or physician verbal dominance. Patients in race-concordant visits rate their physicians as more participatory. Additionally, patients in race-concordant visits have a higher probability of strongly agreeing with the statements "Overall, I was satisfied with this visit" and "I would recommend this physician to a friend." [11]
11. **E**. The Hispanic paradox is sometimes used to describe the findings that Hispanic women in the United States have a lower proportion of peripartum hospitalizations and a lower severe maternal morbidity (SMM) prevalence during hospitalization than Black and White women. Despite having socioeconomic profiles that are comparable to Blacks, Hispanics in the United States have either comparable or improved rates of maternal and birth outcomes compared to White women and improved rates compared to Black women. The healthy immigrant effect (HIE) has been used to explain the Hispanic paradox and hypothesizes that healthier people are more likely to immigrate. This selection process makes immigrants stand out in terms of health levels when compared with the general population in their destination countries. This effect has been noted in studies examining immigrants in Australia, Canada, China, Mexico, the Netherlands, the United Kingdom, and the United States. Consistently, the HIE diminishes the longer the immigrant stays in the destination country. The "salmon" effect is a second explanation for the better health of immigrants and refers to the selective return of unhealthy immigrants. It is hypothesized that less healthy immigrants have a greater tendency to return to their original communities than healthier immigrants. There is less evidence for this explanation [12–14].
12. **D**. The most recent year with statistics for maternal deaths is 2017. Globally, the lifetime risk for a 15-year-old girl dying of maternal causes nearly halved between 2000 and 2017, from 1 in 100 in 2000 to 1 in 190 in 2017. There is wide variation by country. The estimated lifetime risk of maternal mortality for a 15-year-old girl in 2017 ranges from the highest-risk countries of Chad (1 in 15) and South Sudan (1 in 18) to the lowest-risk countries of Italy (1 in 51,300), Poland (1 in 30,300), and Greece (1 in 26,900). In North America (Canada and the United States), the risk is 1 in 3100 [10].

13. **A**. The decreased risk of severe maternal morbidity (SMM) associated with neuraxial analgesia is similar between White women and racial and ethnic minority women and between low-risk and high-risk women. Compared with women without labor neuraxial analgesia, women with labor neuraxial analgesia are more likely to be non-Hispanic White and have private health insurance, premature rupture of membranes, induced labor, or fetal heart rhythm abnormalities. Women with neuraxial labor analgesia are also likely to give birth in a high-volume teaching hospital and in a hospital with a higher utilization of neuraxial techniques. More than one-fifth of the association between neuraxial analgesia and the reduced risk of SMM is mediated through the decreased risk of postpartum hemorrhage [15].
14. **E**. As shown in Fig. 1, the highest percentage of cigarette smokers were mothers classified as non-Hispanic American or Alaska Natives, given CDC data from 2016 (the most recent year available): [16]
15. **C**. The mechanisms whereby racism, economic inequities, and nontraditional gender identities can lead to adverse health and pregnancy outcomes remain uncertain. One concept that is used to delineate the mechanisms that lead to adverse health outcomes is that of allostatic load. Allostatic load represents the cumulative burden of chronic physiological and psychological stress and can be measured by combining multiple biomarkers of systemic function into a single

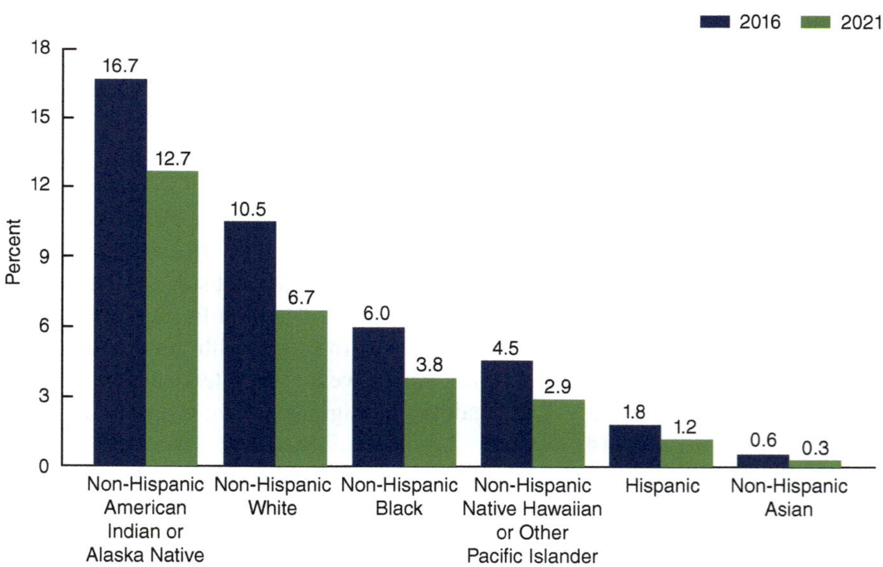

NOTES: Declines for all race and Hispanic-origin groups between 2016 and 2021 and differences between race and Hispanic-origin groups between 2016 and 2021 were significant ($p < 0.05$). Access data table for Figure 3 at: https://www.cdc.gov/nchs/data/databriefs/db458-tables.pdf#3.
SOURCE: National Center for Health Statistics. National Vital Statistics System, Natality.

Fig. 1 Percentage of mothers who smoked cigarettes during pregnancy, by race and Hispanic origin; United States, 2016 and 2021 (CDC) [16]

continuous index score of biologic risk. The markers used reflect the status of the cardiovascular, inflammatory, metabolic, and immune systems. Allostatic load is postulated to be an important cause of disparities in mental health, substance use, and chronic diseases. Women who identify as lesbian or bisexual have an increased allostatic load, which may be a cause of the increased risks of diabetes mellitus, hypertension, venous thromboembolism, myocardial infarction, and stroke. Consideration of elective cesarean section is appropriate for patients with gender dysphoria [17, 18].

16. **B**. Black women have higher rates of comorbid conditions than all other racial and ethnic groups, with 55% of Black women having no comorbidities compared to 67% of White women, 68% of Hispanic women, and 72% of Asian women. Compared to women with no comorbidities (rate = 48.5 per 10,000), there was an increased risk of severe maternal morbidity among women with one comorbidity (rate = 238.6; OR = 5.0), two comorbidities (rate = 379.9; OR = 8.1), and three or more comorbidities (rate = 560; OR = 12.1) [19].
17. **A**. US servicewomen have a higher rate of unintended pregnancy than civilian women. In 2011, the rate for the active-duty military was 72 per 1000 women aged 18–44; the rate for the general population was 45 per 1000 women aged 15–44. TRICARE is the military health insurance program for service members and their families. It covers abortion services only if the pregnancy is the result of an act of rape or incest or if the life of the mother is at risk. TRICARE does not cover services and supplies related to a noncovered abortion, such as counseling, referral, preparation, and follow-up for a noncovered abortion. TRICARE also does not cover abortions for fetal abnormality or for psychological reasons (**B**). Unintended pregnancy rates do not differ between women who were deployed in the previous 12 months and non-deployed women (**C**). There is no significant difference in unintended pregnancy rates in servicewomen who are White, Black, or Hispanic (**D**). The rate of unintended pregnancies per 1000 women is as follows: Air Force 50, Army 68, Coast Guard 32, Marine Corps 125, and Navy 95 (**E**) [20–23].
18. **E**. Except for individuals aged 35 or greater, non-Hispanic Asian parturients have the lowest rates of cesarean deliveries. For all age groups, non-Hispanic Black parturients have the highest rates of cesarean deliveries. These rates of cesarean deliveries are not adjusted for comorbidities [24].
19. **E**. Out of 17.4 obstetric deaths per 100,000 live births in 2018, there were 3.62 homicides per 100,000 live births among females who were pregnant or within 1 year postpartum. Homicide during pregnancy or within 42 days of the end of pregnancy exceeded all the leading causes of maternal mortality (such as hypertensive disorders, hemorrhage, and infection) by more than twofold. There is a significantly elevated homicide risk in the Black population and among girls and younger women (age 10–24 years) for all racial and ethnic subgroups. The perinatal period not only appears to increase the likelihood of experiencing violence, but injuries inflicted on pregnant females are more likely to be fatal. Rates of intimate partner homicide among females outside of the perinatal period were similar across White and Black populations. However, Black

females had a pregnancy-associated intimate partner homicide rate more than three times higher than that of White females and more than eight times higher than that of nonpregnant Black females [25].

20. **B**. Most studies show that Black healthcare providers are more likely to demonstrate no implicit bias than White healthcare providers and other minorities. Bias can exist on both explicit and implicit levels. Explicit bias encompasses our conscious attitudes, which can be measured by self-report. Implicit biases are unconscious and involuntary attitudes and can influence affect, behavior, and cognitive processes. A is false since there is limited, if any, evidence that education in implicit bias improves provider behavior, patient care delivery, and patient outcomes. More research is needed in this area. Higher implicit bias is associated with poorer patient-provider interactions (**C**). The small number of studies published does not consistently show that interventions to reduce implicit bias demonstrate post-intervention reduction in implicit bias (**D**) [26, 27].
21. **B**, **D**, **F**. Investigators at the CDC analyzed pregnancy-related deaths by combining data from 36 states from 2017 to 2019. Pregnancy-related deaths were defined as deaths that occurred during pregnancy, delivery, or up to 12 months postpartum. Although the leading cause of death differed based on race and ethnicity, investigators determined that over 80% of deaths were preventable. The leading causes of death were determined for the following populations: (1) in non-Hispanic Black patients, cardiac conditions (such as vascular heart disease, pulmonary hypertension, hypertensive disorders, and valvular heart disease), (2) in Hispanic and non-Hispanic White patients, mental health conditions (such as suicide or substance use disorder/overdose), and (3) in Asian patients, hemorrhage [28].
22. **D**, **E**. Low birth weight and unemployment were the most harmful indicators of maternal mortality in a county-level study published by the American College of Obstetrics and Gynecology (ACOG). Authors investigated individual vs population health factors that were associated with pregnancy-related mortality. Although several factors, such as maternal age, cesarean delivery, and obesity, contributed to disparities in pregnancy-related mortality, these conditions only partially explained the disparities, leading investigators to conclude that external factors such income inequality and unemployment can have broad and negative impacts on maternal health [29].
23. **B**. In 2021, 1205 women died of maternal causes in the United States compared with 861 in 2020 and 754 in 2019. The maternal mortality rate for 2021 was 32.9 deaths per 100,000 live births, compared with a rate of 23.8 in 2020 and 20.1 in 2019. In 2021, the maternal mortality rate in the United States for non-Hispanic Black (subsequently, Black) women was 69.9 deaths per 100,000 live births, 2.6 times the rate for non-Hispanic White women (26.6) [30, 31].
24. **E**. Healthcare providers have been shown to exhibit implicit biases that mirror those of the general population, that is, implicit positive bias toward White patients and a negative bias toward patients of color. The difference in care and experience in the healthcare system can include differences in wait times, visit

length, and management based on perceived patient adherence and addressing postpartum pain. Despite numerous studies delineating the disparity in care, educational interventions at all levels of training and practice are needed to make physicians aware of their own biases and deliver tools to improve patient care and communication [32–39].

25. **D**. Per the CDC, racial/ethnic disparities were noted during 2016–2018, and there were 41.4 deaths per 100,000 live births for non-Hispanic Black persons. This is 4× the rate of non-Hispanic White persons at 13.7 deaths per 100,000 [40].
26. **C**. Based on the US Department of Health and Human Services/Centers for Disease Control and Prevention MMWR published in September 2019, 13 state maternal mortality review committees showed that 60% of pregnancy-related deaths were preventable. Per the CDC, the definition of preventability is preventable if the committee determines that there was some chance of the death being averted by one or more reasonable changes to the patient, community, provider, health facility, and/or system factors [28].
27. **A**. Mental health conditions are the leading cause of pregnancy-related death in Hispanic women accounting for 24.1% of deaths. Hemorrhage is the second leading cause of death at 21.3%. Cardiac disease/coronary conditions and infection are third with 10.6% of each accounting for peripartum mortality in this population. These trends are similar to the overall population data; however, peripartum hemorrhage contributing to death is considerably higher in Hispanic women than the overall mortality of 13.7% from peripartum hemorrhage [28].
28. **B**. Per the World Health Organization, maternal death is defined as within 42 days of termination of pregnancy. Late maternal death occurs after 42 days but less than 1 year after the termination of pregnancy. They include both direct and indirect maternal/obstetric deaths. The 42 days was chosen for the 6-week postpartum period [41].

References

1. Hoyert DL. Maternal mortality rates in the United States, 2020. NCHS Health E-Stats. 2022. https://doi.org/10.15620/cdc:113967.
2. Sufrin C, Beal L, Clarke J, Jones R, Mosher WD. Pregnancy Outcomes in US Prisons, 2016–2017. Am J Public Health. 2019;109(5):799–805. https://doi.org/10.2105/AJPH.2019.305006. Epub 2019 Mar 21. Erratum in: Am J Public Health. 2020;110(2):e1.
3. Sufrin C, Jones RK, Mosher WD, Beal L. Pregnancy prevalence and outcomes in U.S. jails. Obstet Gynecol. 2020;135(5):1177–83. https://doi.org/10.1097/AOG.0000000000003834.
4. Chambers BD, Baer RJ, McLemore MR, Jelliffe-Pawlowski LL. Using index of concentration at the extremes as indicators of structural racism to evaluate the association with preterm birth and infant mortality-California, 2011–2012. J Urban Health. 2019;96(2):159–70. https://doi.org/10.1007/s11524-018-0272-4.
5. Curtis DS, Fuller-Rowell TE, Carlson DL, Wen M, Kramer MR. Does a rising median income lift all birth weights? County median income changes and low birth weight rates Among births to black and white mothers. Milbank Q. 2022;100(1):38–77. https://doi.org/10.1111/1468-0009.12532. Epub 2021 Oct 5

6. Sheppard AJ, Shapiro GD, Bushnik T, Wilkins R, Perry S, Kaufman JS, Kramer MS, Yang S. Birth outcomes among first nations, Inuit and Métis populations. Health Rep. 2017;28(11):11–6.
7. Shah PS, Zao J, Al-Wassia H, Shah V, Knowledge Synthesis Group on Determinants of Preterm/LBW Births. Pregnancy and neonatal outcomes of aboriginal women: a systematic review and meta-analysis. Womens Health Issues. 2011;21(1):28–39. https://doi.org/10.1016/j.whi.2010.08.005. Epub 2010 Dec 3.
8. Bodnar L, Hutcheon J. Are detailed behavioral, psychosocial, and environmental variables necessary to control for confounding in pregnancy weight gain research? Epidemiology. 2023;34(1):56–63. https://doi.org/10.1097/EDE.0000000000001556.
9. Paradies Y, Ben J, Denson N, Elias A, Priest N, Pieterse A, Gupta A, Kelaher M, Gee G. Racism as a determinant of health: a systematic review and meta-analysis. PLoS One. 2015;10(9):e0138511. https://doi.org/10.1371/journal.pone.0138511.
10. UNFPA, World Health Organization, UNICEF, World Bank Group, the United Nations Population Division. Trends in maternal mortality: 2000 to 2017. Geneva: Estimates by WHO, UNICEF, UNFPA, World Bank Group and the United Nations Population Division. https://www.unfpa.org/publications/trends-maternal-mortality-2000-2017. Accessed 20 Feb 2023.
11. Cooper LA, Roter DL, Johnson RL, Ford DE, Steinwachs DM, Powe NR. Patient-centered communication, ratings of care, and concordance of patient and physician race. Ann Intern Med. 2003;139(11):907–15. https://doi.org/10.7326/0003-4819-139-11-200312020-00009.
12. Kennedy S, Kidd MP, McDonald JT, et al. The healthy immigrant effect: patterns and evidence from four countries. Int Migr Integr. 2015;16:317–32. https://doi.org/10.1007/s12134-014-0340-x.
13. Puschmann P, Donrovich R, Matthijs K. Salmon bias or red herring? Comparing adult mortality risks (ages 30-90) between natives and internal migrants: stayers, returnees and movers in Rotterdam, The Netherlands, 1850–1940. Hum Nat. 2017;28(4):481–99. https://doi.org/10.1007/s12110-017-9303-1.
14. Lu Y, Qin L. Healthy migrant and salmon bias hypotheses: a study of health and internal migration in China. Soc Sci Med. 2014;102:41–8. https://doi.org/10.1016/j.socscimed.2013.11.040. Epub 2013 Nov 28
15. Guglielminotti J, Landau R, Daw J, Friedman AM, Chihuri S, Li G. Use of labor Neuraxial analgesia for vaginal delivery and severe maternal morbidity. JAMA Netw Open. 2022;5(2):e220137. https://doi.org/10.1001/jamanetworkopen.2022.0137.
16. Martin JA, Osterman MJK, Driscoll AK. Declines in cigarette smoking during pregnancy in the United States, 2016–2021. NCHS Data Brief, no 458. Hyattsville, MD: National Center for Health Statistics; 2023. https://doi.org/10.15620/cdc:123360.
17. Ejiogu NI. LGBTQ+ health and anesthesia for obstetric and gynecological procedures. Curr Opin Anesthesiol. 2022;35(3):292–8. https://doi.org/10.1097/ACO.0000000000001134.
18. Lueth AJ, Allshouse AA, Blue NM, Grobman WA, Levine LD, Simhan HN, Kim JK, Johnson J, Wilson FA, Murtaugh M, Silver RM, National Institutes of Health (NIH), Eunice Kennedy Shriver National Institute of Child Health and Human Development (NICHD), Nulliparous Pregnancy Outcomes Study: Monitoring Mothers-to-Be (nuMoM2b), and National Heart, Lung, and Blood Institute (NHLBI) nuMoM2b Heart Health Study (nuMoM2b-HHS). Allostatic load and adverse pregnancy outcomes. Obstet Gynecol. 2022;140(6):974–82. https://doi.org/10.1097/AOG.0000000000004971. Epub 2022 Nov 2.
19. Brown CC, Adams CE, George KE, Moore JE. Associations between comorbidities and severe maternal morbidity. Obstet Gynecol. 2020;136(5):892–901. https://doi.org/10.1097/AOG.0000000000004057.
20. Defense Health Agency: Home | TRICARE. Fall Church, VA: Defense Health Agency; Abortions | TRICARE; 2022. https://tricare.mil/CoveredServices/IsItCovered/Abortions.
21. Grindlay K, Seymour JW, Fix L, Reiger S, Keefe-Oates B, Grossman D. Abortion knowledge and experiences among U.S. servicewomen: a qualitative study. Perspect Sex Reprod Health. 2017;49(4):245–52. https://doi.org/10.1363/psrh.12044. Epub 2017 Nov 15.

22. Grindlay K, Grossman D. Unintended pregnancy among active-duty women in the United States military, 2011. Contraception. 2015;92(6):589–95. https://doi.org/10.1016/j.contraception.2015.07.015. Epub 2015 Sep 4
23. Hamrick JE, Ahmed AE, Witkop CT, Manetz KE, Mancuso JD. Unintended pregnancy among U.S. military active duty servicemembers: estimates for 2018 and trends since 2005. Contraception. 2023;119:109894. https://doi.org/10.1016/j.contraception.2022.09.132. Epub 2022 Oct 13.
24. Agency for Healthcare Research and Quality. 2022 National Healthcare Quality and Disparities Report. 2023. https://www.ahrq.gov/research/findings/nhqrdr/nhqdr22/index.html. Accessed 24 Feb 2023.
25. Wallace M, Gillispie-Bell V, Cruz K, Davis K, Vilda D. Homicide during pregnancy and the postpartum period in the United States, 2018–2019. Obstet Gynecol. 2021;138(5):762–9. https://doi.org/10.1097/AOG.0000000000004567. Erratum in: Obstet Gynecol. 2022 Feb 1;139(2):347.
26. Maina IW, Belton TD, Ginzberg S, Singh A, Johnson TJ. A decade of studying implicit racial/ethnic bias in healthcare providers using the implicit association test. Soc Sci Med. 2018;199:219–29. https://doi.org/10.1016/j.socscimed.2017.05.009. Epub 2017 May 4.
27. Mavis SC, Caruso CG, Dyess NF, Carr CB, Gerberi D, Dadiz R. Implicit bias training in health professions education: a scoping review. Med Sci Educ. 2022;32(6):1541–52. https://doi.org/10.1007/s40670-022-01673-z.
28. Trost SL, Beauregard J, Njie F, et al. Pregnancy-related deaths: data from maternal mortality review committees in 36 US states, 2017–2019. Atlanta, GA: Centers for Disease Control and Prevention, US Department of Health and Human Services; 2022.
29. Barrera CM, Kramer MR, Merkt PT, Petersen EE, Brantley MD, Eckhaus L, Beauregard JL, Goodman DA. County-level associations between pregnancy-related mortality ratios and contextual sociospatial indicators. Obstet Gynecol. 2022;139(5):855–65. https://doi.org/10.1097/AOG.0000000000004749. Epub 2022 Apr 5.
30. Munira Z. Gunja, Evan D. Gumas, and Reginald D. Williams II. In: The U.S. maternal mortality crisis continues to worsen: an international comparison, To the Point (blog), Commonwealth Fund; 2022. https://doi.org/10.26099/8vem-fc65.
31. U.S. Department of Health & Human Services. Centers for Disease Control and Prevention. National Center for Health Statistics. Maternal mortality rates in the United States, 2021. https://www.cdc.gov/nchs/data/hestat/maternal-mortality/2021/maternal-mortality-rates-2021.htm. Accessed 17 Mar 2023.
32. FitzGerald C, Hurst S. Implicit bias in healthcare professionals: a systematic review. BMC Med Ethics. 2017;18:19.
33. Chapman EN, Kaatz A, Carnes M. Physicians and implicit bias: how doctors may unwittingly perpetuate healthcare disparities. J Gen Intern Med. 2013;28:1504–10.
34. Hall WJ, Chapman MV, Lee KM, et al. Implicit racial/ethnic bias among healthcare professionals and its influence on healthcare outcomes: a systematic review. Am J Public Health. 2015;105:e60–76.
35. Yee LM, Liu LY, Sakowicz A, et al. Racial and ethnic disparities in use of 17-alpha hydroxyprogesterone caproate for prevention of preterm birth. Am J Obstet Gynecol. 2016;214:374.e1–6.
36. Butwick AJ, Blumenfeld YJ, Brookfield KF, Nelson LM, Weiniger CF. Racial and ethnic disparities in mode of anesthesia for cesarean delivery. Anesth Analg. 2016;122(2):472–9. https://doi.org/10.1213/ANE.0000000000000679.
37. Cintron A, Morrison RS. Pain and ethnicity in the United States: a systematic review. J Palliat Med. 2006;9:1454–73.
38. Badreldin N, Grobman WA, Yee LM. Racial disparities in postpartum pain management. Obstet Gynecol. 2019;134:1147–53.

39. Hoffman KM, Trawalter S, Axt JR, Oliver MN. Racial bias in pain assessment and treatment recommendations, and false beliefs about biological differences between blacks and whites. Proc Natl Acad Sci USA. 2016;113(16):4296–301. https://doi.org/10.1073/pnas.1516047113. Epub 2016 Apr 4
40. Centers for Disease Control and Prevention. Pregnancy mortality surveillance system. 2022. https://www.cdc.gov/reproductivehealth/maternal-mortality/pregnancy-mortality-surveillance-system.htm.
41. World Health Organization. Infant mortality rate (probability of dying between birth and age 1 per 1000 live births). WHO. https://www.who.int/data/gho/indicator-metadata-registry/imr-details/4622.

Obstetric Care in Developing Countries

Maria Acosta de Gonzalez and Ashley Beem

Questions

1. **A G4P3003 at 26w0d presents to prenatal care reporting extreme fatigue. Upon chart review you notice that the patient has lost 6 pounds from pre-pregnancy weight. Upon examination the patient has decreased skin turgor and has diminished fat tissue. What is the most common diagnosis in developing countries?**
   A. Maternal iron-deficiency anemia
   B. Malaria
   C. Leishmaniasis
   D. Schistosomiasis
2. **What is the most common parasitic infection in pregnancy?**
   A. *Trichuris trichiura* (whipworm)
   B. *Ascaris lumbricoides* (roundworm)
   C. *Entamoeba histolytica*
   D. *Ancylostoma duodenale* (hookworm)
3. **What is the most common cause of pregnancy-related death in low-income countries?**
   A. Ruptured ectopic pregnancy
   B. Pregnancy-induced hypertensive disorders pregnancy
   C. Postpartum hemorrhage
   D. Sepsis

M. A. de Gonzalez
Loma Linda University Health, Loma Linda, CA, USA

A. Beem (✉)
Loma Linda OBGYN Residency Program, Linda School of Medicine, Loma Linda, CA, USA

Riverside University Health System, Moreno Valley, CA, USA
e-mail: a.beem@ruhealth.org

A. C. Sinha, I. F. Pasca (eds.), *Peripartum Care of the Pregnant Patient*,
https://doi.org/10.1007/978-3-031-62756-9_46

4. **Which is the most common cause of intrauterine growth restriction worldwide?**
   A. Preeclampsia
   B. Malaria
   C. Malnutrition
   D. Fetal malformations
5. **What factor/factors plays/play an important role in the high primary cesarean section rate in Latin America?**
   A. Cultural preferences
   B. Lack of access to continuous fetal heart monitoring
   C. Inability to safely titrate oxytocin
   D. All the above
6. **What is the most common dermatosis in pregnant patients in developing countries?**
   A. Gestational pemphigoid (also known as pemphigoid gestations).
   B. Pruritic and urticarial papules and plaques of pregnancy (PUPPP, also known as pruritic eruption of pregnancy and toxemic rash of pregnancy).
   C. Intrahepatic cholestasis of pregnancy.
   D. Impetigo herpetiformis.
   E. Atopic eruption of pregnancy encompasses atopic eczema in pregnancy, prurigo of pregnancy, as well as pruritic folliculitis of pregnancy in earlier classifications.
   F. Scabies.
7. **What is/are the indication/indications for treatment of tuberculosis during pregnancy?**
   A. HIV patients with positive screening test and recent exposure to a patient with active respiratory TB
   B. HIV patients with positive screening test and recent conversion (within 2 years) of a test for TB infection from negative to positive
   C. HIV patients in a high TB transmission setting (countries with incidence more than 500 cases per 100,000)
   D. Active tuberculosis disease
   E. All the above
8. **Which is the most common gynecological cancer in developing countries that can also be seen in pregnant women?**
   A. Cervical cancer
   B. Endometrial cancer
   C. Vulvar cancer
   D. Ovarian cancer
9. **Which country has the highest maternal mortality ratio (MMR)?**
   A. Cambodia
   B. Venezuela
   C. Haiti
   D. South Sudan

10. **What factor/factors contributes/contribute to the high maternal mortality ratios in African countries?**
    A. Poverty
    B. Inadequate access to healthcare
    C. Political unrest
    D. Medical comorbidities
    E. All the above (multifactorial)
11. **Basic Emergency Obstetric Care (BEmOC) facilities in low-income countries can provide the following except:**
    A. Assisted vaginal delivery
    B. Blood transfusion
    C. IV/IM uterotonics
    D. Parenteral anticonvulsants
12. **What is the most common worldwide indication for peripartum ICU admission?**
    A. Preeclampsia
    B. Hemorrhage
    C. Cardiomyopathy
    D. Infections
13. **Uncomplicated malaria in pregnancy should receive which treatment?**
    A. Atovaquone-proguanil
    B. Isoniazid
    C. Sulfadoxine-pyrimethamine
    D. Artemisinin-based combination therapy
14. **What are the WHO estimates for worldwide maternal sepsis rates?**
    A. 2%
    B. 4%
    C. 8%
    D. 16%
15. **What is the most common cause for worldwide maternal sepsis?**
    A. Episiotomy
    B. Blood transfusion
    C. Cesarean section
    D. Manual placental extraction

Answers and Explanations

1. **A**. Up to 52% of parturients in developing countries have iron-deficiency anemia with Hgb levels less than 11 g/dL. Anemia in developing countries may be complicated by acute on chronic malnutrition and depleted reserves of proteins and micronutrients like zinc. With iron supplementation alone, the hematologic system may not have the nutrients necessary to increase hemoglobin production. In countries with limited food reserves, mothers with children at home often prioritize the feeding of children above their own nutrition. These patients

may need admission for nutritional recovery until they can safely be discharged [1].

2. **B**. A very common situation in low- and middle-income countries is parasitic infections, occurring in 24–70% of pregnant women, due to widespread fecal water source contamination. In certain areas this is so common that pregnant patients will take medication to deworm even without an ova and parasite test. This deworming treatment provides maximum coverage against the two biggest families of GI parasites helminths and protozoa. The medication used first line is albendazole for helminths, metronidazole for protozoans, and praziquantel for *Schistosoma*, used mainly in the second and third trimester [2].
3. **C**. Statistics from the WHO show that 99% of the nearly half-million annual worldwide maternal mortalities are from developing countries. These countries have limited access to uterotonic medication necessary to decrease maternal mortality from hemorrhage. Access to oxytocin, methylergonovine, and carboprost is largely unavailable in several low-income countries due to heat lability and the necessity for IV or IM routes. One option that is thermostable and can be given orally, rectally, or vaginally is misoprostol that is more readily available although less effective uterotonic for decreasing postpartum hemorrhage. Malnutrition, home labor and birth, grand multiparity, and limited access to blood products also play an important role in the incidence and ultimate obstetric morbidity and mortality rates in low-income countries [3].
4. **B**. Malaria is a common diagnosis in several countries in equatorial Africa and Latin America where cases are endemic throughout the year. The pathogen *Plasmodium falciparum* (most deadly) is transmitted by mosquito sporozoites. Pregnant patients who become infected commonly develop placental abnormalities with breakdown of syncytiotrophoblasts and abnormal placental development that leads to intrauterine growth restriction (IUGR). Patients with malaria also develop severe anemia decreasing fetal perfusion and further restricting fetal growth [4].
5. **D**. The primary cesarean rate can be as high as 45% in Latin America and some Caribbean countries. Multiple factors play an important role in this reality including patient autonomy and elective primary cesarean section requests for personal reasons. In some countries like Venezuela, higher socioeconomic status patients will request cesarean section because of concerns with sexual dysfunction and distorted vaginal anatomy after a vaginal delivery. Other factors that impact increased cesarean delivery are lack of access to continuous fetal heart monitoring especially in the setting of oligohydramnios, gastroschisis, and IUGR with abnormal Dopplers. Another common scenario is lack of drug pumps that makes titration of oxytocin difficult with higher incidence of intrapartum fetal intolerance to labor [5].
6. **F**. Scabies is highly prevalent in tropical areas with poor access to water, making mothers and children highly susceptible to this infection which can cause streptococcal and staphylococcal superinfections. Fear of receiving treatment as well as the complexity of treatment adds to the 2–6% prevalence of scabies infection in observational studies. To successfully treat scabies patients, patients

need to place the treatment head to toe with permethrin, wash all their clothes with hot water or dryer, rid their house of scabies, and deep clean the mattress they use [6].

7. **E**. Approximately one fourth of the world population has tuberculosis (TB). Pregnancy does not change susceptibility to tuberculosis or conversion from latent to active state. The symptoms of pregnancy mimic those of tuberculosis with increased weakness, weight loss, and shortness of breath. Criteria for the treatment of tuberculosis during pregnancy are active tuberculosis on symptomatic patients with positive sputum acid-fast bacilli smear, positive sputum nucleic acid amplification test, or upper lobe infiltrate in an individual with relevant risk factors. Risk factors include HIV patient and recent exposure to a patient with active respiratory TB [7].
8. **A**. Multiple factors determine the fact that cervical cancer is the most common gynecological cancer in developing countries. One of the most important is lack of access to the HPV vaccine. This is due to low treatment affordability imposed by pharmaceuticals in the country, government restrictions, fear of potential side effects, or lack of coverage from insurance. Other factors include early age to start sexual intercourse, likely in certain countries of Africa where girls that start to menstruate are given in marriage, high incidence of non-appropriately treated HIV, lack of access to Pap smear or visual inspection, and lack of access to HPV DNA testing [8].
9. **D**. As a continent, Africa has the worst maternal mortality ratios, and South Sudan is the country with the highest peripartum mortality with 2054 deaths per 100,000 live births. Out of the top 20 highest maternal mortality ratio countries, 19 are in Africa. For comparison the United States has a maternal mortality ratio of 21/100,000 live births. Italy has a rate of 5/100,000 live births [9].
10. **E**. The African continent has some of the highest maternal mortality rates on the planet. The reasons are variable and multifactorial. The United Nations Sustainable Development Goals are working toward global maternal mortality rates, MMR, lower than 70 per 100,000 births. Socioeconomic status, parity, and living in rural areas influence maternal mortality as well as civil wars, insurgencies, and political upheavals. In addition to obstetric causes such as preeclampsia and postpartum hemorrhage, non-obstetric causes also play a role in maternal mortality. These include conditions such as malaria, tuberculosis, and HIV [10].
11. **B**. Basic Emergency Obstetric Care (BEmOC) facilities have been promoted to address high maternal mortality in low-income countries. These BEmOC facilities provide six signal functions including (1) removal of retained products, (2) assisted removal of the placenta, (3) assisted vaginal delivery, (4) IV/IM antibiotics, (5) IV/IM anticonvulsants, and (6) IV/IM uterotonics. The Comprehensive Emergency Obstetric Care (CEmOC) facilities can provide these six core functions in addition to providing blood transfusion and cesarean delivery [9].
12. **B**. The most common indication for peripartum ICU admission worldwide is hemorrhage which is also one of the most common causes for peripartum mortality. Preeclampsia and hypertensive disorders are also a major factor for ICU

admission. Worldwide variations occur due to social and economic infrastructures that impact maternal healthcare. Maternal mortality is also heavily impacted by the disease patterns and the healthcare infrastructure present [11].

13. **D**. Malaria in pregnancy is associated with an increased risk of abortion, stillbirth, and low birth weight due to placental red cell sequestration and compromised perfusion to the developing fetus. Malaria prophylaxis with sulfadoxine-pyrimethamine in pregnancy is recommended as part of antenatal care in all malaria-endemic areas (**C**) [12]. In the non-obstetric population, atovaquone-proguanil is the recommended antimalarial prophylaxis (**A**) [13]. Isoniazid is a tuberculosis medication (**B**). The WHO recommends all second or third trimester pregnant women infected with *P. falciparum* malaria to be treated with artemisinin-based therapy which includes a combination of short-acting artemisinin (artesunate, artemether, or dihydroartemisinin) and a long-acting antimalarial drug (lumefantrine, piperaquine, mefloquine, or amodiaquine). The short-acting artemisinin component decreases the parasite burden for the first 3 days, and the long-acting component eliminates the remaining parasites and prevents new infections. The PREGACT trial studied uncomplicated *P. falciparum* malaria in pregnant women and revealed cure rates of 94.8 to 99.2% with mild drug-related adverse events. The reported placental malaria rate was highest in the sulfadoxine-pyrimethamine treatment group at 50% and lowest in the dihydroartemisinin-piperaquine group at 27% [12].
14. **B**. Worldwide maternal sepsis is estimated at 5.7 million cases per year. Maternal sepsis occurs in 4.4% of live births with the highest incidence in low- and middle-income countries at 7%. Despite antibiotic prophylaxis recommendations from the WHO, infection remains a leading cause of peripartum mortality, accounting for 10% of deaths from the onset of labor to the 42nd postpartum day [14].
15. **C**. The most common global cause for peripartum infection is cesarean section for which the WHO recommends surgical aseptic techniques and the use of prophylactic antibiotics. Globally, the use of prophylactic antibiotics, with a single dose of first-generation cephalosporin or penicillin, before incision varies widely among institutions, and surgical site infections occur in 2–7% of cesarean sections [15]. Furthermore, the WHO recommends that prophylactic antibiotics be given before skin incision rather than after umbilical cord clamping for women undergoing elective or emergency cesarean although during emergencies the antibiotics are also effective after cord clamping. Antibiotics were also recommended for third-degree or fourth-degree perineal tear after vaginal birth and for manual placental extraction. Postpartum infections after spontaneous and induced abortions account for 34% of deaths in this population [15]. Antibiotics are not recommended for uncomplicated vaginal births, episiotomy, or assisted vaginal birth with forceps or vacuum [14].

References

1. Abu-Ouf NM, Jan MM. The impact of maternal iron deficiency and iron deficiency anemia on child's health. Saudi Med J. 2015;36(2):146–9.
2. Vasconcelos A, Sousa S, Bandeira N, Alves M, Papoila AL, Pereira F, Machado MC. Intestinal parasitic infections, treatment and associated factors among pregnant women in Sao Tome and Principe: a cross-sectional study. J Trop Med. 2022;2022:7492020. https://doi.org/10.1155/2022/7492020.
3. Snelgrove JW. Postpartum haemorrhage in the developing world a review of clinical management strategies. Mcgill J Med. 2009;12(2):61.
4. Chua CLL, Khoo SKM, Ong JLE, Ramireddi GK, Yeo TW, Teo A. Malaria in pregnancy: from placental infection to its abnormal development and damage. Front Microbiol. 2021;12:777343. https://doi.org/10.3389/fmicb.2021.777343.
5. Betran AP, Ye J, Moller AB, Souza JP, Zhang J. Trends and projections of caesarean section rates: global and regional estimates. BMJ Glob Health. 2021;6(6):e005671. https://doi.org/10.1136/bmjgh-2021-005671.
6. Weill A, Bernigaud C, Mokni M, Gil S, Elefant E, Chosidow O. Scabies-infested pregnant women: a critical therapeutic challenge. PLoS Negl Trop Dis. 2021;15(1):e0008929. https://doi.org/10.1371/journal.pntd.0008929.
7. Miele K, Bamrah Morris S, Tepper NK. Tuberculosis in pregnancy. Obstet Gynecol. 2020;135(6):1444–53. https://doi.org/10.1097/AOG.0000000000003890.
8. Ebrahimi N, Yousefi Z, Khosravi G, Malayeri FE, Golabi M, Askarzadeh M, Shams MH, Ghezelbash B, Eskandari N. Human papillomavirus vaccination in low- and middle-income countries: progression, barriers, and future prospective. Front Immunol. 2023;14:1150238. https://doi.org/10.3389/fimmu.2023.1150238.
9. Dahab R, Sakellariou D. Barriers to accessing maternal care in low income countries in Africa: a systematic review. Int J Environ Res Public Health. 2020;17(12):4292. https://doi.org/10.3390/ijerph17124292.
10. Onambele L, Ortega-Leon W, Guillen-Aguinaga S, Forjaz MJ, Yoseph A, Guillen-Aguinaga L, Alas-Brun R, Arnedo-Pena A, Aguinaga-Ontoso I, Guillen-Grima F. Maternal mortality in Africa: regional trends (2000–2017). Int J Environ Res Public Health. 2022;19(20):13146. https://doi.org/10.3390/ijerph192013146.
11. Bajwa SK, Bajwa SJ. Delivering obstetrical critical care in developing nations. Int J Crit Illn Inj Sci. 2012;2(1):32–9. https://doi.org/10.4103/2229-5151.94897.
12. Tarning J. Treatment of malaria in pregnancy. N Engl J Med. 2016;374(10):981–2. https://doi.org/10.1056/NEJMe1601193.
13. Freedman D. Malaria prevention in short-term travelers. N Engl J Med. 2008;359:603–12. https://doi.org/10.1056/NEJMcp0803572.
14. Bonet M, Oladapo OT, Khan DN, Matthews Mathai A, Gülmezoglu M. New WHO guidance on prevention and treatment of maternal peripartum infections. Lancet. 2015;3(11):E667–8. https://doi.org/10.1016/S2214-109X(15)00213-2.
15. Boushra M, Rahman O. Postpartum infection. In: StatPearls. Treasure Island, FL: StatPearls Publishing; 2023. https://www.ncbi.nlm.nih.gov/books/NBK560804/.

Simulation and Educational Principles in Obstetric Anesthesiology

Anju Grewal, Gegal Pruthi, and Hemanth Kumar

Questions

1. **Obstetric phantom developed** by **Angelique Marguerite Le Boursier du Coudray to teach midwives and surgeons used____.**
   A. Animal models
   B. Cloth birth simulators
   C. Hard wood simulators
   D. Leather doll simulators
2. **The medical equivalent of LOFT (Line-Oriented Flight Training), the highest level of simulation in the aviation model, in obstetric care, is:**
   A. TOMS
   B. PediaSIM
   C. US LapTrainer
   D. KISMET
3. **Which one of the following statements is false?**
   A. Successful crisis resource management (CRM) enhances team performance.
   B. Nontechnical skills when added to technical skills improve patient outcomes.
   C. Crisis resource management (CRM) eliminates human error.
   D. Cost and access are main barriers to implementing simulation-based education (SBE).
4. **The debriefing model consists of all the following except:**
   A. Discovery
   B. Deepening
   C. Defusing
   D. Developing

A. Grewal (✉) · G. Pruthi · H. Kumar
Department of Anaesthesiology and Critical Care, AIIMS Bathinda, Bathinda, Punjab, India

A. C. Sinha, I. F. Pasca (eds.), *Peripartum Care of the Pregnant Patient*,
https://doi.org/10.1007/978-3-031-62756-9_47

5. **______ is defined as the potential severity of an event and its subsequent impact on the patient.**

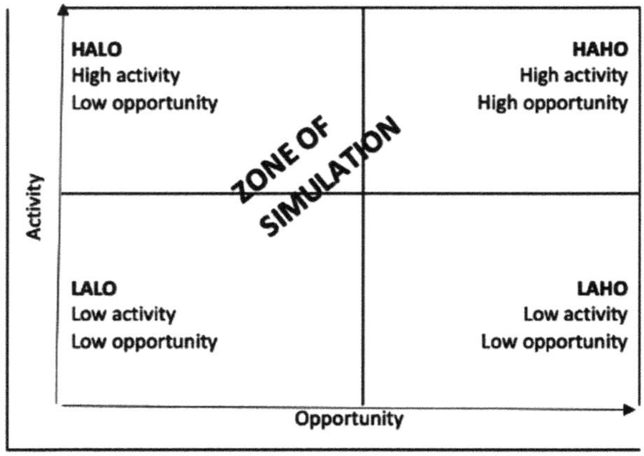

   A. Opportunity
   B. Efficacy
   C. Acuity
   D. Adversity

6. **With respect to the context of the zone of simulation in obstetric anesthesia, opportunity is defined as ____.**

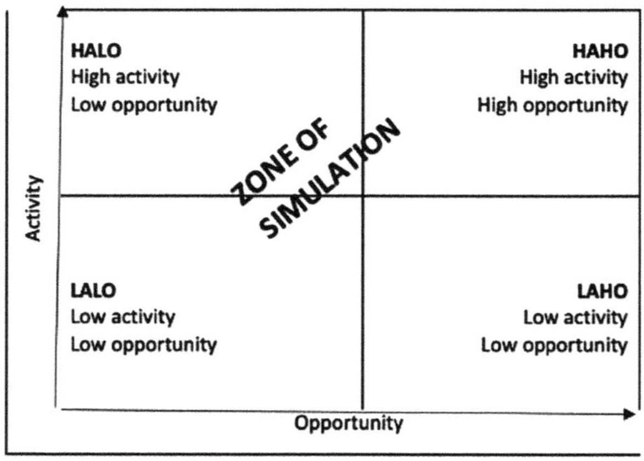

A. Impact of an event on the patient
B. Potential severity of a series of events
C. Frequency in which a certain department or individual is involved in management of the event
D. Threshold for knowledge retention in an individual

7. **Maternal ACLS comes under which zone of simulation?**
   A. High acuity low opportunity
   B. High acuity high opportunity
   C. Low acuity low opportunity
   D. Low acuity high opportunity
8. **A 27-year-old female G2P1L1 with 38 weeks' gestational age must undergo cesarean section in view of fetal bradycardia with meconium-stained amniotic fluid. This simulation in obstetric anesthesia lies in which zone of simulation?**

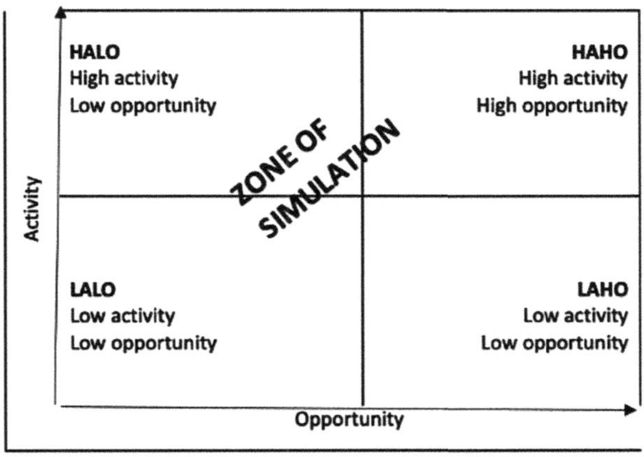

   A. HALO
   B. HAHO
   C. LALO
   D. LAHO
9. **Bloom's cognitive domain does not include the following:**
   A. Understanding
   B. Teaching
   C. Application
   D. Evaluation
E. Synthesis
10. **Which of the following simulations in obstetric anesthesia care has the better outcome?**
   A. High-fidelity manikin-based simulation
   B. Tele simulation-based training
   C. Low-fidelity haptic simulators
   D. Mental imagery training
11. **All the following are true <u>except</u>:**
   A. In situ drills to teach teamwork preserve the culture of safety in obstetric units
   B. Simulation improves the performance of complex procedures such as emergency cricothyroidotomy

   C. A single simulation session does not improve the outcome of the acquisition of technical skills in obstetric anesthesia
   D. Review articles and simulation instructional articles are useful for the spread of simulation in obstetric anesthesia care

12. **The SBAR technique is used for:**
   A. Debriefing of the entire simulation process
   B. Effective communication during emergency cesarean section simulation
   C. Practices of sign-offs and handovers during practice drills
   D. Psychomotor skill training
13. **All the following are drills advocated for use by labor and delivery staff undergoing team training except:**
   A. HELLP syndrome
   B. Anaphylaxis
   C. Failed tracheal intubation
   D. Elective cesarean section
   E. Postpartum hemorrhage
14. **Simulation in obstetric anesthesia helps in the improvement of all the following except:**
   A. Teamwork
   B. Effective communication between workers
   C. Patient and environment safety
   D. Long-term retention of knowledge and skills
15. **Choose the advantage of simulation for research, training, and performance assessment from the following:**
   A. Risk to patients.
   B. The underlying causes of the situation are unknown.
   C. Clinicians do not get exposed to actual medical equipment in manikin-based simulators.
   D. Intrusive recording of simulation sessions is not feasible due to patient confidentiality.
   E. Interpersonal interactions with other clinical staff can be explored.
16. **For the newly joined anesthesia residents, a faculty member wishes to organize an emergent rapid sequence intubation simulation session during the workday. Which of the following debriefing models may be best suited for this scenario**?
   A. Seven-step Team-Guided team self-correction, Advocacy-Inquiry, and Systemic-constructivist (TeamGAINS) model.
   B. Facilitator-guided Promoting Excellence and Reflective Learning in Simulation (PEARLS) model.
   C. Learner-guided diamond debriefing method.
   D. Debriefing would provide limited benefit while practicing.
17. **A first-year anesthesiology resident is paged to code in the PACU. There were no other physicians at that time, and he found the patient to be unresponsive and pulseless. The resident had never run code before. However, fortunately, he carries their ACLS cognitive aid with him in his apron. All**

the following features of the cognitive aids would be helpful to him in this high-acuity situation except:
   A. Color-coded algorithms for different cardiac arrhythmias
   B. Clustering of information into boxes
   C. An unformatted list of steps including complex-level reasoning for each step
   D. Simple illustrations accompanying steps requiring physical measures

18. **All the following depict the best suited characteristics for low-fidelity simulation except:**
   A. Remote areas
   B. Large group of people need to be trained over a short period of time
   C. Limited resources or in situations where a large group of people need to be trained over a short period of time
   D. Institutional setup for already trained healthcare workers

19. **Multidisciplinary obstetric simulated emergency scenarios (MOSES) involve participation of:**
   A. Real obstetric surgeons
   B. Anesthesia providers
   C. Midwives
   D. All the above

Answers and Explanations

1. **B**. With *La Machine (a cloth birth simulator)*, one of the first obstetric phantoms, Madame du Coudray taught thousands of midwives and even physicians [1].
2. **A**. TOMS, Team-Oriented Medical Simulation, emphasizes the combined performance of the whole operating team during critical events [2]. (**B**) PediaSIM is a simulator of a 6-year-old patient with a comprehensive set of clinical features for trauma, nursing, and emergency response. (**C**) LapTrainer is a simple laparoscopic training box. (**D**) KISMET is a knowledge-based system for the simulation of discrete manufacturing operations.
3. **C**. The aim of CRM is to strengthen a system to support human performance throughout (**A**), including in unanticipated events, without eliminating human error [3]. CRM refers to a set of principles dealing with cognitive and interpersonal behaviors that contribute to optimal team performance. Adding nontechnical skills (NTS) to technical skills in simulation (**B**) could improve the patient's outcome. NTS are made up of individual cognitive skills (situation awareness and decision-making), social or behavioral skills (communication, teamwork, leadership, followership, and assertiveness), and personal resource skills (management of stress and fatigue). Simulation-based education is hindered by barriers (**D**).
4. **D**. The debriefing model consists of three Ds: (a) defusing, allowing the training to emotionally decompress after a stressful simulation; (b) discovery, allowing reflective observation of the actions taken during the event; and (c)

deepening, helping the learner connect learning from the simulation to potential changes in clinical practice [4].

5. **C**. Acuity is defined as the potential severity of an event (or a series of events) and its subsequent impact on the patient [5].
6. **C**. Opportunity is defined as the frequency with which a certain department or individual is involved in the management of the event. It represents the y-axis in the zone of the simulation graph [5]. Acuity is defined as the potential severity of an event (or a series of events) and its subsequent impact on the patient. (**A** and **B**) The zone of simulation is the area in which simulation might play an important role in teaching and training necessary skills and may be preferable over other instructional media.
7. **A**. There are four zones of simulation:
   (i) High acuity high opportunity
   (ii) High acuity low opportunity
   (iii) Low acuity high opportunity
   (iv) Low acuity low opportunity

   The given scenario, maternal ACLS, comes under high acuity low opportunity [5].

Opportunity			
Acuity		Low	High
	High	AFE Unexpected PAS Maternal ACLS	Emergent c-section Postpartum hemorrhage
	Low	Skin reaction to antiseptic prep	Nausea during a cesarean delivery

8. **B**. The given scenario is a case of emergency C-section, which comes under the high acuity high opportunity zone of simulation [5].

Opportunity			
Acuity		Low	High
	High	AFE Unexpected PAS Maternal ACLS	Emergent c-section Postpartum hemorrhage
	Low	Skin reaction to antiseptic prep	Nausea during a cesarean delivery

9. **B**. Bloom's six levels of increasing difficulty or depth representing the cognitive domain are as follows [6]:

Bloom's taxonomy of cognitive domain	
1.	Knowledge
2.	Understanding (e.g., putting knowledge into one's own words) (**A**)
3.	Application (e.g., applying knowledge) (**C**)
4.	Analysis (e.g., calling upon relevant information)
5.	Synthesis (e.g., putting it all together to come up with a plan) (**E**)
6.	Evaluation (e.g., comparing and evaluating plans) (**D**)

10. **A**. High-fidelity manikin-based simulation is better than low-fidelity haptic simulators [7]. (**A** and **B**) Tele simulation is useful in reaching remote areas, but the outcome is less retention (**C**). Mental imagery technique enhances the retention capacity when used with other methods of simulation (**D**).
11. **C**. A single simulation session improves the outcome on the acquisition of technical skills in obstetric anesthesia [8]. In situ drills teach teamwork (**A**) to preserve the culture of safety in the obstetric units. Simulation improves the performance (**B**), especially in complex procedures such as emergency cricothyroidotomy. Research works such as review articles and simulation instructional articles (**D**) are useful for the spread of simulation in obstetric anesthesia care.
12. **C**. The SBAR technique, Situation-Background-Assessment-Recommendation technique, is used to practice sign-offs and handovers during practice drills [9].
13. **D**. Elective cesarean section is not a drill usually advocated for labor and delivery staff undergoing team training simulation. Drills advocated for use by labor and delivery staff undergoing team training include profound fetal bradycardia, magnesium sulfate overdose, shoulder dystocia, maternal hemorrhage (**E**), failed tracheal intubation (**C**), anaphylaxis (**B**), amniotic fluid embolism, and severe preeclampsia/eclampsia/HELLP syndrome (**A**).
14. **D**. It has been observed that simulation does not help in long-term retention of knowledge and skills. Simulation in obstetric anesthesia can be divided into four broad uses [10]. The first is training of technical skills including communication skills (**B**), second is training of nontechnical or teamwork skills (**A**), third is evaluation of individual clinical competence, and fourth is evaluation of safety of the clinical environment (**C**).
15. **E**. The advantage of simulation for research, training, and performance assessment is interpersonal interactions with other clinical staff [11]. Teamwork, leadership, and communication training (**E**) can be provided. Many scenarios can be presented, including uncommon critical situations in which a rapid response is needed with no risk to patients (**A**). Participants can see the results of their decisions and actions; errors can be allowed to occur and reach their conclusion. Identical scenarios can be presented to different clinicians or teams. The underlying causes of the situation are known (**B**), and with manikin-based simulators, clinicians can use actual medical equipment (**C**), exposing limitations in the human–machine interface. Intensive and intrusive recording of the simulation session is feasible, including audiotaping, videotaping, and even physiological monitoring of participants. There are no issues of patient confidentiality, and the recording can be preserved (**D**) for research, performance assessment, or accreditation.
16. **B**. Facilitator-guided debriefing provides a host of benefits over learner guidance, such as time efficiency and staying on task when addressing learning objectives [12]. PEARLS (**B**) is a four-phase model building on prior three-phase models and includes a step that allows facilitators and learners to establish a shared mental model before further debriefing. Debriefing models that include a step for addressing emotions set the stage for higher-quality

discussions. No one debriefing model is superior to the rest. However, the advantages and disadvantages of each may help guide the decision of which one to choose in a specific scenario.

17. **C**. An unformatted list of steps including complex-level reasoning for each step will not be helpful in the high-acuity situation.
18. **D**. Low-fidelity simulation might be very useful in remote areas with limited resources or in situations where a large group of people need to be trained over a short period of time [10].
19. **D**. Multidisciplinary obstetric simulated emergency scenarios (MOSES) were developed by the St Bartholomew's Hospital group in the United Kingdom, which involves the participation of real surgeons (rather than actors playing the role of real surgeons), anesthesia providers, and midwives in team training on a high-fidelity simulator [13].

References

1. Scharf JL, et al. *La machine*: obstetric phantoms of Madame Du Coudray… *Back to the roots*. J Med Educat Curri Develop. 2022;9:23821205221090168.
2. Wong AK. Full scale computer simulators in anesthesia training and evaluation. Can J Anesth. 2004;51(5):455.
3. Russ AL, et al. The science of human factors: separating fact from fiction. BMJ Quality Safety. 2013;22(10):802–8.
4. Zigmont, J.J et al. 2011. The 3D model of debriefing: defusing, discovering, and deepening. In Seminars in perinatology (Vol. 35, 2, pp. 52–58). WB Saunders.
5. Rivière E, et al. Twelve tips for efficient procedural simulation. Med Teach. 2018;40(7):743–51.
6. Levine AI, et al. The comprehensive textbook of healthcare simulation. Springer Science & Business Media; 2013.
7. Mahoney B, Luebbert E. Updates on simulation in obstetrical anesthesiology through the COVID-19 pandemic. Anesthesiol Clin. 2021;39(4):649–65.
8. Boet S, et al. Twelve tips for a successful interprofessional team-based high-fidelity simulation education session. Med Teach. 2014;36(10):853–7.
9. Kostoff M, et al. An interprofessional simulation using the SBAR communication tool. Am J Pharm Educ. 2016;80(9):157.
10. Marynen F, et al. Simulation in obstetric anesthesia: an update. Curr Opin Anesthesiol. 2020;33(3):272–6.
11. Gaba DM. Anesthesiology as a model for patient safety in health care. BMJ. 2000;320(7237):785–8.
12. Sawyer T, et al. More than one way to debrief: a critical review of healthcare simulation debriefing methods. Simul Healthc. 2016;11(3):209–17.
13. Freeth D, et al. MOSES: multidisciplinary obstetric simulated emergency scenarios. J Interprof Care. 2006;20(5):552–4.

Statistics

Leonard J. Soloniuk

Questions

1. **You are considering a trial of low-dose naltrexone to patients receiving neuraxial opioids as part of anesthesia for cesarean delivery. You expect no benefit to the mother from this intervention but hypothesize that there will be less respiratory depression and improved neurobehavioral scores for the neonate.**

   To receive Institutional Review Board approval for the study, all the following would be required <u>except</u>:

   A. An animal safety study demonstrating safety using the trial protocol
   B. A human safety study in nonpregnant women demonstrating safety using the trial protocol
   C. Informed consent obtained from the mother
   D. Naltrexone levels to be measured in both umbilical artery and umbilical vein samples of trial participants
   E. Informed consent which should be obtained from the father of the fetus

2. **You are conducting a study comparing epidural lidocaine to epidural chloroprocaine during cesarean deliveries with the primary outcome being severity of back pain after surgery. The surgical times appear to have a normal (Gaussian) distribution, but the mean surgical time for patients who received lidocaine was 38 min, and for patients who received chloroprocaine, it was 44 min.**

   Which would be the correct statistic to compare baseline characteristics and determine the significance of the difference in surgical times?

   A. A chi-squared test, such as the Pearson χ^2 test

L. J. Soloniuk (✉)
Riverside University Health System, Moreno Valley, CA, USA

Loma Linda University, Loma Linda, CA, USA
e-mail: l.soloniuk@ruhealth.org

A. C. Sinha, I. F. Pasca (eds.), *Peripartum Care of the Pregnant Patient*,
https://doi.org/10.1007/978-3-031-62756-9_48

B. One-sample t-test
C. Two-sample t-test
D. Standardized mean difference (SMD)

3. **A study was performed on patient–physician race concordance and its effect on six measures of patient-centered communication and three measures of patient satisfaction.**

   What statistical method should be used to minimize the risk of a false positive result?

   A. The comparison p value of 0.006 (i.e., 0.05/9) should be used in evaluating the results of statistical tests (Bonferroni correction).
   B. Each measure should be considered an independent study and be analyzed independently of the other measures.
   C. Pearson correlation coefficients should be calculated for each of the nine measures.
   D. Linear and logistic regression with generalized estimating equations should be used to assess the presence, strength, and statistical associations between race concordance and the outcome variables.

4. **In a standard format report of a medical trial, the first paragraph of the report covers the following:**

   A. The significance of the topic studied
   B. The background on the topic studied
   C. The rationale for the study
   D. The study aims or objectives
   E. The primary study hypothesis and, if any, the secondary study hypotheses

5. **You are designing a clinical trial to determine if intrathecal dexmedetomidine given after inadvertent dural puncture reduces the duration of post-dural puncture headache. You decide to use as the outcome variable the number of days with a headache after the procedure with the patients divided into two groups, dexmedetomidine and control (no medication).**

   The appropriate statistic for evaluating the outcome of the trial would be:

   A. One- or two-tailed t-test
   B. Analysis of variance (ANOVA)
   C. Poisson regression or negative binomial regression
   D. A chi-squared test, such as the Pearson χ^2 test

6. **A randomized trial was performed comparing the incidence of bradycardia after phenylephrine versus norepinephrine when used to prevent and treat spinal-induced hypotension in women undergoing cesarean delivery with spinal anesthesia.**

   There were a control group given phenylephrine and a treatment group given norepinephrine. The outcome variable was the finding of bradycardia or no bradycardia.

What is an appropriate statistical test for determining whether there is a statistically significant difference between the two groups?

A. One- or two-tailed t-test
B. Analysis of variance (ANOVA)
C. Poisson regression or negative binomial regression
D. A chi-squared test, such as the Pearson χ^2 test

7. **A study was performed to observe gastric emptying after the administration of 400 mL of a preoperative carbohydrate drink provided 2 h before elective cesarean delivery.**

   The cross-sectional area (CSA) of the antrum was measured with ultrasonography and was monitored with serial measurements at seven different times during the next 120 min.

   To decide when the CSA returned to baseline and when there was no statistically significant difference from baseline, which one of the following statistical methods should be used?

   A. Descriptive statistics
   B. Two-tailed t-test
   C. Analysis of variance (ANOVA)
   D. Poisson regression or negative binomial regression
   E. A chi-squared test, such as the Pearson χ^2 test

8. **A trial of a new treatment thought to reduce the risk of postpartum hemorrhage is stopped early because a preplanned interim analysis showed benefit meeting a prespecified stopping rule based on the O'Brien–Fleming method. The interim analysis shows that the estimated benefit corresponds to a hazard ratio of 0.62, which is unexpectedly better.**

   Which of the following statements is most likely true?

   A. If the trial were continued, the hazard ratio is likely to be superior to 0.62.
   B. If the trial were continued, there is a significant possibility that the treatment benefit would not meet statistical significance.
   C. With a preplanned interim analysis with additional looks at the data, to maintain the criterion of $p < 0.05$, a higher bar needs to be used for the interim analysis.

9. **A noninferiority study was performed comparing the onset times of epidural extension for cesarean deliveries between chloroprocaine and a mixture of lidocaine, epinephrine, sodium bicarbonate, and fentanyl.**

A noninferiority margin of 180 s was chosen so that if epidural extension with chloroprocaine took more than 180 s longer, it would not be considered noninferior.

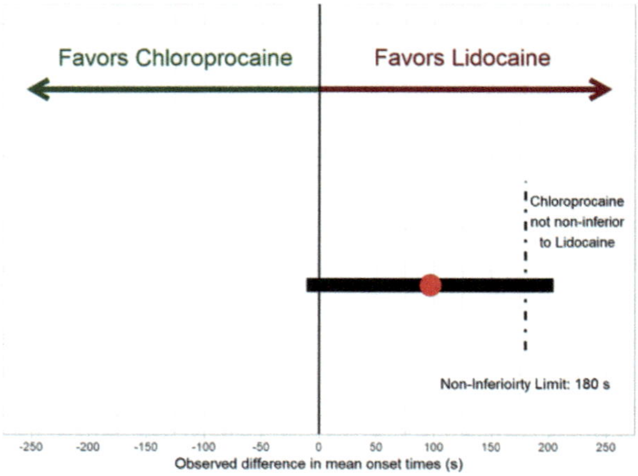

The study finds that the lidocaine arm had a mean onset that was 97 s faster than the chloroprocaine arm, with a 90% confidence interval (CI) of −10.6 to 204 s faster.

The best interpretation of these results would be:

A. Because the mean difference in time was less than the noninferiority limit, chloroprocaine was considered noninferior
B. Because the confidence interval includes no difference between the treatments, the two treatments would be considered equivalent
C. Because the confidence interval includes a difference greater than the noninferiority limit, chloroprocaine would be considered inferior
D. Because the confidence interval includes a difference greater than the noninferiority limit, chloroprocaine cannot be considered noninferior

10. **Compared to explanatory trials, which of the following statements about pragmatic clinical trials is correct?**
    A. Expert clinicians are used to deliver the care.
    B. Inclusion criteria focus on selecting patients who are most likely to respond to the therapy.
    C. Clinical care during the trial is focused on providing the intervention in settings that allow expert aftercare.
    D. The focus of the trial design is on external validity compared to internal validity.
11. **You read with interest a report of a clinical trial evaluating the efficacy and duration of analgesia of a single spinal injection of bupivacaine, fentanyl, and morphine for labor pain. The report describes that the patients who received spinal analgesia had a mean pain-free period of 238.96 (95% confidence interval of 217.08 to 260.84) min. If you were to replicate this study, what would be the probability that the second study would find a mean pain-free period between 217.08 and 260.84 min?**
    A. 95%
    B. 83.4%

C. 5%
D. 2.5%

12. **You read with interest an article that describes a study looking at the risk of bradycardia between phenylephrine and norepinephrine (NE) when used to treat hypotension after spinal anesthesia. The study hypothesis is that NE is associated with less bradycardia, with the null hypothesis being that the agents are associated with equal rates of bradycardia.**

    The authors found that the incidence of bradycardia was lower with the use of NE, with a *p* value of <0.001.

    The best interpretation of this p value is:

    A. The effect size of using norepinephrine was much greater than if the p value was 0.05
    B. The study hypothesis has a >99.9% chance of being true
    C. A p value of <0.001 indicates a high probability that the results are clinically significant
    D. There is less than a 0.1% chance that the data are consistent with the null hypothesis

13. **Mean, median, and mode are summary statistics used to describe data. Which of the following statements about these statistics is correct?**

    A. The mean represents the 50th centile of the data.
    B. The mode is the most frequently used measure of central tendency.
    C. The mean is the middle observation of the group of data.
    D. Statistical inference about population means is easier than for population medians.

14. **You are interested in the risk of postdural puncture headache after epidural placement using air vs. liquid for loss-of-resistance technique. You review a meta-analysis of studies exploring this question. The study calculates an I^2 statistic for the comparisons between the studies used in the meta-analysis.**

    For a calculated I^2 of 0%, which of the following statements is most correct?

    A. There is a large amount of heterogeneity between the findings of the studies in the meta-analysis.
    B. The result is highly statistically significant.
    C. A single summary statistic will not adequately describe the results.
    D. Any variability in population estimates is explained by chance.

15. **You are comparing a new way of teaching obstetric anesthesia to an older way of teaching, and you are using an exit pass/fail test as your way of evaluation. You compile the following data:**

	Residents who passed	Residents who failed	Pass rate	Pass/fail rate
New way of teaching	50	30	62.5%	1.67
Old way of teaching	20	25	44.4%	0.8

When comparing the new way to the old way, which of the following statements is correct?

A. Both the odds ratio and relative risk are 2.09, i.e., 1.67/0.8.
B. The relative risk is not relevant for these data.
C. The relative risk is 1.41, i.e., 62.5%/44.4%.
D. The hazard ratio is 0.67, i.e., (100% to 62.5%)/(100% to 44.4%).

16. **Based on this table, which represents Type I error?**

	The null hypothesis is actually true	The null hypothesis is actually false
You reject the null hypothesis	A	B
You accept the null hypothesis	C	D

A. Cell A
B. Cell B
C. Cell C
D. Cell D

17. **You examine emergency cesarean deliveries at your institution by hour of the day. You find that they happen with equal frequency at any hour. You want to calculate the chances that multiple emergency sections can occur in the same hour.**

The distribution of the number of emergency cesarean deliveries per hour would be a:

A. Normal distribution
B. Gaussian distribution
C. Binomial distribution
D. Poisson distribution

18. **You are doing a power analysis for a study that you are planning. You hypothesize that administering epidural dexmedetomidine at the beginning of the second stage of labor will result in better pain scores. You are calculating what your sample size should be for the study.**

Your projected sample size would be less if:

A. You wanted a higher-powered study with a β of 0.9 rather than 0.8
B. You estimate the variability of outcomes to be high, rather than low
C. You choose an outcome that is a dichotomous variable (e.g., "worked," "didn't work"), rather than a continuous variable (e.g., the scale on a satisfaction instrument)
D. The relative risk of success with the treatment will be 1.5 rather than 1.25

19. **You are considering a study evaluating blood pressure values as calculated continuously by a noninvasive device compared with oscillometric blood pressure monitoring. Your statistician recommends using a Bland–Altman plot for analysis of the data.**

Which of the following diagrams represents a Bland–Altman plot?

A.

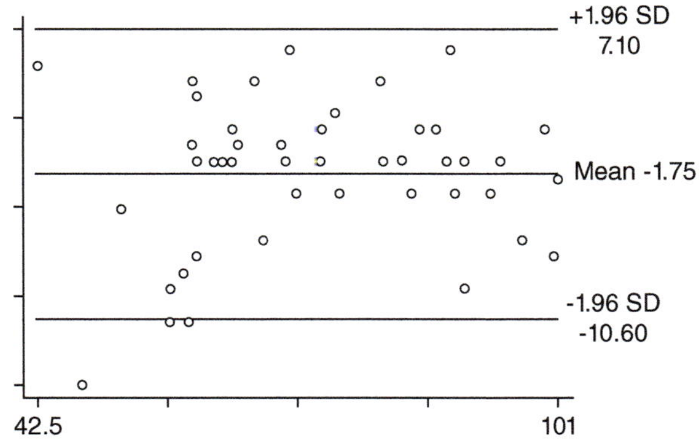
+1.96 SD
7.10
Mean -1.75
-1.96 SD
-10.60
42.5
101

B.

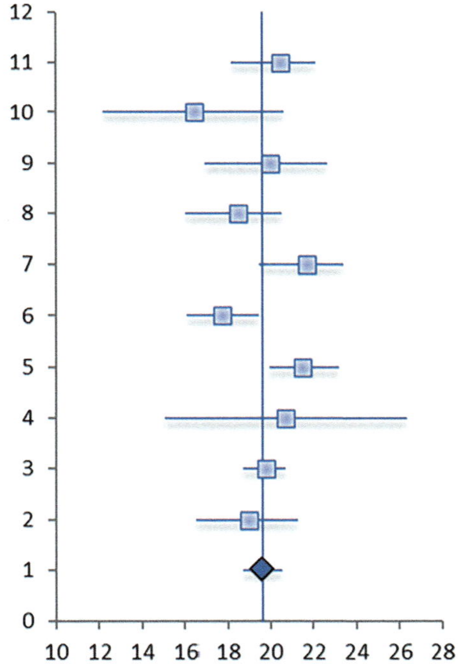
12
11
10
9
8
7
6
5
4
3
2
1
0
10 12 14 16 18 20 22 24 26 28

C.

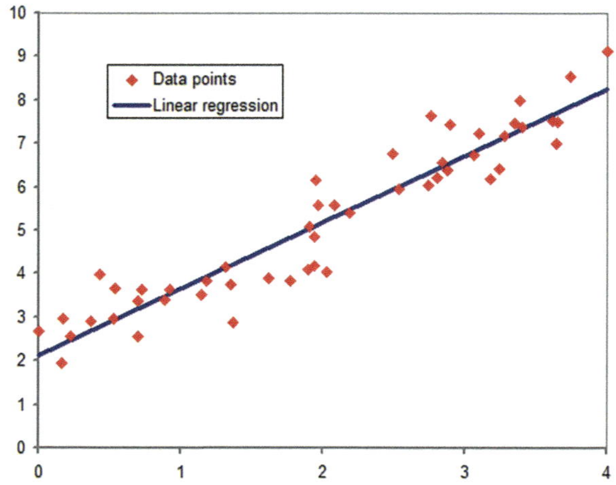

D.

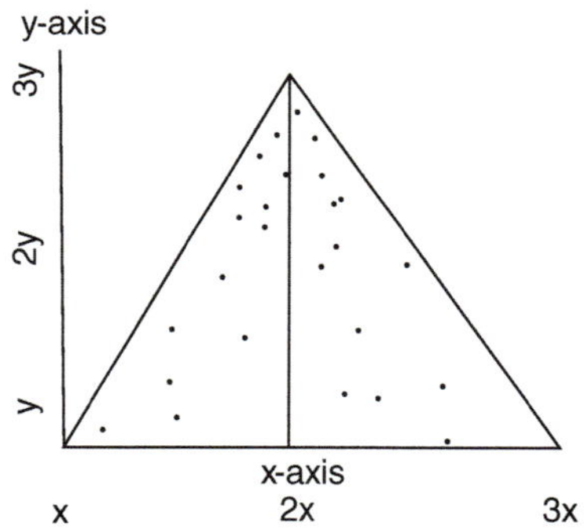

Answers and Explanations

1. **D**. An animal and human safety study would be required before exposing pregnant patients to a medication (**A**, **B**). If the research poses benefit solely to the fetus, the pregnant patient and the father need to give consent except if the father is incapacitated, unavailable, or incompetent (**C**, **E**). There is no specific requirement for any component of a study involving parturients and fetuses, such as measuring blood levels in this case (**D**). There is guidance from the US Department of Health and Human Resources on the safe inclusion of pregnant individuals in clinical trials, addressing maternal consent and documenting preexisting data on intervention safety. For safety studies, the regulations require

that "where scientifically appropriate, preclinical studies, including studies on pregnant animals, and clinical studies, including studies on nonpregnant women, have been conducted and provide data for assessing potential risks to pregnant women and fetuses." Regarding consent, "if the research holds out the prospect of direct benefit solely to the fetus then the consent of the pregnant woman and the father is obtained." There are limited exemptions for paternal consent [1].

2. **D**. A chi-squared test evaluates whether two (or more) categorical variables are significantly different (a categorical variable divides observations into mutually exclusive classes, such as surgical time <40 min and surgical time ≥40 min). It is used to test study results, not to compare baseline characteristics (**A**). A one-sample t-test evaluates whether the mean of a population has a value specified in a null hypothesis. These tests are used to evaluate study results, not to compare baseline characteristics (**B**). A two-sample test evaluates whether the means of two populations are equal. These tests are used to evaluate study results, not to compare baseline characteristics (**C**). A standardized difference—or standardized mean difference (SMD)—is the mean difference between groups divided by the standard deviation of either the control group (called Glass's delta) or the combined groups (called Cohen's d). SMDs of 0.2, 0.5, and 0.8 are considered small, medium, and large, respectively (**D**) [2–5].
3. **A**. When multiple hypotheses are being tested in a clinical trial, there is an increased risk of false positive results (**A**). If the risk of a false positive result for each outcome is 5% ($p = 0.05$), evaluating the results of 9 outcome measures with $p = 0.05$ for each outcome would give a possibility of a false positive outcome for the entire study of 9 * 5% or 45%. To correct for testing multiple hypotheses, the simplest approach is the Bonferroni correction, in which the significance threshold is set at α (usually 5%) divided by the number of hypothesis tests. Of the nine results, only results with p values smaller than the adjusted significance criterion ($p = 0.006$) were considered statistically significant (**A**). Treating each measure as an independent study increases the risk of false positive results (**B**). The Pearson correlation coefficient measures the strength of the correlation between two continuous variables. This would not be appropriate since patient–physician race concordance is a categorical variable and not a continuous variable. Additionally, it would not correct for testing multiple hypotheses simultaneously (**C**). With linear and logistic regression with generalized estimating equations, the goal is to produce reasonable estimates of model parameters, along with standard errors. Model parameters are estimates of the values of variables that describe the population studied. Although useful, this approach does not account for the increased risk of false positives with multiple hypothesis testing (**D**) [6, 7].
4. **A**. According to Tom Vetter in his article "In the Beginning-There Is the Introduction-and Your Study Hypothesis," the first paragraph of a report with a standard format covers the significance of the topic, including the pathophysiology, epidemiology, and impact of the clinical condition studied (**A**). The second paragraph provides the background on the topic, including the most pertinent

previous studies and their key findings (**B**). The third paragraph defines the rationale for the study. The rationale can be structured around the "FINER" acronym, Feasible, Interesting, Novel, Ethical, and Relevant (**C**). The fourth paragraph lists the study aims or objectives (**D**). The fifth and final paragraph states the primary study hypothesis and, if any, the secondary study hypotheses (**E**) [8].

5. **C**. The number of days with a headache is an example of a "count variable." The values of the result will be discrete (0 days, 1 day, 2 days, …) and not continuous. Other examples of countable quantities include hospital length of stay, the number of intraoperative cardiac arrests per 100,000 operations, or the number of postoperative infections. The values of count variables are nonnegative whole numbers (0, 1, 2, …), and the distribution is usually markedly skewed, with many values being relatively low and few being high. A count variable usually does not have a normal (Gaussian) distribution. T-tests assume a normal (Gaussian) distribution for the data. They are also used with continuous variables, not categorical (discrete) values. Therefore, they are not appropriate for this study (**A**). ANOVA provides a statistical test of the difference between two or more means. It is used to analyze continuous variables, not categorical variables, and, so, is not appropriate to use to analyze this study (**B**). To analyze count data, the prototypical approach is to use Poisson regression to determine whether there is a statistically significant difference between outcome count variables. Poisson regression is a special case of the more general negative binomial regression (**C**). Pearson's chi-squared test is used to determine whether there is a statistically significant difference between expected frequencies and the observed frequencies in one or multiple categories. This is not appropriate for this study design (**D**) [9, 10].
6. **D**. The outcome variables can be displayed in a 2 × 2 contingency table. The outcome variables are categorical variables, with a binary outcome of bradycardia or no bradycardia. They are not continuous variables. T-tests assume a normal (Gaussian) distribution for the data. They are used with continuous variables, not categorical (discrete) values. Therefore, t tests are not appropriate here. If the outcome were heart rate (a continuous variable), a t-test may be appropriate (**A**). ANOVA provides a statistical test of the difference between two or more means. It is used to analyze continuous variables, not categorical variables, and, so, is not appropriate to use to analyze this study (**B**). Poisson regression is typically used to analyze "count" data and is therefore not appropriate to analyze the results of this study. A count variable is a variable that records the number of occurrences of an outcome. It takes on positive, integer values (such as 0, 1, 2, …) (**C**). Pearson's chi-squared test is used to determine whether there is a statistically significant difference between expected frequencies and the observed frequencies in one or multiple categories. This test would be a logical choice to use to analyze this study (**D**) [2, 11, 12].
7. **C**. Descriptive statistics (such as count, mean, standard deviation) describe the sample values. They contrast with inferential statistics, which use the sample data to make inferences about the population. Inferential statistics, such as the other methods listed, would be more appropriate to answer the question about

return to baseline (**A**). Two-tailed t-tests determine the statistical significance of the means of two samples. Since there are seven comparisons proposed (baseline CSA with the CSAs found at six different times), this would not be an adequate test (**B**). ANOVA provides a statistical test of the differences between two or more means. It generalizes the t-test for testing more than the means of two samples. This would be appropriate for this study (**C**). Poisson regression is typically used to analyze count data and is therefore not appropriate to analyze the results of this study (**D**). Pearson's chi-squared test is used to determine whether there is a statistically significant difference between expected frequencies and the observed frequencies in one or multiple categories. This would not be appropriate for this study (**E**) [12–14].

8. **C**. Some clinical trials have periodic preplanned analyses to determine if the trial should be stopped early because of unexpected great benefit or futility.

   Trials can also be halted early, even without a preplanned analysis, because of unexpected patient harm, lack of patients, or inadequate resources to continue the trial. It can be difficult to interpret the implications of these trials.

   Stopping early allows more effective use of patient, clinician, and institutional resources. It presents the ethical benefit of not exposing patients to less effective therapy or not allowing access to more effective therapy.

   When a trial is stopped early because of unexpected benefit, the true treatment effect is likely to be lower than the estimate produced by the interim analysis (**A**). When a preplanned interim analysis brings an early end to the trial, the higher statistical bars used make it likely that continuing the trial would show the same result as stopping early (**B**). When multiple looks at the data are made, tighter standards must be used to maintain the same significance as only one look (**C**) [15].

9. **D**. Treatments can be compared with superiority trials, equivalence trials, or noninferiority trials. The differences between these types of trials may appear subtle, but these separate types require different trial designs and different statistical analyses and have different implications.

   If a superiority trial produces results that show no significant difference between the groups studied, it does not follow that the trial demonstrates equivalence. To demonstrate equivalence, carefully chosen equivalence margins must be determined before the trial begins, and the trial must show that the differences found are likely within the equivalence margins.

   Negative noninferiority trials—trials that do not meet criteria for determining noninferiority (i.e., the null hypothesis is not rejected)—are often misreported in publications. One study found "spin" (misreported findings in negative trials) in 75% of negative noninferiority oncology trials. To show noninferiority, the confidence interval cannot include the noninferiority limit (**A**). Equivalence cannot be demonstrated by a noninferiority trial (**B**). Inferiority cannot be demonstrated by a noninferiority trial. The strongest statement that can be made from a negative trial is that noninferiority is not demonstrated (**C**). If the confidence interval includes the noninferiority limit, noninferiority has not been demonstrated (**D**) [16–18].

10. **D**. An explanatory trial seeks to isolate the effect of the intervention being tested. The trial design focuses on selecting a homogenous group of patients with carefully detailed care and aftercare.

    A pragmatic trial seeks information about how an intervention would work in "the real world." The trial design focuses on selecting patients who are representative of patients likely to be offered the therapy with care administered by clinicians who normally treat the targeted condition. Aftercare would be representative of the usual aftercare offered to patients outside the trial.

    A pragmatic trial generates data that will be more useful in guiding clinical practice. To minimize variability, an explanatory trial uses expert or carefully trained clinicians. A pragmatic trial would have care administered by clinicians who usually care for the condition being studied (**A**). A pragmatic trial would include a variety of patients with the condition being studied and who would be offered the therapy being studied (**B**). A pragmatic trial would use the type of aftercare that is typically available for patients (**C**). External validity refers to how valid it is to apply the result of a research study to situations outside the context of the study. Pragmatic trials attempt to maximize the external validity of the study (**D**) [19].
11. **B**. The replication interval is different from the confidence interval (**A**). When studies are replicated, the 95% confidence interval (CI) of the means in the original study will capture 83.4% of future replication means (**B**) [20–22].
12. **D**. Accurate interpretation of p values can be subtle. A p value is the probability that, using a specified statistical model, a statistical summary of population data (such as a difference in incidence of bradycardia in all patients) would be equal to or more extreme than the observed value. A p value does not measure effect size. In hypothesis testing, the p value is affected by factors such as effect size, power, sample size, and measurement precision (**A**). A p value reflects the compatibility of the data with the null hypothesis, not the truth of the null hypothesis. It is a statement about the data, not the clinical truth (**B**). P values reflect the statistical analysis of the data, not the clinical significance. A very low p value can be associated with a finding that is not clinically significant (**C**). The p value reflects how compatible the data are with the null hypothesis (**D**) [4, 11, 23].
13. **D**. Summary statistics are part of the reduction of data to a meaningful summary to gain understanding and make useful predictions. Mean, median, and mode are measures of central tendency, also called measures of location. The median represents the 50th percentile of the data (**A**). The mode is frequently not reported as it is usually not useful in describing data sets (**B**). The median is the middle observation of the group of data (**C**). Mathematically, it is easier to make statistical inferences about means than about medians and modes (**D**) [24].
14. **D**. A low I^2 of 0% indicates that there is no observed heterogeneity between the studies being compared (**A**). The I^2 statistic impacts the clinical interpretation of the result, analyzing the variability between studies. It does not reflect statistical significance (**B**). With an I^2 of 0%, there is low variability between studies, and the result can be described adequately with a single summary statistic (**C**). The low I^2 suggests that any variability between the studies is explained by chance (**D**) [25, 26].

15. **C**. The odds ratio is 2.09, but the relative risk is calculated differently (**A**). The relative risk is a relevant way of presenting the results of this study (**B**). The hazard ratio is not relevant for categorical outcomes but for time-to-event outcomes (such as survival time) or continuous variable outcomes. For time-to-event variables, the hazard ratio is calculated by assessing outcomes over the entire curve of outcomes over time (**D**).

    When assessing how much of an impact an intervention has, the effect size, there are several measures that can be reported. For categorical outcome variables, such as in this question with the outcomes of pass/fail, the odds ratio and the relative risk are frequently used.

    The odds ratio is the ratio of two odds. In this case, the odds ratio is the ratio of the odds of passing with the new way of teaching (50:30 or 1.67) to the odds of passing with the old way of teaching (20:25 or 0.8).

    The relative risk is the ratio of two probabilities. In this example, the relative risk is the ratio of the probability of passing with the new way of teaching (62.5%) to the probability of passing with the old way of teaching (44.4%) (**C**).

    Odds and probabilities are related. Probabilities can range from 0 to 1 (0% to 100%). Odds can range from 0 to infinity [27].
16. **A**. A study result is positive when the null hypothesis is rejected. Box A is where the null hypothesis is true, but you reject it. This represents a false positive, and a Type I error is committed (**A**). Box B is where the null hypothesis is false and, correctly, you reject it. This is a true positive (**B**). Box C is where the null hypothesis is true, and you accept it. This is a true negative (**C**). Box D is where the null hypothesis is false, but you accept it. This is a false negative, a Type II error (**D**).

    Care needs to be taken when thinking about these concepts because there is a tendency to analyze studies in terms of the study hypothesis ("the study groups are different") rather than the null hypothesis ("the study groups are the same") [28].
17. **D**. A normal, or Gaussian, distribution describes the distribution for a continuous variable (such as the mean arterial pressure) (**A**). A Gaussian, or normal, distribution describes the distribution for a continuous variable (such as the mean arterial pressure) (**B**). A binomial distribution is a distribution created by an outcome variable that has two mutually exclusive outcomes. For example, the distribution of the number of cesarean deliveries per month that have >1000 mL blood loss would be a binomial distribution (**C**). When an event has an equal chance of occurring in any given time frame, then the count of the number of events per time frame has a Poisson distribution [10, 29].
18. **D**. Achieving a higher power requires a larger sample size (**A**). Highly variable outcomes require larger sample sizes (**B**). Binary (dichotomous) outcome variables, in general, require higher sample sizes than continuous outcome variables (**C**). The higher the expected treatment effect (such as higher odds ratios, relative risks, and hazard ratios), the smaller the projected sample size needed (**D**).

The power of the study is the probability that the study will have a Type II (false negative) error. Prior to starting the trial, the desired power is used to calculate the sample sizes needed.

The estimated sample size needed depends on multiple factors including the strength of the treatment effect expected, the amount of variability in the outcome variable, the desired significance level (p value), and the desired power of the study [28].

19. **A**. The Bland–Altman plot was used to visually compare two methods of measurement. The mean of each pair of test results is plotted on the x-axis. On the y-axis, the paired absolute difference between the results is plotted. A horizontal line is drawn for the mean difference (which is the estimated bias between the measurements). Two more horizontal lines are drawn to show the lower and upper limits of agreement, defined as the mean difference ± 1.96 times the standard deviation of the total differences (**A**). The next diagram shows a forest plot. A forest plot displays the studies showing the likelihood measures along with confidence intervals (**B**). The next diagram shows a scattergram (scatter plot) that displays the relationship between a continuous independent variable and a continuous dependent variable (**C**). The fourth diagram shows a funnel plot that is used to examine studies in a meta-analysis for publication bias. A dot for each study is placed with the value of the outcome variable on the x-axis, and the precision of the study (the inverse of the standard error) is plotted on the y-axis (**D**) [30, 31].

References

1. US Department of Health & Human Services. Additional protections for pregnant women, human fetuses and neonates involved in research. https://www.hhs.gov/ohrp/regulations-and-policy/regulations/45-cfr-46/common-rule-subpart-b/index.html. Accessed 26 Feb 2023.
2. Schober P, Vetter TR. Chi-square tests in medical research. Anesth Analg. 2019;129(5):1193. https://doi.org/10.1213/ANE.0000000000004410.
3. Schober P, Vetter TR. Correct baseline comparisons in a randomized trial. Anesth Analg. 2019;129(3):639. https://doi.org/10.1213/ANE.0000000000004211.
4. Schober P, Bossers SM, Schwarte LA. Statistical significance versus clinical importance of observed effect sizes: what do P values and confidence intervals truly represent? Anesth Analg. 2018;126(3):1068–72. https://doi.org/10.1213/ANE.0000000000002798.
5. Andrade C. Mean difference, standardized mean difference (SMD), and their use in meta-analysis: as simple as it gets. J Clin Psychiatry. 2020;81(5):20f13681. https://doi.org/10.4088/JCP.20f13681.
6. Cooper LA, Roter DL, Johnson RL, Ford DE, Steinwachs DM, Powe NR. Patient-centered communication, ratings of care, and concordance of patient and physician race. Ann Intern Med. 2003;139(11):907–15. https://doi.org/10.7326/0003-4819-139-11-200312020-00009.
7. Schober P, Vetter TR. Adjustments for multiple testing in medical research. Anesth Analg. 2020;130(1):99. https://doi.org/10.1213/ANE.0000000000004545.
8. Vetter TR, Mascha EJ. In the beginning-there is the introduction-and your study hypothesis. Anesth Analg. 2017;124(5):1709–11. https://doi.org/10.1213/ANE.0000000000002028. Erratum in: Anesth Analg. 2017;125(1):366.

9. Schober P, Vetter TR. Count data in medical research: Poisson regression and negative binomial regression. Anesth Analg. 2021;132(5):1378–9. https://doi.org/10.1213/ANE.0000000000005398.
10. Coxe S, West SG, Aiken LS. The analysis of count data: a gentle introduction to poisson regression and its alternatives. J Pers Assess. 2009;91(2):121–36. https://doi.org/10.1080/00223890802634175.
11. Sharkey AM, Siddiqui N, Downey K, Ye XY, Guevara J, Carvalho JCA. Comparison of intermittent intravenous boluses of phenylephrine and norepinephrine to prevent and treat spinal-induced hypotension in cesarean deliveries: a randomized controlled trial. Anesth Analg. 2019;129:1312–8.
12. Popivanov P, Irwin R, Walsh M, Leonard M, Tan T. Gastric emptying of carbohydrate drinks in term parturients before elective cesarean delivery: an observational study. Int J Obstet Anesth. 2020;41:29–34. https://doi.org/10.1016/j.ijoa.2019.07.010. Epub 2019 Aug 6.
13. Haskins SC, Kruisselbrink R, Boublik J, Wu CL, Perlas A. Gastric ultrasound for the regional anesthesiologist and pain specialist. Reg Anesth Pain Med. 2018;43(7):689–98. https://doi.org/10.1097/AAP.0000000000000846.
14. Schober P, Vetter TR. Analysis of variance in medical research. Anesth Analg. 2020;131(2):508–9. https://doi.org/10.1213/ANE.0000000000004839.
15. Viele K, McGlothlin A, Broglio K. Interpretation of clinical trials that stopped early. In: Livingston E, Lewis R, editors. JAMA guide to statistics and methods. McGraw Hill; 2020.
16. Sharawi N, Bansal P, Williams M, Spencer H, Mhyre JM. Comparison of chloroprocaine versus lidocaine with epinephrine, sodium bicarbonate, and fentanyl for epidural extension anesthesia in elective cesarean delivery: a randomized, triple-blind, noninferiority study. Anesth Analg. 2021;132(3):666–75. https://doi.org/10.1213/ANE.0000000000005141.
17. Schober P, Vetter TR. Noninferiority and equivalence trials in medical research. Anesth Analg. 2020;131(1):208–9. https://doi.org/10.1213/ANE.0000000000004783.
18. Ito C, Hashimoto A, Uemura K, Oba K. Misleading reporting (spin) in noninferiority randomized clinical trials in oncology with statistically not significant results: a systematic review. JAMA Netw Open. 2021;4(12):e2135765. https://doi.org/10.1001/jamanetworkopen.2021.35765.
19. Loudon K, Treweek S, Sullivan F, Donnan P, Thorpe KE, Zwarenstein M. The PRECIS-2 tool: designing trials that are fit for purpose. BMJ. 2015;350:h2147. https://doi.org/10.1136/bmj.h2147.
20. Vetter TR, McGwin G Jr, Pittet JF. Replicability, reproducibility, and fragility of research findings-ultimately, caveat emptor. Anesth Analg. 2016;123(1):244–8. https://doi.org/10.1213/ANE.0000000000001398.
21. Chauhan G, Samyal P, Pathania AA. Single-dose intrathecal analgesia: a safe and effective method of labor analgesia for parturients in low resource areas. Ain-Shams J Anesthesiol. 2020;12:23. https://doi.org/10.1186/s42077-020-00075-w.
22. Cumming G, Williams J, Fidler F. Replication, and researchers' understanding of confidence intervals and standard error bars. Underst Stat. 2004;3:299–311.
23. Wasserstein RL, Lazar NA. The ASA statement on p values: context, process, and purpose. Am Stat. 2016;70(2):129–33. https://doi.org/10.1080/00031305.2016.1154108.
24. Carlin JB, Doyle LW. 2: describing and displaying data. J Paediatr Child Health. 2000;36(3):270–4. https://doi.org/10.1046/j.1440-1754.2000.00494.x.
25. Schier R, Guerra D, Aguilar J, Pratt GF, Hernandez M, Boddu K, Riedel B. Epidural space identification: a meta-analysis of complications after air versus liquid as the medium for loss of resistance. Anesth Analg. 2009;109(6):2012–21. https://doi.org/10.1213/ANE.0b013e3181bc113a.
26. Murad MH, Montori VM, Ioannidis JP, Jaeschke R, Devereaux PJ, Prasad K, Neumann I, Carrasco-Labra A, Agoritsas T, Hatala R, Meade MO, Wyer P, Cook DJ, Guyatt G. How to read a systematic review and meta-analysis and apply the results to patient care: users' guides to the medical literature. JAMA. 2014;312(2):171–9. https://doi.org/10.1001/jama.2014.5559.
27. Kallogjeri D, Piccirillo JF. A simple guide to effect size measures. JAMA Otolaryngol Head Neck Surg. 2023;149(5):447–51. https://doi.org/10.1001/jamaoto.2023.0159.

28. Mascha EJ, Vetter TR. Significance, errors, power, and sample size: the blocking and tackling of statistics. Anesth Analg. 2018;126(2):691–8. https://doi.org/10.1213/ANE.0000000000002741. Erratum in: Anesth Analg. 2018.
29. Viti A, Terzi A, Bertolaccini L. A practical overview on probability distributions. J Thorac Dis. 2015;7(3):E7–E10. https://doi.org/10.3978/j.issn.2072-1439.2015.01.37.
30. Vetter TR, Schober P. Agreement analysis: what he said, she said versus you said. Anesth Analg. 2018;126(6):2123–8. https://doi.org/10.1213/ANE.0000000000002924.
31. Frassanito L, Sonnino C, Piersanti A, Zanfini BA, Catarci S, Giuri PP, Scorzoni M, Gonnella GL, Antonelli M, Draisci G. Performance of the hypotension prediction index with noninvasive arterial pressure waveforms in awake cesarean delivery patients under spinal anesthesia. Anesth Analg. 2022;134(3):633–43. https://doi.org/10.1213/ANE.0000000000005754.

Research Methods

Christopher Patty and Jessica Chan

Questions

1. **The Institutional Review Board (IRB) has the authority and responsibility to evaluate which of the following?**
   A. The scientific merit of a proposed research study.
   B. Compliance with federal research regulations.
   C. The ethical treatment of human subjects in a proposed research study.
   D. All the above are correct.
   E. B and C only.
2. **The Revised Common Rule (2019) removes significant special protections required of vulnerable persons from which of the following populations?**
   A. Prisoners
   B. Children
   C. Pregnant women
   D. Refugees
3. **Where therapeutic research studies are considered, the strongest level of evidence for practice can be obtained from the following:**
   A. Expert opinion or "first principles"
   B. Systematic reviews of homogeneous randomized controlled trials (RCTs)
   C. Case series
   D. Outcomes research and ecological studies
4. **When developing your research question, which of the following frameworks would provide the most useful guidance?**

C. Patty (✉)
Kaweah Delta Health Care District, Visalia, CA, USA
e-mail: CPatty@KaweahHealth.org

J. Chan
Kaweah Health Medical Center, Visalia, CA, USA
e-mail: jechan@kaweahhealth.org

A. C. Sinha, I. F. Pasca (eds.), *Peripartum Care of the Pregnant Patient*,
https://doi.org/10.1007/978-3-031-62756-9_49

   A. FINER (**F**easible, **I**nteresting, **N**ovel, **E**thical, **R**elevant)
   B. SMART (**S**pecific, **M**easurable, **A**chievable, **R**elevant and **T**imely)
   C. OKR (**O**bjectives and **K**ey **R**esults)
   D. PICO (**P**opulation, **I**ntervention, **C**omparison, **O**utcome)
   E. Both A and D
5. **An important strength of the case–control study design is as follows:**
   A. Reduction of sampling bias
   B. Facilitation of the study of multiple outcomes
   C. Efficiency for the study of rare outcomes
   D. Estimation of incidence and prevalence of disease
6. **You have developed the research question "Does eating more fish during pregnancy increase the risk of fetal mercury toxicity?". In this research question, the amount of fish eaten represents:**
   A. The independent variable
   B. The confounding variable
   C. The dependent variable
   D. The interval variable
7. **You plan to assemble a research team and conduct a systematic review of RCTs. You want to register this review to improve its quality and transparency. You will register the protocol for your systematic review at which of the following databases?**
   A. ClinicalTrials.gov
   B. PROSPERO
   C. National Institute for Health and Care Research (NIHR)
   D. EQUATOR Network
8. **You are collecting data for a research study designed to describe attitudes toward weight gain in pregnancy among persons of differing ethnic and cultural backgrounds. You have reached a point where you have collected enough data to draw your conclusions, and new information will not change these conclusions. The research term for this point is:**
   A. Maturation
   B. Grounding
   C. Data overload
   D. Saturation
9. **The research question is "Do Latinas in the United States have higher rates of gestational diabetes than Whites, African Americans, or Asian Americans?". What existing database might enable you to determine race-specific rates of gestational diabetes at low cost of time and money?**
   A. Healthy People 2030
   B. NHANES (National Health and Nutrition Examination Survey)
   C. National Obesity Database
   D. ACOG (American College of Obstetricians and Gynecologists)
10. **An investigator is interested in conducting a randomized controlled trial (RCT) for the purpose of seeking a new marketing indication for an**

existing FDA-approved drug. The most appropriate clinical trial phase for this type of investigation is a:
   A. Phase 1 trial
   B. Phase 2 trial
   C. Phase 3 trial
   D. Phase 4 trial

11. **For a normal distribution, what is the percentage of data points that would be within one standard deviation (SD) from the mean?**
   A. 50%
   B. 68%
   C. 75%
   D. 95%

12. **A 28-year-old female enters the OB-GYN office for a follow-up on a test result regarding HPV. The patient asks the OB-GYN, "What are the chances that I do not have HPV?" Which of the following epidemiological parameters best answers the patient's question?**
   A. Positive predictive value (PPV)
   B. Negative predictive value (NPV)
   C. Sensitivity
   D. Specificity

13. **Investigators would like to start a study comparing phenylephrine and ephedrine on systolic blood pressure (SBP). What level of measurement would best represent systolic blood pressure (SBP) for statistical analysis?**
   A. Nominal
   B. Interval
   C. Ordinal
   D. Structural

14. **Investigators would like to compare postoperative nausea and vomiting (PONV) in parturients who underwent C-section. Researchers grouped the patients into two: patients who underwent general anesthesia and patients who underwent spinal anesthesia. What study design best describes this situation?**
   A. Meta-analysis
   B. Case series
   C. Case–control study
   D. Cohort study

15. **Researchers would like to quantify postoperative pain after spinal anesthesia. In the recovery room, patients were given a piece of paper with a line with one end describing unbearable pain and the other end no pain. Patients were asked to mark their pain level on the line. Which of the following best describes this method?**
   A. Visual analog scale
   B. Open-ended questions
   C. Likert scale
   D. Wong–Baker scale

Answers and Explanations

1. The correct answer is **D**. The IRB has an obligation to evaluate scientific merit (**A**) if it is to remain in compliance with federal regulations (**B**) and research ethics (**C**). Choice **E** is incorrect [1].
2. The correct answer is **C**. The previous Common Rule (in place for almost 30 years) had considered pregnant women a vulnerable population for almost all human subjects research (HSR). The 2019 revision removed most special protections for pregnant women to encourage their inclusion in research if the study could benefit the fetus or if the risk to the fetus is minimal and leads to important biomedical knowledge. Protections for prisoners (**A**), children (**B**), and refugees (**C**) remain essentially unchanged [1].
3. The correct answer is **B**. Systematic reviews of RCTs with homogeneity produce the strongest level of evidence for practice [2]. Expert opinion (**A**) represents the lowest level of strength of evidence, and case series (**C**) or outcomes research (**D**) represents intermediate levels.
4. The correct answer is **E**. Both the PICO framework (**D**) and the FINER model (**B**) are widely utilized (often together) in the development of researchable questions [3]. The SMART (**A**) and OKR (**C**) frameworks are used in more generic goal setting.
5. The correct answer is **C**. A major strength of this study design is the rapid yield of information from a relatively small number of participants [3]. The other possible answers **A**, **B**, and **D** represent major weaknesses of the case–control study design.
6. The correct answer is **A**. The independent variable (cause) is what we expect will influence the dependent variable (**C**, effect). A confounding variable (**B**) affects the relationship between other variables [4], and the term "interval variable" (**D**) is incorrect.
7. The correct answer is **B**. The International Prospective Register of Systematic Reviews, better known as PROSPERO, is a database of systematic review protocols in health and social care. ClinicalTrials.gov (**A**) is a registry of FDA-regulated research, NIHR is the largest funder of research in the United States, and the EQUATOR Network (**D**) is a repository of research writing guidelines.
8. The correct answer is **D**. Saturation in qualitative research means that a point is reached where additional data will not change the properties examined. **A**, **B**, and **C** are not correct; they are nonsensical confounders.
9. The correct answer is **B**. NHANES is a (US) population-based study repository, and data are available to any researcher at a nominal cost [3]. The data include variables such as self-reported clinical history of gestational diabetes. Healthy People 2030 (**A**) is a health promotion resource, the National Obesity Database (**C**) is a future project of the United Kingdom, and ACOG (**D**) is a professional organization with limited nonmember resources.
10. The correct answer is **C**. A phase 3 trial can be used to develop new drug indications by comparing it with standard treatments [5]. A phase 1 trial (**A**)

investigates drug safety and side effects, a phase 2 trial (**B**) investigates drug effectiveness and safety, and a phase 4 trial (**D**) investigates safety in the general population.

11. The correct answer is **B**. One standard deviation (SD) from the (+/−) mean equals 68%. The value within two standard deviations (SD) from the mean is 95% while 99.7% is the value within three standard deviations (SD) from the mean [6]. Choices **A**, **C**, and **D** are incorrect.
12. The correct answer is **B**. Negative predictive value (NPV) is the likelihood of not having the disease given a negative test result [7]. Choices **A**, **C**, and **D** are incorrect. Sensitivity is the probability of ruling out the disease, and specificity is the probability of ruling in the condition. Positive predictive value (PPV) is the likelihood of having the disease given a positive test result.
13. The correct answer is **B**. The interval variable is a quantitative variable that not only has a clear ordering of the values on a scale, but also these values on the scale are equally spaced apart. In this scenario, SBPs of 150 and 160 mmHg have a 10 mmHg difference and are meaningful to measure. Choices **A** and **C** are incorrect. Choice **D** is a confounder. Nominal variable has no ordering to the categories (e.g., hair color). Ordinal variables have an order, but the differences between the categories are not equally spaced apart. For example, for the American Society of Anesthesiologists (ASA) classification, ASA 2 is larger than ASA 1, but the difference between ASA 1 and 2 is not equally spaced apart when compared to the difference between ASA 2 and 3.
14. The correct answer is **D**. Cohort studies determine if the exposure plays a role in the outcome [1]. Answers **A**, **B**, and **C** are incorrect. A meta-analysis is a study that combines data from multiple studies. Case series typically report a condition or treatment for a couple of patients. A case control study determines if the patient with the outcome is associated with the exposure.
15. The correct answer is **A**. The visual analog scale involves patients making a handwritten spot on a line along the continuum between two extreme categories (e.g., pain scale). Choices **B** and **C** are incorrect. Open-ended questions involve participants freely answering the questions with fewer limits. A Likert scale is used to quantify beliefs and attitudes by providing patients with questions and asking them to select a response that best represents their belief (e.g., strongly disagree, disagree, neutral, agree, strongly agree). Response **D** is a confounder.

References

1. Amdur RJ, Bankert EA. Institutional review board: member handbook. Jones & Bartlett Learning; 2022.
2. Centre for Evidence Based Medicine. http://www.cebm.net. Accessed 10 Mar 2023.
3. Hulley. Designing clinical research. 4th ed. Philadelphia, PA: Lippincott, Williams & Wilkins; 2013.
4. NIH National Library of Medicine, Finding and Using Health Statistics. https://www.nlm.nih.gov/nichsr/stats_tutorial/cover.html. Accessed 10 Mar 2023.

5. NIH clinical research trials and you: the basics. https://www.nih.gov/health-information/nih-clinical-research-trials-you/basics. Accessed 16 Mar 2023.
6. Bruce N, Pope D, Stanistreet D. Quantitative methods for health research: a practical interactive guide to epidemiology and statistics. Wiley; 2009.
7. Gordis L. Epidemiology. Saunders Elsevier; 2009.

Further Reading

Amdur RJ, Bankert EA. Institutional review board: member handbook. Jones & Bartlett Learning; 2022.

Gordis L. Epidemiology. Saunders Elsevier; 2009.

Hulley. Designing clinical research. Fourth ed. Philadelphia, PA: Lippincott, Williams & Wilkins; 2013.

Obstetric Anesthesia and Perioperative Care: The Perioperative Surgical Home

Brandon Ngo and Gary Stier

Questions

1. **Which of the following statements best describes the Perioperative Surgical Home model of care?**
   A. The PSH model of care is focused primarily on the care provided to a patient following discharge from the hospital.
   B. The PSH model of care is focused primarily on the preoperative phase of care.
   C. The PSH model of care is a patient-centered, physician-led whole-health model that focuses on the entire perioperative continuum, from the decision to operate to 90 days after hospital discharge.
   D. The PSH model of care focuses primarily on the intraoperative phase of care.
2. **The implementation of the Perioperative Surgical Home model of care has resulted in which of the following patient outcomes?**
   A. Improved quality of care.
   B. Shorter hospital length of stay.
   C. Improved patient satisfaction.
   D. All the above are true.
3. **A 25-year-old G2P1 female had an epidural catheter placed for labor. During the epidural procedure, a dural puncture occurred. After the**

B. Ngo
UC Riverside School of Medicine, Riverside, CA, USA
e-mail: Brandon.Ngo@medsch.ucr.edu

G. Stier (✉)
Anesthesiology, Internal Medicine, Critical Care/Loma Linda University, Loma Linda, CA, USA

Riverside University Health System Medical Center, Moreno Valley, CA, USA
e-mail: g.stier@ruhealth.org

A. C. Sinha, I. F. Pasca (eds.), *Peripartum Care of the Pregnant Patient*,
https://doi.org/10.1007/978-3-031-62756-9_50

vaginal delivery, the patient complained of the classical signs of a postdural puncture headache (PDPH). Which of the following is not effective medication for PDPH?

A. Acetaminophen
B. Caffeine
C. Barbiturates
D. Sumatriptan

4. **The enhanced recovery after obstetric surgery (EROS) pathway includes all the following interventions except:**
   A. Early mobilization
   B. Clear liquids in the immediate recovery period
   C. Regular diet beginning 8 h after surgery
   D. Chewing gum to decrease the time to first flatus and a bowel movement
5. **Which of the following statements is true for healthy female patients in labor?**
   A. A platelet count should be routinely obtained.
   B. Clear liquids are allowed up to 2 h prior to expected surgery.
   C. The ingestion of solid food is allowed for patients expected to have a vaginal delivery.
   D. A blood crossmatch is indicated for patients expected to have an operative delivery.
6. **Gestational diabetes mellitus is associated with all the following except:**
   A. Gestational hypertension
   B. Obesity
   C. Family history of type 2 diabetes mellitus
   D. Adverse pregnancy outcomes
7. **Which of the following choices regarding anesthetic care for cesarean delivery is included within the 2016 ASA Practice Guidelines for Obstetric Anesthesia?**
   A. Do not delay the initiation of spinal anesthesia to administer a fixed volume of IV fluid (preloading).
   B. Ephedrine should be utilized in preference to phenylephrine for the management of intraoperative hypotension.
   C. A cutting-bevel spinal needle is recommended in preference to use of a pencil-point spinal needle for spinal anesthesia.
   D. Intermittent parenteral opioids are recommended over the use of neuraxial opioids for postoperative pain management.
8. **Regarding hypertensive disorders of pregnancy, all the following statements are true except:**
   A. Gestational hypertension (GH) is defined as an elevation of blood pressure ≥140/90 in a previously normotensive patient
   B. Preeclampsia is a multisystem disorder characterized by the new onset of hypertension and proteinuria after the first 20 weeks of pregnancy
   C. Systolic blood pressure consistently ≥145/90 should be treated
   D. Hydralazine is an acceptable medication for the treatment of high blood pressure

9. **Predictors of chronic pain following childbirth include all the following except:**
   A. Prenatal anxiety and poor physical function
   B. Delivery by cesarean section
   C. Preexisting chronic pain
   D. All the above are true
10. **Regarding the use of nonsteroidal anti-inflammatory drugs (NSAIDs) after both vaginal and post-cesarean delivery, which of the following statements is true?**
   A. When co-administered with opioids, NSAIDs produce a modest opioid-sparing effect.
   B. Ibuprofen, a nonselective NSAID, causes renal artery vasodilation.
   C. NSAIDs should not be used while breast-feeding due to significant transfer of the medication to breast milk.
   D. In addition to analgesic effects, NSAIDs have both anti-inflammatory and antipyretic properties.
11. **Following cesarean section, acceptable discharge criteria include all the following except:**
   A. No intravenous fluid requirement
   B. Severe postoperative pain requiring regular use of oral opioids
   C. Hemodynamic stability
   D. Absence of ongoing medical problems
12. **Smoking during pregnancy is associated with all the following adverse outcomes except:**
   A. Fetal growth retardation
   B. Respiratory complications
   C. Increased risk of preeclampsia
   D. Impaired wound healing
13. **Transitional care management (TCM) is the management of patient transitions between settings of care, including safely returning the patient back to their prior residence. Which of the following statements is/are true with respect to TCM?**
   A. TCM involves activities focused on care coordination, including the post-discharge follow-up clinic appointment.
   B. TCM includes ensuring patient education and engagement.
   C. TCM involves the identification and documentation of any health problems during hospitalization that are associated with poor outcomes following discharge.
   D. All the above statements are correct.
14. **Nausea and vomiting are commonly encountered symptoms during cesarean delivery. All the following statements related to perioperative nausea and vomiting are true except:**
   A. Intraoperative maternal hypotension from regional anesthesia is a common cause

B. Fluid preloading and lower limb compression are effective in reducing the incidence of intraoperative maternal hypotension
C. The use of corticosteroids, such as dexamethasone, has been found to reduce the postoperative incidence of nausea and vomiting
D. A multimodal approach to reducing the incidence of postoperative nausea and vomiting following cesarean delivery includes the use of combination antiemetic agents

15. **Patients with a severe β-lactam allergy (e.g., anaphylaxis, angioedema, respiratory distress, or urticaria) may be given which of the following preoperative prophylactic antibiotics?**
A. Clindamycin
B. Amoxicillin
C. Penicillin
D. None of the above

16. **Which alcohol-based antiseptic agent is best utilized to perform preoperative surgical site skin preparation to prevent surgical site infections following cesarean delivery?**
A. Iodine-alcohol
B. Chlorhexidine-alcohol
C. Povidone-iodine (Betadine)
D. Hydrogen peroxide

17. **Enhanced recovery after surgery (ERAS) is a standardized perioperative care pathway tailored to a specific surgical procedure. All the following statements concerning the use of an ERAS pathway are true <u>except</u>:**
A. ERAS pathways have been shown to reduce hospital length of stay
B. ERAS pathways have been shown to reduce perioperative complications
C. ERAS pathways have not been shown to reduce overall health system costs
D. ERAS is a tool for process management

18. **Regarding anemia in pregnancy, all the following statements are correct <u>except</u>:**
A. Iron deficiency is the most common cause of anemia in pregnancy
B. Iron-deficiency anemia during the first trimester of pregnancy increases the risk for preterm delivery
C. Iron-deficiency anemia during the second and third trimesters of pregnancy has been demonstrated to result in adverse perinatal outcomes
D. Daily oral iron supplementation in pregnancy decreases the risk for maternal anemia

19. **Regarding risk factors for venous thromboembolic events (VTEs) in pregnancy, which of the following statements is <u>false</u>?**
A. The highest risk for VTE occurs during the first trimester.
B. VTE is associated with a previous history of thromboembolism.
C. VTE is associated with obesity.
D. Hypertensive disorders increase the risk of VTE during pregnancy.

20. **Which of the following statements regarding postoperative implementation of a multimodal analgesia strategy is <u>false</u>?**

A. The goal of a multimodal analgesic approach is to achieve adequate analgesia with minimal side effects balanced by minimal risk to the neonate.
B. There is a strong emphasis on the use of nonopioid analgesic medications.
C. NSAIDs and low-dose aspirin should be avoided if breast-feeding.
D. Oral opioid medications should be used only for breakthrough pain that is not adequately relieved with nonopioid medications.

Answers and Explanations

1. **C**. The Perioperative Surgical Home (PSH) model is a patient-centered, physician-led, team-based model of care that guides the patient throughout all phases of the surgical journey, from the decision to operate through the preoperative, intraoperative, postoperative, and transitional care phases, ending 90 days after hospital discharge. The PSH model provides a framework that better aligns a complex microsystem of providers and processes, including clinicians, administrators, ancillary services, health information technology (HIT), and the patient, with the goal of reducing care fragmentation that often contributes to adverse outcomes and higher costs. The PSH model has the goal of achieving the Quadruple Aim: better patient outcomes, decreased cost, improved patient satisfaction, and enhanced provider satisfaction [1].
2. **D**. The successful implementation of the Perioperative Surgical Home (PSH) model of care within a healthcare organization has been demonstrated to produce the following outcomes in comparison with the traditional fragmented episode of surgical care: reduced length of hospital stay; reduced incidence of hospital-acquired conditions; reduced readmissions; reduced episode of care costs; improved patient satisfaction; and a reduction in the use of skilled nursing facilities [2].
3. **D**. Epidural blood patches remain the definitive treatment for PDPH; however, before choosing an invasive procedure (epidural), conservative management is often recommended. Initial treatment regimens center on counteracting the loss of cerebrospinal fluid through puncture in the dura and cerebral vasodilation. Proposed treatment modalities include hydration therapy, strict bed rest, supine positioning, prone positioning, and tight-fitting abdominal binders. Although there may be some temporary relief, there remains little evidence to support any of the conservation measures mentioned in a meaningful reduction of symptoms of a PDPH. There is some limited evidence that medical therapies such as NSAIDS, caffeine, barbiturates (butalbital), and gabapentinoids reduce pain scores from PDPH. Randomized control trials as well as a Cochrane review have not shown sumatriptan to be efficacious for PDPH [3].
4. **C**. The enhanced recovery after surgery (ERAS) pathway was first reported over 20 years ago in patients undergoing colorectal surgery. The demonstrated success of an ERAS pathway has since led to the adoption of the ERAS framework within different specialties for a variety of surgical procedures, including cesarean section. In general, an enhanced recovery pathway is an

evidence-based, multimodal, integrated care plan for perioperative care that reorganizes care around the surgical episode. The goal is to combine multiple evidence-based interventions, each of which may have a small impact in isolation, into a coordinated, standardized pathway with beneficial effects on reducing the surgical stress response and with a goal of early return of function. For the best outcomes, ERAS pathways require collaboration and care coordination between providers, ancillary healthcare services, health information technology (HIT), and the patient. The ERAS pathway, including EROS, not only includes standardized orders but also addresses optimal patient preparation, intraoperative management, and early postoperative care, combined with an overall assessment of clinical pathway compliance and a review of outcomes. Included within the postoperative care phase of the EROS pathway are the following: removal of the urinary catheter immediately after surgical end; early mobilization; clear liquids in the immediate postoperative period; resumption of a regular diet within 2 h after surgery; nausea and vomiting prophylaxis with fluids and antiemetic mediations; and chewing gum. This approach has been demonstrated to result in less morbidity, less need to remain in the hospital, less variability between practitioners, and lower resource use [4, 5].

5. **B**. The updated 2016 ASA Practice Guidelines for Obstetric Anesthesia focus on the anesthetic management of pregnant patients during labor, vaginal delivery, cesarean delivery, and selected aspects of postpartum care and analgesia. In the updated guidelines, a routine platelet count is not necessary for a healthy parturient; solid foods should be avoided in laboring patients; patients undergoing elective surgery (e.g., cesarean delivery) should undergo a fasting period for solids of 6–8 h; clear liquids are allowed for uncomplicated laboring patients and up to 2 h before the induction of anesthesia for those undergoing elective surgery; and a routine blood crossmatch is not necessary for healthy parturients for vaginal or operative delivery [6].
6. **A**. The diagnosis of gestational diabetes applies to a patient with diabetes mellitus or glucose intolerance that is first diagnosed during pregnancy, depending on the screening and diagnostic strategies utilized. The diagnosis of gestational diabetes mellitus (GDM) is made when the fasting plasma glucose level is ≥92 mg/dL or following an oral glucose tolerance test, the plasma glucose is ≥180 mg/dL at 1 h and ≥153 mg/dL at 2 h. The risk of GDM is increased in the following instances: prior history of GDM; age >35 years; obesity; family history of type 2 diabetes mellitus; history of polycystic ovarian syndrome; and history of macrosomic babies or stillbirths. GDM has not been found to be associated with gestational hypertension. Patients with GDM have a recurrence rate of GDM of 35–70% in subsequent pregnancies [7].
7. **A**. The 2016 ASA Practice Guidelines for Obstetric Anesthesia updated the previous guidelines published in 2007. The guidelines focus on the anesthetic management of pregnant patients during labor, vaginal delivery, cesarean delivery, and selected aspects of postpartum care and analgesia. Many updated recommendations were included within the 2016 guidelines. Among the many recommendations offered, a sampling of key statements included the following:

a routine platelet count is not necessary for a healthy parturient; a routine blood crossmatch is not necessary for a healthy uncomplicated parturient for vaginal or cesarean delivery; do not delay the initiation of spinal anesthesia to administer a fixed volume of intravenous fluid; either IV ephedrine or phenylephrine may be used for treating hypotension during neuraxial anesthesia; a pencil-point spinal needle should be used instead of a cutting-bevel spinal needle to minimize the risk of postdural spinal puncture headache; and neuraxial opioids are recommended in preference to intermittent injections of parenteral opioids for postoperative analgesia after neuraxial anesthesia for cesarean delivery [6].

8. **C**. Hypertensive disorders of pregnancy include chronic hypertension, chronic hypertension with onset of preeclampsia, preeclampsia, eclampsia, and gestational hypertension. Gestational hypertension (GH) is defined as a blood pressure (BP) of ≥140/90 mmHg on two occasions (at least 4 h apart) after 20 weeks of gestation in a previously normotensive woman, without the presence of proteinuria or other clinical features (thrombocytopenia, impaired renal or kidney function, pulmonary edema, or new-onset headache) suggestive of preeclampsia. Preeclampsia is a heterogeneous disorder characterized by the development of new-onset hypertension and new-onset proteinuria after 20 weeks of pregnancy. The goal of therapy is to keep the blood pressure below 160/110 mmHg; treatment is therefore warranted for a systolic blood pressure ≥160 mmHg. Acceptable antihypertensive medications to achieve treatment goals in preeclamptic patients include labetalol (IV/PO), hydralazine (IV), and nifedipine (IV/PO) [8].
9. **D**. Persistent pain following vaginal or cesarean delivery is well established. In fact, approximately one out of ten women who deliver by cesarean section reports chronic pain at 1 year after delivery. Risk factors for the development of prolonged postdelivery pain include the following: induction of labor; the magnitude of the acute pain score after delivery; delayed functional recovery; prolonged use of opioid medications (cesarean delivery was predictive of longer use of opioids compared with vaginal delivery); prenatal anxiety and poor physical function; and history of pregnancy-related and prepregnancy back pain. Finally, obesity has been associated with persistent postpartum back pain [9].
10. **D**. Nonsteroidal anti-inflammatory drugs (NSAIDs) reduce inflammatory reactions by inhibiting cyclooxygenase (COX) enzymes. Due to these beneficial properties (including fever reduction), this drug class has been an important component of perioperative multimodal analgesia strategies. NSAIDs are particularly effective for use following cesarean delivery, and when combined with opioids, NSAIDs produce a significant opioid-sparing effect, with reports of up to a 50% reduction in the required opioid doses. With respect to postoperative pain management, NSAIDs are most effective when administered at fixed intervals rather than as needed. Nonselective NSAIDs (i.e., inhibit both COX-1 and COX-2 isoenzymes) inhibit platelet function, cause renal arterial vasoconstriction, and produce gastrointestinal irritation; as such, caution must be exercised when considering the use of these medications in patients with risk factors.

NSAIDs are very minimally transferred to breast milk, so NSAIDs can be given to breast-feeding mothers to manage postdelivery pain [10].

11. **B**. Traditional discharge criteria following surgical procedures include the absence of a need for intravenous fluids, absence of fever, and wound infection; additional criteria for discharge readiness include the ability to safely ambulate, acceptable pain control, hemodynamic stability, no evidence of bleeding, and the ability to urinate. Discharge opioid medications are acceptable as discharge medications; however, opioids should rarely be required for adequate pain control once discharged [4].
12. **C**. Smoking is associated with an increased incidence of preterm labor, spontaneous fetal loss, placental abruption, small for gestational age fetus, adverse pulmonary effects (e.g., mucus volume and clearance, bronchitis), and a reduced risk of preeclampsia. Smoking cessation in early pregnancy, compared to stopping tobacco use later in pregnancy, is associated with a reduced risk of fetal growth retardation [11].
13. **D**. Transitional care management (TCM) is care coordination. Within the context of perioperative care, TCM begins with the preoperative assessment process and ends at a set time frame following hospital discharge (typically 30–90 days after discharge). The primary goal of TCM is to ensure successful transitions from one care setting to another care setting. Components of TCM include patient engagement; caregiver engagement; early identification of medical comorbidities and institution of medical optimization and prevention strategies; patient education; discharge planning (including medication reconciliation); creation of individualized care plans, including easy access to healthcare and community services; communication with the care providers who will be taking care of the patient; and arranging for timely follow-up. Effective TCM programs have resulted in reduced hospital length of stay, reduced discharge to a skilled nursing facility, fewer hospital readmissions, and improved patient satisfaction [12].
14. **C**. The overall incidence of nausea and vomiting associated with the use of regional anesthesia for cesarean delivery is very common. One of the primary causes of nausea and vomiting is maternal hypotension following the use of spinal anesthesia and is associated with a higher level of spinal block. Nausea and vomiting place the patient at an increased risk of aspiration, so ensuring that the patient is awake and able to protect the airway is essential. Nausea and vomiting are also associated with reduced patient satisfaction and longer hospitalization. Preemptive management techniques include fluid preloading, aggressive treatment of hypotension using either ephedrine or phenylephrine, lower limb compression, and use of antiemetic medications. Institution of a multimodal emetic approach is recommended; 5-HT3 antagonists (e.g., ondansetron), dopamine antagonists (e.g., metoclopramide, droperidol), propofol, and midazolam are medications that can be considered in a multitiered approach to avoid or reduce postoperative nausea and vomiting. Corticosteroids such as dexamethasone have been found to reduce only intraoperative nausea and vomiting and not postoperative nausea and vomiting [13].

15. **A**. Patients with a severe β-lactam allergy (e.g., anaphylaxis, angioedema, respiratory distress, or urticaria) may be given a combination of clindamycin (900 mg) plus an aminoglycoside (5 mg/kg) 60 min prior to the start of the cesarean delivery [14].
16. **B**. Surgical site infection (SSI) is a leading cause of nosocomial infections in hospitalized patients. In particular, post-cesarean infectious complications can occur in up to 20% of patients. The occurrence of an SSI in a patient following cesarean delivery is associated with increases in the length of hospitalization, readmission risk, hospital cost, and burden on the patient and family. In studies comparing preoperative skin antiseptic agents, chlorhexidine-alcohol was demonstrated to be more efficacious in the prevention of surgical site infection (SSI) after cesarean delivery than the antiseptic agents povidone-iodine and iodine-alcohol [15, 16].
17. **C**. Enhanced recovery after surgery (ERAS) arose out of Europe as a pathway to promote the rapid recovery of a patient after colorectal surgery. The original consensus article appeared in 2005 and described 17 evidenced-based interventions that, when implemented together, not only reduced the hospital length of stay but also had a positive effect on patient outcomes, including better pain control, more rapid return of gut function, and earlier ambulation. ERAS pathways have since been adopted for a variety of surgical procedures, including gynecologic surgery and cesarean sections. With the institution of all components of the pathway, a variety of beneficial outcomes have been achieved. Outcome benefits include reduction in hospital length of stay, reduced postoperative complications (e.g., wound infections), reduction in the use of hospital resources and cost, enhanced patient satisfaction, and reduced readmissions. The rate of adherence with components of an ERAS pathway is an excellent tool for process improvement [13].
18. **C**. Physiologic anemia of normal pregnancy results from the disproportionate increase in plasma volume (by 50%) and red cell mass (by 30%); this increase in plasma volume/red cell mass ratio results in physiologic anemia during pregnancy. However, other causes of anemia during pregnancy must be ruled out. Iron deficiency is the most common cause of pathologic anemia during pregnancy, becoming more significant as pregnancy progresses. Iron deficiency that occurs during the first trimester increases the risk of preterm delivery and low birth weight; however, there is a paucity of evidence to suggest that anemia during the second and third trimesters is associated with adverse perinatal outcomes. Administration of daily oral iron supplementation during pregnancy reduces the risk of maternal anemia, although clear evidence for such treatment improving perinatal outcomes is lacking. The risk of postpartum blood transfusion is associated with the presence of anemia during pregnancy [17].
19. **A**. Pregnant women are at an increased risk of VTE during pregnancy compared to nonpregnant women. The risk of VTE is highest during the first week postpartum. Risk factors for VTE in pregnancy include a previous history of VTE, thrombophilic disorders (e.g., factor V Leiden mutation), obesity, hypertensive

disorders, tobacco use disorder, older age, immobility, heart disease, blood transfusion, postpartum infection, and multiple pregnancy [18].

20. **C**. The concept of the implementation of postoperative multimodal analgesia strategies involves the use of a variety of medications with differing mechanisms of action with the goal of producing synergistic clinical effects in treating acute postoperative pain. The multimodal analgesia approach emphasizes the foundational use of nonopioid medications while minimizing the use of opioids. As such, opioids should only be utilized for significant breakthrough pain poorly controlled with nonopioids. While the primary goal of multimodal analgesia is effective pain control, other intended benefits of opioid-sparing analgesic strategies are reduction in maternal clinical side effects (e.g., interference with infant care, respiratory depression, cognitive changes, constipation) and minimal transfer of drugs to breast milk; thus, medications such as NSAIDs and low-dose aspirin, which are insignificantly transmitted to breast milk, are safely administered in breast-feeding parturients. Medications included within multimodal analgesic strategies include acetaminophen, celecoxib (or ibuprofen), gabapentin, short-acting opioids (used sparingly and only for breakthrough pain), and ketamine for severe pain [19].

References

1. ASA PSH Implementation Guide. PSH learning collaborative: roadmap to success; 2021. Accessed asahq.org/psh.
2. Garson L, Schwarzkopf R, et al. Implementation of a total joint replacement-focused perioperative surgical home: a management case report. Anesth Analg. 2014;118:1081–9.
3. Katz D, Beilin Y. Review of the alternatives to epidural blood patch for treatment of postdural puncture headache in the parturient. Anesth Analg. 2017;124:1219–28.
4. Adshead D, Wrench I, et al. Enhanced recovery after elective Caesarian section. BJA Educ. 2020;20:354–7.
5. Nelson G, Altman A, et al. Guidelines for postoperative care in gynecologic/oncology surgery: enhanced recovery after surgery (ERAS) society recommendations-part II. Gynecol Oncol. 2016;140:323–32.
6. ASA Practice Guidelines for Obstetric Anesthesia. An updated report by the American Society of Anesthesiologists Task Force on obstetric anesthesia and the Society of Obstetric Anesthesia and Perinatology. Anesthesiology. 2016;124:270–300.
7. Wissler RN. Endocrine disorders. In: Chestnut D, Wong C, editors. Chestnut's OB anesthesia: principles and practice. 6th ed. p. 1056–87.
8. Smiley R, Meng M-L. Pregnancy-associated diseases. In: Hines R, Jones S, editors. Stoelting's anesthesia and co-existing disease. 8th ed. Philadelphia, PA: Elsevier Publishers; 2022. p. 697–712.
9. Ansari J, Flood P. Chronic pain during and after pregnancy. In: Chestnut D, et al., editors. Chestnut's obstetric anesthesia: principles and practice. 6th ed. Philadelphia, PA: Elsevier Publisher; 2020. p. 1033–56.
10. George RB, Carvalho B, et al. Postoperative analgesia. In: Chestnut D, et al., editors. Chestnut's obstetric anesthesia: principles and practice. 6th ed. Philadelphia, PA: Elsevier Publisher; 2020. p. 627–70.

11. Leffert L. Substance use disorders. In: Chestnut D, et al., editors. Chestnut's obstetric anesthesia: principles and practice. 6th ed. Philadelphia, PA: Elsevier; 2020. p. 1248–73.
12. Naylor MD, et al. Components of comprehensive and effective transitional care. J Am Geriatr Soc. 2017;65:1119–25.
13. Macones G, Caughey A, et al. Guidelines for postoperative care in cesarean delivery: enhanced recovery after surgery (ERAS) society recommendations (part 3). Am J Obtet Gynecol. 2019;221(247):e1–9.
14. Reiff E, Habib A, et al. Antibiotic prophylaxis for cesarean delivery: a survey of anesthesiologists. Anesth Res Pract. 2020;2020:3741608. https://doi.org/10.1155/2020/3741608.
15. Tuuli M, Liu J, et al. A randomized trial comparing skin antiseptic agents are cesarean delivery. N Engl J Med. 2016;374:647–55.
16. Luwant A, Saha P, et al. Chlorhexidine-alcohol versus povidone-iodine as preoperative skin antisepsis for prevention of surgical site infection in cesarean delivery-a pilot randomized control trial. Trials. 2021;22:540.
17. Mhyre J. Hematologic and coagulation disorders. In: Chestnut D, et al., editors. Chestnut's obstetric anesthesia: principles and practice. 6th ed. Philadelphia, PA: Elsevier publisher; 2020. p. 1088–94.
18. Toledo P. Embolic disorders. In: Chestnut D, et al., editors. Chestnut's obstetric anesthesia: principles and practice. 6th ed. Philadelphia, PA: Elsevier publisher; 2020. p. 937–42.
19. George R, Carvalho B, et al. Postoperative analgesia. In: Chestnut D, et al., editors. Chestnut's obstetric anesthesia: principles and practice. 6th ed. Philadelphia, PA: Elsevier publisher; 2020. p. 627–33.

Index

A. C. Sinha, I. F. Pasca (eds.), *Peripartum Care of the Pregnant Patient*,
https://doi.org/10.1007/978-3-031-62756-9

D

T

GPSR Compliance

The European Union's (EU) General Product Safety Regulation (GPSR) is a set of rules that requires consumer products to be safe and our obligations to ensure this.

If you have any concerns about our products, you can contact us on ProductSafety@springernature.com

In case Publisher is established outside the EU, the EU authorized representative is:

Springer Nature Customer Service Center GmbH
Europaplatz 3
69115 Heidelberg, Germany

Batch number: 10732076

Printed by Printforce, the Netherlands